Philosophy and Medicine

Volume 123

The Philosophy and Medicine series is dedicated to publishing monographs and collections of essays that contribute importantly to scholarship in bioethics and the philosophy of medicine. The series addresses the full scope of issues in bioethics, from euthanasia to justice and solidarity in health care. The Philosophy and Medicine series places the scholarship of bioethics within studies of basic problems in the epistemology and metaphysics of medicine. The latter publications explore such issues as models of explanation in medicine, concepts of health and disease, clinical judgment, the meaning of human dignity, the definition of death, and the significance of beneficence, virtue, and consensus in health care. The series seeks to publish the best of philosophical work directed to health care and the biomedical sciences.

More information about this series at http://www.springer.com/series/6414

I dedicate this book to the memory of my deceased mother who, after many years of suffering and increasing frailty, was in the end granted the sudden, painless death she had always hoped for.

Contents

1 Introduction

Today, end-of-life care and palliative medicine garner great attention in medicine, in the public sphere and in politics. There is hardly another field in modern healthcare that exhibits a similar dynamic and resonates so strongly in society. Thousands of hospices, palliative care units and other facilities for the terminally ill and dying have been created over the past decades and their number continues to grow. Today, more and more people can finish their days in dignity and without unbearable physical pain, professionally cared for by nurses and doctors trained in palliative medicine. Palliative medicine has become a field in its own right, with national and international associations for those specialized in it and scientific and professional journals featuring articles on the subject published by the hundreds every year.[1]

The field is widely considered a very young phenomenon.[2] Its beginnings are usually dated to the 1960s or 1970s. At that time, Cicely Saunders founded St Christopher's Hospice in London, which would serve as the model for countless similar institutions in the years that followed.[3] Soon after, the first palliative care unit in a modern hospital was opened in Montreal under the direction of Balfour

[1] For global surveys see David Clark, End-of-life care around the world. Achievements to date and challenges remaining, in: Omega 56 (2007), pp. 101–10; Economist Intelligence Unit, The quality of death. Ranking end-of-life care across the world, 2010 (www.eiu.com/sponsor/lienfoundation/qualityofdeath); Stephen R. Connor and Maria Cecilia Sepulveda Bermedo (eds), Global atlas of palliative care at the end of life, WHO: Worldwide Palliative Care Alliance 2014.

[2] See e.g. Susanne Ringskog and Danuta Wassermann, Hastening the end of life. History, research and current Swedish and international debate on the issue of euthanasia, Stockholm: National Center for Suicide Research and Prevention of Mental Ill-Health 2000, p. 86: "The palliative medicine takes its start in London, in 1967"; or Lavi, The modern art of dying (2005), p. 6: "in previous centuries the medical doctor would leave the bedside when it was clear that the patient was hopelessly ill".

[3] Du Boulay, Cicely Saunders (1984); Mary Campion, Ein Hospiz entsteht: von Pionierinnen der Hospizbewegung, Straubing: Attenkofer 1997.

M. Stolberg, *A History of Palliative Care, 1500–1970*, Philosophy and Medicine 123,
DOI 10.1007/978-3-319-54178-5_1

Mount.[4] These recent developments are well known and have often been described. Here and there, historians have traced the origins of palliative medicine and the hospice back at bit further, to the late nineteenth century. However, historians have been virtually unanimous that palliative medicine is recent phenomenon and linked to the rise of modern biomedicine and intensive care. Some authors have even given reasons why hospices and specialized palliative medical care could not have their place before the nineteenth century. "It was only modern medicine," argues Nicolaus Eschenbruch for instance, "that made it [...] possible to delineate at all 'dying' as a longer, defined phase of life, and thereby the object of the work of the hospice." In earlier times, dying was "either short, hardly predictable and brutal" or "a long infirmity that was seen as God-given and simply a part of life." It was, in this view, only thanks to the new therapeutic possibilities of modern medicine that the dying process could "move from something omnipresent that was to be taken as a matter of course to a more clearly defined phase of life."[5]

It takes only a brief look at older medical writing and of personal testimonials and other sources that reflect everyday practice and daily life in earlier centuries to see that such assessments bypass the historical realities and indeed turn them on their heads. As this book will show, palliative care is definitely not an invention of the nineteenth or twentieth century. Its history goes back much further. The physician's obligation to continue to assist the severely ill and dying when all hope for a cure was lost was widely recognized from the end of the Middle Ages at the latest. The practicalities of nursing and treating these patients were dealt with in medical literature beginning in the late sixteenth century using terms like *cura palliativa* and, with a view to the terminally ill and dying, *euthanasia medicinalis* in numerous texts and they were put to use at the sickbed.[6]

This early interest in the alleviation of the suffering of the dying is surprising only at first glance. Precisely because the means available in pre-modern medicine were very limited according to today's standards, the question was in many ways even more urgent than it is today as to how the suffering of fatally ill and dying patients was to be at least alleviated. Numerous case histories by pre-modern physicians confirm this over and again. They give vivid accounts of the agonies that many patients suffered in the final months and weeks of their lives if they were suffering and dying of cancer, consumption or dropsy, at the time the three most commonly discussed and widely feared terminal illnesses among adults. They describe cancer patients whose screams of pain echoed through the rooms day and night and whose

---

[4] Balfour Mount and J. Andrew Billings, What is palliative care? in: Journal of palliative medicine 1 (1998), pp. 73–81, here p. 73.

[5] Nicholas Eschenbruch, Ein besseres Sterben? Die Entstehung der modernen Hospizbewegung und ihre historischen Voraussetzungen, in: Praxis 93 (2004), pp. 1265–7; along similar lines: Student, Geschichte (2007).

[6] See the surveys in Hoffmann, Inhalt (1969) and Stolberg, "Cura palliativa" (2007b).

ulcerous, decomposing tumors let off an unbearable stench.[7] The agonizing, convulsive coughing of consumptive patients often lasted hours, exhausted them and robbed them of their sleep. In the end, they struggled for breath or suffered from "terrifying constriction."[8] Indeed, the "most frightening fear of death with a constant danger of suffocation" took hold of the patient, as C. W. Hufeland in the early nineteenth century described the suffering of a patient who fell into "pure desperation."[9] Death from suffocation was also the fate of many dropsical patients.

Medical case histories and similar accounts torments of dying patients also make it clear that the major ethical questions surrounding the medical treatment of moribund and dying patients that are widely discussed today were no less agonizing to deal with in the seventeenth and eighteenth centuries. Was the doctor allowed in obviously hopeless cases to contribute deliberately and actively to a curtailing of suffering and life? Was he allowed to risk that his efforts to alleviate the agonizing complaints of dying patients might accelerate the coming of death? And above all: Was he allowed to at least forgo further healing attempts, even if this meant risking that certain patients would die who perhaps still had a chance? Some modern authors have claimed that in earlier times this question was hardly asked because doctors could not effectively influence the course of a disease anyway. "In the past," wrote Hazel Biggs for example, "the question of inappropriately prolonging life was not a consideration. Rather, people would have died for want of effective medical care."[10] Yet this is an anachronistic misjudgment. Certainly, seen from today's perspective, the available remedies would have offered little prospect of prolonging a patient's life, but that is not the point here. From the perspective of the physicians and patients of that time, medicine was very well in the position to maintain and prolong life. Accordingly, the question of whether or not such an attempt to prolong life continued to make sense in desperate cases was, as we will see, discussed in great detail.

Against this backdrop, this book will take the long view and trace the history of terminal care from the late Middle Ages to the present. My examination will link two major research questions.

First, I will investigate the theoretical discussion and the everyday practice of terminal care, as carried out by doctors, nurses and attendants. I will trace both the change and the continuity in the medical debates about this topic. I will sketch out the history of institutional care for terminally ill and dying patients and throw a new light on the historical roots of the hospices for the dying and the palliative care units

[7] See e.g. Olaus Borrichius, Olai Borrichii itinerarium 1660–1665. The journal of the Danish Polyhistor Ole Borch. Ed. by H. D. Schepelern, vol. 1, Copenhagen–London: Reitzels Forlag and Brill 1983, p. 69, on the case of a woman with terrible abdominal pain who, for the 3 weeks before her death, could no longer eat but only scream and moan terribly ("per tres integras hebdom[adas] ante mortem nihil cibi assumpsit, ejulavit tantum et horrendo gemitu vociferata est")

[8] Friedrich Benjamin Osiander, Über die Entwicklungskrankheiten in den Blüthenjahren des weiblichen Geschlechts, part 1, Tübingen: Bey dem Verfasser 1817, pp. 117–8, on the case of a female consumptive patient, around 18 years old, who, in the end, only hoped to die as quickly as possible.

[9] Hufeland, Enchiridion medicum (1837), p. 853.

[10] Hazel Biggs, Euthanasia, death with dignity and the law, Oxford–Portland: Hart 2001, p. 2.

today. Drawing on personal accounts as well as on works of fiction, I will also try to arrive at least at a rough understanding of the experience of dying and of terminal care from the perspective of patients and their families.

Second, I will trace the changes that have taken place with regard to the perception and handling of the major ethical dilemmas that, for centuries, have quite consistently arisen from caring for fatally ill and dying patients, from the question of deliberately shortening a person's life to the communication of an unfavorable or fatal prognosis. In so doing, I will not just look at theoretical and normative texts and debates but also draw on sources that reflect the actual practice of doctors and nurses at the sickbed. This has often been neglected in histories of medical ethics but it is crucial for our historical understanding. What people—including physicians—do in ordinary life can differ substantially from what they should do according to abstract norms.

The geographic reach of my study is quite wide as well. I will concentrate on central and western Europe and in particular on the German-speaking areas, England and France. Where it seems important for an understanding of global developments, I will also take a look at the developements elsewhere, in Europe and North America.[11]

This broad temporal and geographic scope inevitably calls, at the same time, for a focusing in terms of content. This is not a comprehensive account of the social and cultural history of death and dying, in the style of Philippe Ariès's acclaimed work.[12] I will largely limit myself to an analysis of the approaches taken by doctors and nurses who cared for the terminally ill and dying and to the ethical questions and of debates that arose in this context. Moreover, in my attempt to sketch out the broad developmental stages, I will necessarily have to generalize. Inevitably my overview can do justice to the different social, cultural and political contexts in the different countries only to a limited extent. I will be mentioning differences from time to time between countries, religious denominations and social classes when it came to dealing with dying and death. However, systematic comparisons and in-depth examinations of long-term developments in specific national and confessional contexts, like those of Karen Nolte and Jason Szabo for nineteenth-century Germany and France, will have to be left to future studies. I should also point out from the start that the National Socialist "euthanasia" programs, the organized mass-murder of chronically sick patients, will only be mentioned in passing. These crimes have not only been extensively researched by others already; they also targeted the terminally ill and dying only exceptionally and marginally. The victims were above all

[11] A comparative analysis of non-western cultures, as interesting as it would be, is beyond the scope of this book.

[12] Ariès, Western attitudes (1974); idem, L'homme devant la mort; Ariès relied primarily on literary and visual sources, seeking evidence for a "better" way of dying in previous centuries and hardly mentions palliative care. For more recent and nuanced analyses of the cultural history of death and dying see e.g. Mischke, Umgang (1996); Hugger, Meister Tod (2002); Richter, Der phantasierte Tod (2010).

psychiatric patients, those with mental and physical disabilities and other chronically ill people for whom an imminent death caused by illness could hardly be expected.

Regardless of such limitations, I firmly believe that the following attempt at an overview is not only justifiable but, given the current state of research, is greatly needed. The developments since around 1960 have been described many times. We have David Clark, in particular, to thank for valuable work in this regard.[13] For the preceding decades beginning around 1870 there have been some studies on the leading protagonists and early facilities for the care of terminally ill and dying patients.[14] Covering especially the time from the late nineteenth century onward, Milton Lewis, in 2007, presented the first monographic overview for Anglo-Saxon countries, in which he summarized the existing research and added new insights, especially for Australia, from his first-hand study of sources.[15] For France, Ann Carol studied the medical literature on death in the period between 1800 to about 1960, dedicating attention to the question of apparent death and the medical handling of corpses as well as a chapter to pain management and another to ethical debates.[16] Pat Jalland in her book *Death in the Victorian Family* also dealt with the medical approach to the terminally ill in nineteenth-century England.[17] Jason Szabo in his abovementioned book, and on the basis of extensive source studies, traced the handling of incurables in nineteenth-century France.[18] Supported by a wide corpus of handwritten and printed sources, ranging from medical case studies to private diaries, Karen Nolte has recently studied terminal care in Germany in the first half of the nineteenth century, taking into account the perspectives of medicine, nursing and pastoral care.[19] However, a comprehensive, transnational analysis of the historical developments in the treatment of terminally ill and dying patients has yet to be undertaken. So far, little is known about the time before the late nineteenth century, in particular, when it comes to the medical and nursing practice in the treatment of the dying, and thus the long-term continuities and processes of change in this regard have escaped

---

[13] Clark, Cradled to the grave? (1999); idem, From margins (2007); see also idem, History, gender and culture in the rise of palliative care, in: Sheila Payne, Jane Seymour and Christine Ingleton (eds), Palliative care nursing. Principles and evidence for practice, Buckingham: Open University Press 2004, pp. 39–54; idem, H. A. M. J. ten Have and Rien Janssens, Palliative care service developments in seven European countries, in: H. A. M. J. ten Have and David Clark (eds), The ethics of palliative care. European perspectives, Buckingham: Open University Press 2002, pp. 34–51; see also Mielke, Sterben und Tod (2006), esp. pp. 113–20; Stoddard Holmes, "The grandest badge" (2003); Buck, Rights of passage (2005); J. Seymour, D. Clark and M. Winslow, Pain and palliative care: the emergence of new specialties, in: Journal of pain & symptom management 29 (2005), pp. 2–13; Hayley and Sachs, A brief history (2005).

[14] Humphreys, "Undying spirits" (1999); Humphreys, Last summons (2001); Hughes and Clark, "A thoughtful and experienced physician" (2004).

[15] Lewis, Medicine (2007).

[16] Carol, Les médecins (2004), esp. pp. 47–127.

[17] Jalland, Death (1996), esp. pp. 77–97, chapter on "Death and the Victorian doctors".

[18] Szabo, Incurable (2009).

[19] Nolte, Todkrank (2016).

us as well. The further back we go in time, the patchier our knowledge. The title of a recent book by Harold Y. Vanderpool, *Palliative care. The 400-year quest for a good death* might suggest that he has filled this gap.[20] Vanderpool's book, which offers a useful collection of sources for the more recent past, devotes only a few pages to the demand for and practice of palliative care before 1800, however, presenting and paraphrasing a handful of texts which deal with these issues, at least in a wider sense. The title of his book refers to Francis Bacon's famous call on physicians to help dying patients die a "good death." As we will see, this call had been preceded by at least 200 years of writing on—and the actual practice of—palliative care on the sick and dying.

The history of the ethical debates surrounding the care for terminally ill and dying patients has been significantly better researched.[21] The mass murders of sick people during the Nazi era, euphemistically characterized as "euthanasia," and the ethical debates about voluntary euthanasia that preceded this, beginning around 1870, have been studied and described in hundreds of works.[22] In addition, for the time before 1870, there have been several overviews. These overviews are limited in large part to presenting and analyzing theoretical, normative texts, however,[23] and offer only very limited insight into the actual day-to-day practice at the deathbed.[24] Based on such sources, it has been widely assumed, for example, that active euthanasia only became the subject of medical debate around 1900. But sources that reflect ordinary medical practice make it clear that the deliberate shortening of the life and suffering of the terminally ill was discussed, supported and practiced by some doctors as early as 1800.[25]

A major goal of mine, in writing the book, was, professedly, to give those who work in palliative medicine today or who advocate for it a deepened sense of its history and thus also a sense of the historically grown identity of their discipline. Of course, historical research on a topic like palliative care that is of outstanding importance today carries a certain risk. It can entice us to view and evaluate historical events all too one-sidedly from today's perspective. In the literature on the history of palliative medicine, there has been many an example of such anachronistic misjudgments, and I briefly want to address the most common ones:

Some writers have described palliative care as nothing new because pre-modern medicine lacked effective treatments and hence was inherently limited to a

---

[20] Vanderpool, Palliative care (2015).

[21] For thorough recent accounts and useful collections of sources, see Cavina, Andarsene (2015); Benzenhöfer, Der gute Tod (2009) and idem, Euthanasia; and Grübler, Quellen (2007) and idem, Euthanasie (2011).

[22] See below for biographical information.

[23] Schleiner, Medical Ethics (1995); Bergdolt, Gewissen (2004); for the early modern period in particular, see Pohl, Unheilbar Kranker (1982); Elkeles, Aussagen (1979); and Brand, Ärztliche Ethik (1977).

[24] An exception is the recent book by Nolte, Todkrank (2016).

[25] Michael Stolberg, Two pioneers of active euthanasia around 1800, in: The Hastings Centre report 38 (2008), n. 6, pp. 19–22.

palliative approach to illnesses.[26] Equating "palliative" with "ineffective" reflects a rather strange understanding of the meaning of "palliative care", however, and it is particularly perplexing coming from authors who work in the field. From today's standpoint, the treatment of illnesses before 1850 or even around 1900 was indeed largely ineffective However, as mentioned above, doctors and laypeople were convinced that the proper medication and treatment could and frequently did save a sick person's life. In the numerous favorable outcomes that were experienced under a physician's care, they saw unmistakable proof of the effectiveness of medical therapy. The fact that we would attribute this recovery, in most cases, to the natural course of the illness and to placebo effects is irrelevant here. What is more, many commonly used pre-modern treatment procedures such as bloodletting, the use of drastic evacuants and mercury preparations did not have a "palliative" effect in any sense, neither in terms of the intentions at the time nor according to today's understanding. Rather than alleviating subjective complaints, they were frequently unpleasant or painful and weakened the patient and were only tolerated because there was a hope of healing.

Another example of widespread anachronism is the history of the hospice. Just because they carried the same name medieval pilgrims' hospices and early modern hospitals for the poor and invalid known as *hospices* in French have often summarily been declared precursors of modern hospices for the dying. However, as we will see, care for the dying was in no way their primary task.

Such anachronistic misperceptions can be avoided by careful historical analysis. At the same time, with the necessary caution and in the consciousness that any view of history is inevitably informed by the current context, historical research that proceeds from today's problems and questions is not only legitimate: It can also be very fruitful. Historians who attempt to describe phenomena and developments of the past exclusively through the eyes of those living at the time, using their terminology and concepts, will not do justice to the very task of historiography, which is to present history in such a way that the readers as people of their time can understand it and can perhaps even, thanks to the historical insight, arrive at a better understanding of the present. In this regard, the history of palliative medicine is not essentially different from many other historical undertakings. Whether we write histories of kings or executioners, of dancing or smoking, of honor or rape—to name just a few examples from the wide range of subjects that have been addressed in recent cultural-historical research—the professions, objects, activities or concepts that are referred to always call forth numerous associations and value judgments that reflect our experience today. And it is often precisely from the friction between then and now that the similarities and differences and with them what is specific for each period come into sharper focus in all their intricate detail.

[26] H. Pichlmaier, Palliativmedizin (editorial), in: Zentralblatt für Chirurgie 123 (1998), p. 619; P. D. Wall, 25 volumes of "Pain" (editorial), in: Pain 25 (1986), pp. 1–4; Derek Doyle, Geoffrey Hanks and Nathan I. Cherny, Introduction, in: iidem (eds): Oxford textbook of palliative medicine, 3rd edn, Oxford: Oxford University Press 2005, pp. 3–8; Derek Doyle, The provision of palliative care, in: ibid., pp. 41–53, here p. 41.

A big challenge for the historian wanting to write a history of end-of-life care and the related ethical dilemmas is finding suitable sources. In this book, I will draw on a wide range of printed and manuscript sources. Nevertheless, given the broad chronological and geographic scope of my analysis, my choice of sources will inevitably be selective and, when it comes to manuscript sources, sometimes reflect chance discoveries that I made in the course of my ongoing search for illuminating archival material. The public medical discourse about terminal care and the medical and ethical issues that it raised are relatively easy to reconstruct. Here we can draw on numerous printed sources. It is significantly more difficult to gain insights into the everyday medical and ethical practice with terminally ill and dying patients. Medical case histories offer valuable information in this regard, for example the large collection of medical *Observationes* published by the Dutch town physician Pieter van Foreest.[27] Further, as Werner F. Kümmel has shown, the pre-modern funeral sermons contain, despite their highly normative and idealizing character, valuable information on the care given by doctors and nurses in the days and weeks before death.[28] Once hospitals and hospices providing care for the dying were established, annual reports are helpful for an understanding of the care they provided. Not least of all, I will be drawing on numerous handwritten sources that are reflective of everyday life, for example private medical journals and notebooks, in which physicians expressed what they thought about the questions at hand, at times with unusual candor.[29]

The ways in which sick people and their relatives experienced palliative care and how they responded to the ethical issues that arose as death approached are particularly difficult to uncover. Occasionally patients described how they battled with their illness in letters or even autobiographies[30]—Albrecht von Haller and Madame de Graffigny are two impressive examples here[31]—but even then, such descriptions are cut short with the onset of the dying process. In the educated classes, the last days and hours of a dying person were sometimes described by relatives or friends or—as in the case of Philipp Melanchthon or the Count of Mirabeau—by the attending physician in letters to friends and family, or recounted in a funeral sermon or in

[27] Foreest, Observationum (1603–1606).

[28] Kümmel, Leichenpredigten (1984).

[29] A particularly rich source of this kind are, for the sixteenth century, the extensive notebooks of the Bohemian physician Georg Handsch, with altogether about 4.000 pages, which have survived in the Österreichische Nationalbibliothek in Vienna; cf. Michael Stolberg, Empiricism in sixteenth-century medical practice: The notebooks of Georg Handsch, in: Early science and medicine 18 (2013), pp. 487–516.

[30] The experience of dying patients plays a very marginal role e.g. in Lachmund's and Stollberg's extensive survey of German patient autobiographies from the late eighteenth to the early twentieth centuries [Lachmund and Stollberg, Patientenwelten (1995)]; although she has unearthed some interesting new sources in an archive of personal diaries Karen Nolte [Nolte, Todkrank (2016)], has ultimately come to the same conclusion.

[31] Haller, Briefe (1923); Graffigny, Correspondance (1985–2016); on Mme de Graffigny's experience of her illness and of her medical care see also Judith Oxfort, Meine Nerven tanzen. Die Krankheiten der Madame de Graffigny (1695–1758), Cologne: WiKu-Verlag 2010.

a handwritten or published *historia mortis*. The latter was a fairly popular genre, especially in Pietist circles before 1800. Pietism, which developed into a very influential movement within Protestantism in the eighteenth century, extended the Lutheran tradition of recording last words to include detailed descriptions of the last disease. When a Pietist was seen and described as having died in an exemplary, pious manner this was taken as a strong sign that he or she would enter the New Jerusalem.[32] Obviously, great caution must be applied when we use such reports as sources for the actual circumstances, leave alone the personal experience of dying. It is often all too obvious how the authors of these reports were interested in emphasizing the heroic courage and/or the profound piety with which the deceased looked death in the eye. Yet occasionally the descriptions are so concrete and detailed that the personal experiences of the dying and their relatives, the physical changes and the medical treatment come into focus.

Literary depictions form an important complementary source for a historical examination of the experience of death from the point of view of the sick and their relatives and for the perception and evaluation of ethical dilemmas in dealing with the dying. Naturally, the particularities of creative, literary writing must be kept in mind. Poems, stories, novels and plays—and the same is true for autobiographies—follow literary conventions and they are in our case unavoidably shaped by the dominant norms and images of a “good” death. Literary depictions of course accentuate the cultural cogency of these norms and images. Without a doubt they helped form an image of dying in the minds of those who had only had limited experience with death. Not least of all, the belletristic literature of the late nineteenth and twentieth centuries—and perhaps other literature as well—is relevant to the present study because it at times took up the ethical conflicts and portrayed them in a literary manner.

This book is divided into two main sections, followed by a conclusion that highlights some of the overarching features and developments. The first part is dedicated to the time from the late Middle Ages to the turn of the nineteenth century. In view of the current state of research it enters largely unknown territory. Proceeding from the oldest known uses and definitions of the term “palliative” in the fourteenth and fifteenth centuries, it outlines the growing medical attention paid to the *cura palliativa* and traces how medical writing from the mid-seventeenth century, using key words such as *euthanasia medicinalis,* increasingly began to deal specifically with the treatment of the dying. It shows how physicians dealt with the sick and dying and how they addressed the difficult ethical questions that sometimes arose from their treatment. It describes traditional practices such as the centuries-old custom of suddenly removing pillows, whereby one attempted, according to numerous accounts, to shorten the life and suffering of the dying. Drawing on exemplary personal accounts, it also attempts to reconstruct the subjective experience of those affected and their families.

The second part of the book looks at the time from the late eighteenth century to around 1970. It describes how the medical care of the severely ill and especially the

[32] Cf. Gleixner, Pietismus (2005), pp. 195–9.

dying enjoyed widespread attention and was treated by numerous writers, until about 1850, but then retreated into the background for almost a century. It outlines the growing attention paid to nursing in the nineteenth century and presents the most important medications and surgical procedures that were put to use in palliative medical care. It looks into the increasingly charged ethical debates, especially about the question of shortening life, and it presents the first doctors who made a case for active euthanasia around 1800. It also describes in detail, and with occasional glances back at the preceding centuries, the profound changes in the institutional care of terminally ill and dying patients and traces the emergence of independent institutions for such people, some of which can be seen as direct precursors of the modern hospice. It describes the circumstances in which sick people lived out their last days—at home, in hospital or in the new institutions for incurable and moribund patients—and how those affected and their families experienced death and how they dealt with it. Finally, it traces the developments in the years after the World War II and the beginnings of the modern hospice movement. Because these developments and their protagonists have been described in many publications and have been the subject of detailed historical research, my account of the time after 1945 will be limited to the tracing the major, essential developments. It will nevertheless draw on previously unknown sources such as the a detailed travel report, in which Sylvia Lack, the medical director of the first US-American hospice, described the conditions in the in-patient institutions for terminally ill and dying patients in Great Britain at the time.

The conclusion, looks at long-term changes: the growing place of terminal care from the late Middle Ages until about 1850, its marginalization in the following hundred years and its renaissance after World War II. Under the headings "medicalization," "taboo" and "stigma" it then follows three central dimensions of terminal care over time.

An earlier, German-language version of this book was published by Mabuse-Verlag in Frankfurt in 2011, under the title *Die Geschichte der Palliativmedizin. Medizinische Sterbebegleitung von 1500 bis heute* and I was pleased to find that it met with a great response well beyond historical circles. This English-language version has been restructured in part and revised with additions from further sources and recent publications by other scholars. At the same time, in view of the different anticipated readership, I have shortened and sometimes entirely omitted passages concerned primarily with developments in German-speaking areas. A selected bibliography lists the most important and most often cited works, and the shortened references in the footnotes point to this bibliography. For all other works and unprinted sources, the footnotes provide a complete entry.

Acknowledgements Important preliminary work for this book came from the research project "Alltagsgeschichte der medizinischen Ethik" ("History of Medical Ethics in Everyday Life") financed by the Fritz Thyssen-Foundation, which I directed from 2004 to 2006, as well as from a second project funded by the Deutsche Forschungsgemeinschaft (DFG) on the history of palliative medicine. In the context of this second project and under my direction, Hannes Langrieger explored in great detail the history of in-patient palliative medical care prior to 1914 and published case studies of two of these institutions—the homes for incurables in Bamberg and Regensburg.[33] The extensive source material on further institutions, which he found in his archival research but chose not to publish himself, has been used in this study and is attributed to him in the relevant footnotes. For the same DFG-project, Katrin Max took on the task of studying the care of the terminally ill and dying in medicine and nursing between 1880 and 1945 as represented in medical and literary sources.[34] Her book, which came out in 2013, about tuberculosis in Thomas Mann's *The Magic Mountain* and other German-language works of that time offers a wealth of material on the literary depiction of incurable diseases.[35]

33 Langrieger, Ein Platz (2008); idem, Medizinische Versorgung (2010).

34 Cf. Max, Literarische Texte (2008).

35 Max, Liegekur (2013).

Part I

The Early Modern Period (1500–1800)

2 Caring for Terminally Ill Patients

Early modern medical writers frequently discussed the learned physician's professional duties and his appropriate conduct at the sickbed.[1] Some issues were contentious but the authors were virtually unanimous on one point: It was the doctor's duty to care not just for those who could become well again but also for incurable and terminally ill patients; in fact, the doctor's concern with the welfare of these patients was seen as central among his medical obligations.[2] An ulcerated breast cancer, for example, was considered incurable by many authors, and attempting a radical cure was seen as harmful rather than beneficial. Leaving the patient without any help, however, Daniel Sennert, for example, argued in his oft-quoted work on medical practice would be "inhumane" ("inhumanum").[3] At first glance, this position seems to be at odds with that upheld by the ancient authorities. After all, the Hippocratic writings maintained that physicians must not treat incurably ill patients,[4] and Roman authors endorsed this prohibition. According to the encyclopedist Celsus, who was still quoted frequently during the early modern period, the physician needed to know which illnesses were incurable, which were difficult and which easy to treat. Those illnesses that he could not successfully fight he was best not to touch at all.[5] Yet, early modern physicians found other passages in the Hippocratic writings in which the treatment of incurable patients was not rejected but expressly described

[1] Castro, Medicus politicus (1662); Hoffmann, Medicus politicus (1738); cf. Elkeles, Aussagen (1979).

[2] E.g., Codronchi, De christiana ratione (1591), p. 24; Augenius, Epistolarum (1602), fol. 87v.

[3] Daniel Sennert, Opera omnia, Lyon 1656, p. 758.

[4] Hippokrates, Peri technes, in: idem, Œuvres complètes d'Hippocrate. Ed. by Émile Littré (Repr. Amsterdam 1978), Paris: Baillière 1839–1861, vol. 6, pp. 2–26, here 12–14.

[5] Celsus, De medicina libri octo. Ed. by Johannes Antonides van der Linden, Leiden: Elsevier 1657, pp. 282–3 (book 5, ch. 26.1).

M. Stolberg, *A History of Palliative Care, 1500–1970*, Philosophy and Medicine 123,
DOI 10.1007/978-3-319-54178-5_2

as the physician's task.[6] Thus, Guido Guidi, who practiced in the sixteenth century, concluded that Hippocrates had asked physicians to treat incurable diseases rather than not. Guidi argued that, for example, in the case of cancer, the patient's suffering could be diminished considerably and his life prolonged even though he could often not be cured.[7]

In the eyes of the early modern authors, the ancient authorities were not a suitable model in this regard anyway. They were pagans who were ignorant of Christian teaching. The stories of healing in the New Testament as well as the life stories and legends of Christian saints, by contrast, described individuals who were incurably ill and condemned to severe physical suffering as especially worthy subjects of divine healing and Christian *caritas*. The commandment to love one's neighbor, thought the papal physician Paolo Zacchia, expressing what seems to have been the view of many medical practitioners of the seventeenth century, made it a physician's duty to at least slow down the progression of the disease and to ease the suffering when treating a patient who was incurably ill.[8] This medical duty to show concern for incurable and dying people was impressed upon students of medicine and physicians in training already. Celebrating the conferral of a doctorate in 1580, Laurent Joubert explained that the newly awarded doctoral hat was a symbol of the hope that a physician must never lose and went on to state that those who thought desperate cases should not be touched lacked humanity.[9]

The question of medical care for patients who no longer had any prospect of healing arose predominantly with three diseases that were diagnosed quite frequently at the time: cancer, consumption and dropsy. With good reason, many considered cancer the most terrible disease of all. The diagnosis was made often, even back in the sixteenth and seventeenth centuries. Sufferers frequently experienced harrowing, interminable pain and exhausting sleeplessness. Added to this were the decomposing, festering ulcers, the revolting excretions, and the unbearable stench.

Cancer, in the early modern period, was experienced primarily as a female disease, because the large majority of those diagnosed with cancer were women. In retrospect, this can be explained by the fact that, at the time, the diagnosis of "cancer" was largely based on palpatory findings and visual examination from the outside. The eye and the palpating hand, however, were inevitably more or less limited to detecting tumors that were near the skin surface or were at least connected to it through one of the orifices. This was above all the case in breast cancer and to some degree also in uterine cancer, which sometimes could be palpated or announced itself

[6] Renate Wittern, Die Unterlassung ärztlicher Hilfeleistung in der griechischen Medizin der klassischen Zeit, in: Münchener medizinische Wochenschrift 121 (1979), pp. 731–4; Heinrich von Staden, Incurability and hopelessness. The Hippocratic corpus, in: Paul Potter (ed.), La maladie et les maladies dans la collection hippocratique. Actes du VIe Colloque International Hippocratique, Québec: Les Éditions du Sphinx 1990, pp. 75–112; Plinio Prioreschi, Did the Hippocratic physician treat hopeless cases? in: Gesnerus 49 (1992), pp. 341–50.

[7] Guido Guidi, De curatione generatim, in: idem, Opera omnia sive ars medicinalis (separate page numbering), Frankfurt: Typis et sumptibus Wechelianorum 1626, p. 121.

[8] Zacchia, Quaestiones (1651), pp. 392–3.

[9] Laurent Joubert, Oratio de praesidiis futuri excellentis medici, Geneva: Stoer 1580, p. 15.

with bloody or purulent discharge. Until the eighteenth century, these two kinds of cancer represented the large majority of documented cancer diagnoses. The—perceived—much higher incidence of cancer in women, especially following menopause, also accorded with the early modern understanding of female physiology and could be taken to confirm it, in turn. In contrast to men, women required a monthly "natural cleansing," to rid themselves of impure, acrimonious and toxic substances that constantly accumulated in their bodies. When the monthly cleansing ceased at a certain age, these harmful substances accumulated in the body. They could harden and finally develop into painful cancerous tumors, which sooner or later formed ulcers through which they discharged the cancerous matter, at least in part.[10]

The diagnosis of "consumption" or "phthisis" could refer, in the literal sense of the word, to "consuming", "emaciating" diseases in general. In practice, however, it was mainly used for progressive chronic chest or lung complaints. Considering the night sweats and the agonizing and at times bloody coughing that were described as typical symptoms, we would probably diagnose many of these cases as pulmonary tuberculosis today. In some of the cases, however, the patients may, in retrospect, have suffered from lung cancer, other severe chronic diseases of the lungs, or hidden cancerous tumors in other inner organs and even liver or metabolic diseases, all of which share the common feature of severe weight loss.

The early modern notion of "consumption" was closely related to that of the "hectic fever" or *febris hectica*, which was associated with a hastened consumption of vital heat and its substrate, the "radical moisture" or *humidum radicale*. Like the light of an oil lamp whose oil was running low, life's light was thought to go out when this vital moisture was used up. With hectic fever, this happened at an accelerated pace and the body began melting down its own substance. According to contemporary doctrine, experienced uroscopists were even able to tell that this was the case by identifying fat in the urine. In the case of pulmonary consumption, people also assumed acrimonious, sharp, irritating morbid matter, which the body tried to eliminate through expectoration. This morbid matter was taken to be so acrimonious and sharp that it could even eat away the walls of the blood vessels and lead to severe hemorrhage.[11]

In nineteenth-century literary accounts of consumption, we often find it associated with ideas of spiritual elevation and refinement.[12] However, when we read contemporary medical descriptions of the illness, the brutal, violent changes in the body that typically went along with consumption become startlingly clear. It shared the symptoms of emaciation and weakness with other, less common diseases such as diabetes, where the "vital powers were slowly exhausted."[13] Quite often, pulmonary consumption also went along with severe diarrhea. The prolonged violent coughing attacks that many consumptive patients suffered from were excruciating. Yet, what shaped the perception of dying from these diseases, and the fear of them, was an increasing short-

[10] Michael Stolberg, A woman's hell? Medical perceptions of menopause in preindustrial Europe, in: Bulletin of the history of medicine 73 (1999), pp. 408–28.

[11] Stolberg, Experiencing illness (2011), pp. 147–9.

[12] Cf. Sontag, Illness (1978); Pohland, Sanatorium (1984), pp. 146–51.

[13] Watson, Grundgesetze (1851), p. 73.

ness of breath that culminated in "extreme agony and fear of death."[14] Likewise feared were bloody coughs and hemorrhaging that could lead to sudden death.

A third, commonly diagnosed disease that was feared for its long-term fatal outcome was dropsy. Dropsy, today, is seen merely as a symptom that may point to a large number of illnesses, ranging from heart or liver diseases to kidney failure and protein deficiency. Early modern doctors and their patients, by contrast, understood and treated dropsy as a separate clinical entity. The cause was often seen in an excessive accumulation of watery liquid in the entire body or specifically in the abdomen, a condition which we still refer to as *ascites* today. If the water was mixed with air or foul vapors, it was referred to as "wind dropsy" or *tympanites*.[15]

Among the prominent, agonizing symptoms of dropsy some were similar to those of consumption: shortness of breath—including serious choking fits—and a progressive loss of strength. In other respects, the way the disease was visualized and the associations it evoked were contrary to those of consumption. The prevailing imagery here was that of a bloated, bulging belly and body, not a wasted frame of skin and bones. For a long time, the medical literature even considered dropsy to be closely related to the pathological changes concomitant with excessive corpulence, *obesitas nimia*.[16]

There were several other illnesses that, at least in their advanced stages, were often considered incurable. Besides leprosy, which played only a minor role from the seventeenth century onward, these were above all different types of paralysis and severe joint complaints, blindness and deafness, as well as falling sickness and madness. However, in contrast to cancer, consumption and dropsy, these illnesses tended to take a course of several years or decades and were only rarely the immediate cause of death.

When addressing incurable diseases, the medical writers of the day routinely underlined that they required a therapeutic approach that differed from common procedure in essential respects. Usually, as the famous Italian doctor Vettore Trincavelli wrote, it was the task of the physician to "eliminate the illness" and, not only to his mind, this implied attacking its causes.[17] In the early modern period, this standard approach to the treatment of diseases was called "curative" (*curatoria*),[18] "true" (*vera*) or "radical" (*radicalis,* in the sense of going to the roots of the illness). By the sixteenth century, this "curative" approach only rarely still aimed at re-establishing a disturbed balance of the humors and qualities. Instead, early modern doctors attributed most diseases to preternatural, morbid humors or other corrupted,

[14] Ibid., p. 76.

[15] Stolberg, Experiencing illness (2011), pp. 152–3.; Maximilian Hader, Würzburg, is currently working on a thesis about early modern notions of dropsy.

[16] Michael Stolberg, "Abhorreas pinguedinem". Fat and obesity in early modern medicine (c. 1500–1750), in: Studies in the history and philosophy of science 43 (2012), pp. 370–8.

[17] Vettore Trincavelli, Consilia medica. Basel: Waldkirch 1587, consilium X.

[18] E.g., Heinrich Christoph Alberti, De scorbuto, germanice Von dem Scharbock. Exponit Johann Henricus Schmoller, Erfurt: Groschius 1692, pp. 22–3. Other authors used "curare" in the general sense of "treating" or "taking care" and "sanare" for successful cures.

foul or otherwise harmful substances. A "true", "radical" treatment consequently aimed at rendering harmless the morbid matter that was the assumed cause of the illness and/or eliminating it from the body. Thus, evacuative means such as blood-letting or cupping along with a wide variety of emetics and laxatives as well as sudorifics formed the basis of almost every therapy. These were complemented with numerous remedies that were thought to act more or less specifically on certain diseases or morbid substances.[19]

In the case of incurable and dying patients, by contrast, a primarily causal therapy, which attacked the disease at its roots, was found to be futile and often harmful. Here, alleviating the patient's suffering became the principal concern. The patient's symptoms were often so grave, the famous Leiden clinician Franciscus Sylvius (1614–1672) explained, that the doctor had to try to control them without paying any heed to the illness itself. If, for instance, a great loss of blood and other bodily fluids or intense pains exhausted the vital spirits, or else if excessive flatulence or winds pushed the diaphragm upwards and hindered breathing, these complaints had to be addressed and, if necessary, the actual cause of the disease left untouched for the time being.[20] In fact, according to a frequently voiced warning, attempting a radical, curative treatment in such cases even harbored the risk of worsening the illness or killing the patient.

The classic example was breast cancer.[21] A much-quoted aphorism by Hippocrates already warned of treating it aggressively.[22] In his commentary on the Hippocratic aphorisms, Galen used this as a starting point for his theoretical considerations about basic forms of medical treatment.[23] Sometimes the doctor fought the causes of a disease in order to eliminate it. Sometimes, he limited himself to alleviating suffering. Here Galen used the terms *paregorein* (soothing) and *prainein* (alleviating), which Dioscorides, antiquity's great pharmacological authority, had already used to describe medicines that had only an alleviating effect.[24]

---

[19] For a survey of major early modern disease concepts see Stolberg, Experiencing illness (2011), pp. 89–153.

[20] Franciscus Sylvius, De methodo medendi, in: idem: Opera medica. Geneva: Apud Samuelem de Tournes 1681, pp. 34–62, here p. 37.

[21] Biblioteca Lancisiana, Rome, Ms. 259 Tom III, fols 46r–48r, consilium by Giovanni Maria Lancisi, 29 January, 1707, for a nun with ulcerating breast cancer.

[22] Hippokrates, Aphorismoi, in: idem, Œuvres complètes d'Hippocrate. Ed. by Émile Littré (Repr. Amsterdam 1978), Paris: Baillière 1839–1861, vol. 4, pp. 458–609, here p. 572, Aphorism 6.38.

[23] Galen, Opera omnia. Ed. by C. H. Kühn, vol. 18. Leipzig 1822 (Repr. Hildesheim: Olms 1964), pp. 59–61.

[24] Pedanius Dioskurides, De materia medica libri quinque. Ed. by Curtius Sprengel (= Medicorum graecorum opera quae extant, vol. 25), Leipzig: Cnobloch 1829, e.g., vol. 1, p. 37. In another passage, Galen distinguished even more precisely "paregoric" medicines which mitigated the symptoms and, at the same time, fought the disease itself, and "prainonta", which had no effect on the disease itself but only alleviated the pain. (Galen, Opera omnia. Ed. by C. H. Kühn, vol. 13, p. 707); see also Aretaios, Aretaei Cappadocis opera omnia. Ed. by Karl Gottlob Kühn (= Medicorum graecorum opera quae extant, vol. 24), Leipzig: Cnobloch 1828, p. 331 (On chronic diseases, book 2, ch. 3); Oribasius, Œuvres complètes. Ed. and transl. by Charles Daremberg and Cats Bussemaker, Paris: Imprim. impériole 1851–76, vol. 2, pp. 741–2 ("paregorika").

2.1 *Cura palliativa.* Archeology of a Modern Term

Early modern doctors were familiar with the distinction between radical and alleviating therapy and *paregorica* was a common designation for remedies that served to ease the suffering rather than cure the disease.[25] It can be found well into the nineteenth century in the medical literature[26] and in medical dictionaries and encyclopedias, in Latin or in vernacular variants such as *parégoriques*. Some authors preferred to speak of remedies as *mitigantia, mitigativa* or *mitigatoria* in this context[27] and accordingly recommended a *cura mitigativa* or a *cura blanditiva,* a "blandishing cure."[28]

Developing alongside the others since the late Middle Ages, another term came to the fore, however, the *cura palliativa.* The earliest occurrence that I have so far been able to identify dates from the mid-fourteenth century. In an introductory chapter to his *Chirurgia* (from around 1363) Guy de Chauliac (1298–1368) named three exceptional situations in which the doctor could forgo radical, causal treatment and be content with a "cura larga, praeservativa, et palliativa": First, this applied to diseases such as leprosy that by their very nature were incurable; second, if the patient rejected a causal, curative treatment that in principle could be pursued or did not follow the doctor's instructions; and third, if the curative treatment would likely result in greater harm than was caused by the illness itself, for instance if the doctor was able to stop troublesome hemorrhoids from bleeding but the body required the regular bleeding to rid itself of impure, harmful matter that otherwise made it sick.[29]

---

[25] For an early account of the history of the term see Johann Konrad Dieterich, Iatreum hippocraticum: continens narthecium medicinae veteris et novae; ex nobilioribus medicis, tam veteribus, quam recentioribus, jucunda verborum serie, juxta ductum aphorismorum Hippocratis ita compositum, ut et aliarum facultatum studiis queat inservire, Ulm: Balthasar Kühnen 1661, p. 936; in the eighteenth century, expressions like "effectum paregoricum" were still in use (e.g., Oberlin, De opio 1752, p. 22).

[26] See e.g. Jacques Houllier, De morborum internorum curatione libri. With annotations by Ludovicus Duretus, Venice: Apud Iacobum Maceum 1572, fol. 136r.

[27] ÖNB, Cod. 11200, fol. 33r (Georg Handsch, "mitigativa"); Bartholomaeus Castellus, Lexicon medicum graecolatinum […] ex Hippocrate, et Galeno desumptum. Messanae: Typis Petri Breae 1598, p. 307; Emmanuel Stupanus, Lexicon medicum graeco-latinum compendiosiss[imum] a Bartholomaeo Castello Messanense inchoatum. Basel: Impensis Joh. Jacobi Genathi 1628, p. 263; Adrianus Ravesteinus, Lexicon medicum graeco-latinum a Bartholomaeo Castello Messanense inchoatum, Rotterdam: apud Arnoldum Leers 1651, pp. 371–2; Stephanus Blancardus, Lexicon novum medicum graeco-latino-germanicum, Leiden: apud Boutesteyn et Luchtmans 1690, p. 475; Ibid., 5th edn, Halle – Magdeburg 1718, p. 246; Sylvius, Praxeos medicae idea (1695), pp. 89–90, "De indicatione urgente, quibusdam mitigatoria dicta"; Louis-Jacques Bégin et al., Dictionnaire des termes de médecine, chirurgie, art vétérinaire, pharmacie, histoire naturelle, botanique, physique, chimie, Paris: Baillière, Crevot and Béchet 1823, p. 446 ("parégorique"); Dictionnaire des sciences médicales, vol. 39, Paris: Panckoucke 1819, p. 285 ("parégorique", "paregoricus").

[28] Cardano, De malo medendi usu (1536), pp. 8–9.

[29] Guy de Chauliac, Chirurgia, Leiden: apud Sebastianum de Honoratis 1559, fols a2(v)-a3(v); cf. Guy de Chauliac, Guigonis de Caulhiaco inventarium sive chirurgia magna. Ed. by Michael R. McVaugh, vol. 1: text, Leiden 1997.

Guy de Chauliac's *Chirurgia* was the most important late medieval overview publication of surgery, and it was widely circulated, sometimes in vernacular translations. Among the many extant copies are manuscripts written in German, French, Provençal, Catalan, English, Dutch and Italian. Most likely it is one of these manuscripts that the first vernacular use of the term "palliative" can be found. The earliest use of the term in the vernacular that I have been able to discover is in two Middle English manuscripts of the *Chirurgia* that can be dated roughly to the time around 1425 and to the second quarter of the fifteenth century respectively. Here, the chapter about the treatment of cancerous ulcers explicitly speaks of the "cure paliatyf," or "cure palliatif," and also uses the verb form "to palliate."[30] In later vernacular editions of Guy de Chauliac's work, which are based on older manuscripts, the term can also be found where one would expect it. Laurent Joubert's 1579–80 French translation of the *Chirurgia,* for example, provides a very literal rendering of the above-quoted section: "une curation large, preservative & palliative."[31]

Other authors as well adopted the term at this time. An English edition of the *Chirurgia* by Giovanni da Vigo (ca. 1450–1525) from 1543 presents the oldest vernacular use of the term "palliative" in a printed work known today. Writing about the treatment of cancer, da Vigo contrasted the "eradicatyue cure" with a "palliatyue cure."[32] The use of strong medication, wrote da Vigo, might kill the patient, while gentle remedies might allow the patient's life to be prolonged and indeed "some health recouered in palliynge the canker".[33] In his treatise on cancerous nasal polyps, he consequently suggested refraining from the use of powerful, acrid remedies. It was better "to appalliate it by gentle medicines." With a "palliatyve cure," the patient's life could be prolonged without much pain.[34] In an appendix on *The Interpretation of Straunge [sic!] Words* we also find, attached to this work in 1563, the oldest known attempt at a definition: "A cure palliative is, when a disease is cloked for a reason, not perfytlye healed."[35] In 1574, the surgeon Franciscus Arcaeus wrote that in the case of festering breast cancer, a "palliative" cure was the only choice because whatever else one did would result in considerable harm.[36]

[30] Guy de Chauliac, The Cyrurgerie of Guy de Chauliac. Ed. by M. S. Ogden, London et al.: Oxford University Press 1971, p. 302, based on Bibliothèque nationale, Paris, Ms. anglais 25; Guy de Chauliac, The Middle English translation of Guy de Chauliac's treatise on ulcers. Book IV of the Great Surgery. Part I: Text. Ed. by Björn Wallner, Stockholm: Almquist & Wiksell 1982, p. 37 and p. 39, based on a manuscript in the New York Academy of Medicine.

[31] Guy de Chauliac, La grande chirurgie. Ed. by Laurent Joubert, Lyon: Estienne Michel 1580 (printer's mark: 1579).

[32] Vigo, Chirurgerye (1543), fol. 43v: "we wyll speake of his cure aswel eradicatyue as palliatyue".

[33] Ibid., fol. 44v.

[34] Ibid., fols 56r–57v.

[35] Ibid., no page numbering.

[36] Franciscus Arcaeus, De recta curandorum vulnerum ratione libri II, Antwerp: Plantin 1574, pp. 99–101 and p. 102 (explanation of the term "cura palliativa", probably by Alvarus Nonnius); the same passage can be found in the English edition of 1588 (idem, A most excellent and compendious method of curing woundes in the head, and in other partes of the body, London: by Thomas East for Thomas Cadman 1588, pp. 36r–v and 37r–v ("cura palliativa—a palliative cure").

It was probably no coincidence that the term "palliative" was first introduced in medical vocabulary by surgeons such as Guy de Chauliac and Giovanni da Vigo. Surgery occupied a remarkable and so far overlooked place in the early history of palliative medicine. Surgeons' attempts to achieve a radical cure in serious diseases was attended by a particularly high risk of a fatal outcome. Moreover, given the usually excruciating pain, an operation without the patient's consent was hardly conceivable. When the patient refused the procedure or the risk seemed too high, the surgeon had to be satisfied with a treatment that was "only" palliative, even if he saw a realistic chance for a complete cure.

In writings about medical practice and in consultation letters as well, the term came into use around that time at the latest. An unidentified early sixteenth-century writer noted in his personal medical notebook, "Cura cancri est palliatio," adding a recipe designed to maintain and "palliate" the cancer so it would not soften and corrupt.[37] Around 1550, in the notebooks of the Bohemian physician Georg Handsch, the notion recurs in a number of passages. For instance, we find a recipe for an ointment for the "palliation" of leprosy ("ad palleationem leprae") and a German definition of the "palliative cure" ("cura palliativa").[38] In 1574, the Aretino physician and anatomist Laurentius Ricciardus wrote about a patient with a nasal ulcer that the majority of the Venetian doctors and surgeons who had been consulted had considered as cancerous. While one of the doctors voiced some hope, the others declared the complaint incurable and recommended only a "curationem paleativam [sic], et praeservativam" rather than a curative one.[39] When a cancer had ulcerated, as the Basel professor Felix Platter taught his students around 1590, all treatment was palliative, "omnis cura est palliativa".[40]

As these quotes indicate, terms such as *palliatio* and *cura palliativa* became more and more established in common medical parlance during the late sixteenth century.[41] An important contribution in this respect was the widely circulated collection of medical case histories, by the Dutch physician Pieter van Foreest (1522–1597), which continued to be quoted for centuries.[42] Foreest gave several explicit

[37] Universitätsbibliothek Erlangen, Ms. 979, fol. 111r, "Ad conservandum cancrum et palliandum ne mollificetur"; according to a contemporary entry at the beginning, the manuscript was given as a gift to Johannes Oberndorffer in 1531, which would mean that the notes were written before.

[38] ÖNB, Cod. 11200, fol. 4v, and Ibid., Cod. 9666, fol. 43v.

[39] Staatsbibliothek Bamberg, Ms. JH msc. med. 9, Nr. 8, undated account of the results of a medical consultation on a 83-year-old patient, in response to an epistolary request by the Nürnberg surgeon Volcher Coiter, October 25, 1574 (Ibid., Nr. 9).

[40] Landesbibliothek Stuttgart, Cod med. 4° 10, student notes by Konrad Zinn, fol. 238v.

[41] Another example is Franciscus Arcaeus, De recta curandorum vulnerum ratione libri II Antwerp: Plantin 1574, p. 94 (on the pallliative treatment of breast cancer).

[42] Foreest, Observationum medicinalium (1603–1606); on this genre, which became very popular in the early modern period, see Pedro Laìn Entralgo, La historica clinica. Historia y teoria del relato patografico, Barcelona: Salvat Editores 1961; Michael Stolberg, Formen und Funktionen ärztlicher Fallbeobachtungen in der Frühen Neuzeit (1500–1800), in: Johannes Süßmann, Susanne Scholz and Gisela Engel (eds): Fallstudien: Theorie – Geschichte – Methode, Berlin: Trafo-Verlag 2007, pp. 81–95; Gianna Pomata, A word of the empirics: The ancient concept of observation and its recovery in early modern medicine, Annals of science 65 (2011), pp. 1–25.

accounts of a "palliative" therapy. They include the case of a 70-year-old woman from Delft, whom he treated in 1560 for a cancerous ulcer on her breast.[43] He declared the woman's complaint incurable and inoperable and, after administering a gentle laxative, treated the breast "with palliation, as they call it" ("ad palliationem ut vocant") using a locally applied remedy. The ulcer, for the time being, did not grow and the woman lived for some time longer. In other cases, Foreest even emphasized the superiority of a palliative approach to more drastic measures. For example, he advised another female patient not to take any local remedies that would promote an ulceration of the cancer. Among less learned healers, this was a common procedure at the time. It was hoped that the body would rid itself of the cancerous matter with the festering ulcer acting as a conduit. Instead, Foreest in this case recommended laxatives and bloodletting, apparently in order to evacuate the cancerous matter from the body in ways that would not provoke the cancer. Afterward, the patient was to use external remedies for the "palliation of the cancer" ("iis topicis uteretur quae ad palleationem cancri facerent"). The woman, however, disregarded his advice and went instead to a healer, an *empiricus,* who opened her breast. An ulcer developed and the woman began to feel worse and worse. Suffering terrible pain, she finally died a miserable death.[44]

Foreest likewise advised another woman with breast cancer that was not yet open not to irritate the cancer unnecessarily. She, too, went to see a healer, a woman who successfully made the wound fester—doubtlessly with the hope of evacuating the cancerous morbid matter and thus eliminating the cancer. Yet, the consequences were devastating. According to Foreest, the sick woman's arms became swollen. She gave off a stench that was so offensive that people could hardly bear being in her presence. In the end, she ruefully returned to Foreest but it was too late. All he could do was provide a temporary palliative treatment ("palliatione ad tempus in ea usi sumus") by administering remedies for her pain and the sore skin.[45]

Foreest also used this terminology in his surgical *Observationes*, which were published only after his death. With chronic fistulas, he explained, very much in the tradition of Guy de Chauliac, it was at times necessary to "palliate, as they say" ("palliare ut dicunt"), if they were in an adverse location, if the patient was too weak for a surgical procedure or rejected it, or else if there was a risk that the fistula would get worse because of the surgery. He wrote that this kind of "palliation" ("istam palliationem") had already been recommended by Avicenna and Arnau de Vilanova.[46] Elsewhere we find his account of a 60-year-old patient suffering from a festering cancerous tumor of the eye. With the aim of "palliating" and strengthening the eye ("palliandi et roborandi oculum"), the attending surgeon had, among other things,

[43] Foreest, Observationum medicinalium (1603–1606), Buch 16: De pectoris pulmonisque vitiis ac morbis: Et decimusseptimus De cordis ac quibusdam mammillarum affectibus, Leiden 1603 (orig. 1593), pp. 482–6.

[44] Ibid., p. 485.

[45] Ibid.

[46] Foreest, Observationum chirurgicarum (1601), pp. 333–43, esp. p. 343.

prescribed an "unguentum palliativum exsiccans," that is a desiccating palliative ointment that would consume the tumor and prevent its further growth.[47]

Following Foreest's *Observationes,* "palliative" treatment was increasingly mentioned in similar contexts by other doctors as well. Henricus ab Heer, for instance, wrote about a *cura palliativa,* which, in 1605, he administered to a 70-year-old woman with abdominal cancer.[48] Soon after, Paolo Zacchia (1585–1659) of Rome discussed in general terms the treatment "that is called palliative" ("quae palliativa dicitur"), naming it the third basic form of treating illness, the other two being the preventive and the curative treatment. In Hamburg, the Portuguese doctor Roderigo da Castro (ca. 1550–1627) recommended the use of "paleativa [sic]," if a breast cancer had progressed so far that surgery was no longer possible.[49] Daniel Sennert in his influential *Practica Medicina* contrasted the "true" treatment of breast cancer, which aimed at its removal, with the "palliative, as it is called," which "flattered" the cancer, alleviated it, so that the sick person could lead her life and not suffer from her complaints as much.[50]

In the second half of the seventeenth century, the leading medical dictionary of the day *Lexicon Medicum Graeco-Latinum,* established by Bartolommeo Castelli, adopted the term *palliatio* as a separate keyword.[51] Its definition, which was avowedly in the tradition of Foreest, was rendered almost verbatim in English in Robert James's famous dictionary:

> "Palliatio, palliativa cura, it is called by the doctors, when, in the case of desperate and incurable illnesses and with a fatal infaust prognosis, certain remedies are administered which soothe the pain or other burdensome symptoms, as in the case of cancerous ulcers, cancerous fistulas etc."[52] Stephanus Blancardus, in his medical dictionary, also provided some Dutch equivalents, namely "plaats-middelen"—presumably referring to "place", i.e. to local remedies—and "streel-middelen", probably derived from the Dutch word "strelen" for "to alleviate" or "to caress".[53]

---

[47] Ibid., pp. 343–8.

[48] Heer, Observationes (1645), pp. 180–1.

[49] Zacchia, Quaestiones (1651), pp. 392–3.

[50] Daniel Sennert, Opera omnia, Lyon 1656, p. 758.

[51] Jacobus Pancratius Bruno, Castellus renovatus, hoc est., Lexicon medicum, quondam a Barth. Castello Messanensi inchoatum, Nürnberg: Sumtibus Johan. Danielis Tauberi 1682, pp. 875–6: "Palliatio, palliativa cura, vocatur medicis, quando in morbis desperatis et incurabilibus, praemisso prognostico eventus funesti, quaedam remedia mitigantia vel dolorem, vel alia symptomata urgentia adhibentur, ut, in cancris ulceratis, fistulis cancrosis, aliisque."

[52] Robert A. James, A medicinal dictionary, including physic, surgery, anatomy, chymistry, and botany, vol. 3, London: printed for T. Osborne 1745.

[53] Stephanus Blancardus, Lexicon novum medicum graeco-latinum, Leiden: apud Cornelium Boutesteyn and Jordaanum Luchtmans 1690, p. 475.

In 1692, the oldest known monographic treatise about theory and practice of palliative care was published in Erfurt: Elias Küchler's dissertation *De Cura Palliativa.*[54] In its approximately 30 pages, we find the first thorough analysis of the term and a comprehensive exposition of the different aspects and elements of a palliative treatment. The author explained that protracted, chronic diseases and especially those associated with old age often did not allow for a complete, radical cure. The work of someone who knew how to deal with such incurable diseases in a palliative way, however, was as valuable to the health of the sick person as the work of someone who eradicated curable diseases by their roots. Küchler distinguished three types of palliative treatment:

1. a concealing "dissimulating" treatment that cloaked or compensated physical deficiencies or blemishes. To Küchler, this included, for example, cosmetics used to cover undesirable skin alterations, prostheses to replace lost body parts, plastic surgery that (imperfectly) replaced a destroyed nose, belts for bulging abdominal hernias, as well as the deliberate, surgical creation of an artificial opening for the bladder to empty into the intestine in cases where bladder stones made it impossible for the bladder to empty via the urethra.
2. an alleviating "mitigating" treatment used in particular with painful complaints. Here the doctor relied on remedies such as henbane, hemlock and above all opium, which diminished the perception of pain and eased cramps. A "mitigating" treatment could sometimes be carried out in concert with the third type of palliative treatment.
3. a causal treatment that "suspended" or "restricted" the medical condition itself. While this kind of treatment was not able to eliminate the cause of the illness and therefore not the illness itself, it still counteracted it and slowed it down. In this way, febrile diseases for example could be treated with specific fever remedies such as China bark, camphor or gentian, which restored free breathing for people with life-threatening diseases. Further, Küchler, referring to Sylvius, who had shown this with consumption, explained that with illnesses that were chronic, hereditary or age-related, the doctor could make the morbid matter less harmful or acrid, or less viscous and thus easier to excrete; and he could support its excretion with gentle "expelling" remedies. Cancerous ulcers and fistulas could be fought with external means. With renal colic, the passing of the stones could be facilitated using antispasmodic, relaxing remedies that widened the urethra. Stones that blocked the internal urethral orifice could at least temporarily be pushed back into the bladder using a catheter.

[54] Küchler, De cura palliativa (1692); early modern medical dissertations were often written by the professor, who was usually named on the title page as the "promotor" or "praeses", but sometimes also by the doctoral student or by both. Since Küchler did not even mention the "praeses" on the frontispiece and referred repeatedly to "my teacher" ("praeceptor meus") in the text he probably wrote the dissertation at least largely himself.

According to Küchler, palliative treatment, understood correctly, made the complaint easier to bear, for the patient himself but also for the people around him—and it could even prolong life.[55] However, Küchler also warned of the dangers of an unintentional palliative treatment, a "cura palliativa erronea," which was found above all in the practice of the *empirici*. According to Küchler, they treated, for instance, febrile diseases with specific remedies, which, they believed, fought the disease itself. These remedies might alleviate symptoms temporarily but without expelling the true cause of the disease, the morbid matter as such. The harmful, morbid matter remained in the body and as a result patients developed even worse complaints such as dropsy, joint pains, emaciation, spasms, paralysis or at least general lethargy and weakness.

Several years later, in Jena, Philipp Friedrich Schmeltzer, studying with Georg Wolffgang Wedel, defended a doctoral thesis with the same title, *De Cura Palliativa*.[56] The notion of as "palliative" treatment, the author explained, was part of everyday medical parlance.[57] As this form of treatment did not aim at the elimination of the causes of disease as such, it might be criticized for missing the mark and thus being unworthy of the rational physician. Using a wealth of examples, he went on to illustrate that grounds for a palliative treatment had to be established very carefully to avoid forgoing a promising curative treatment in favor of the said palliative treatment. Yet, there were cases where a palliative treatment was indispensable. For example, in most cases of cancer, a palliative treatment that kept the disease from becoming even wilder and spreading further was far superior to an aggressive treatment.[58]

In Erfurt in 1742, Georg Ludwig Rosa submitted his dissertation on the *curatio palliativa*.[59] He wrote that in contrast to a "true" therapy, this treatment was understood to mean an alleviation or elimination of symptoms, regardless of any known or hidden true causes of the illness, to be used when the art of medicine was unable to eliminate these.[60] He held that there were essentially three reasons to reject a causal treatment: Some diseases were inherently incurable; secondly, in certain cases—and here he named breast cancer, longstanding, persistent ulcers of the legs and anal fistulas—treatment stood to cause more harm than the disease itself; and thirdly, there were diseases whose cause was simply not known and could therefore not be fought.[61]

---

[55] Ibid., p. 8 and p. 32.

[56] Wedel, De cura palliativa (1703); the frontispiece carries the erroneous date 1603. As in many early modern medical dissertations (see note on Küchler above), it is not clear whether the "praeses", Wedel, wrote the text or his student, Schmeltzer. The quality and the depth of this work make Wedel the much more probable author in this case, however.

[57] Ibid., p. 4 ("toto die ita medicorum filios loqui").

[58] Ibid., p. 24.

[59] Rosa, De curatione palliativa (1742); Rosa clearly identifies himself as the author ("auctor").

[60] Ibid., p. 6 and p. 41.

[61] Ibid., p. 6.

The "palliative" care of illness increasingly found its place even in introductory works for medical students. For example Herman Boerhaave , likely the most influential clinician teaching in Europe in the early eighteenth century, dedicated a whole chapter of his *Institutiones medicae* to the *curatio palliativa,* offering doctors in training a broad spectrum of remedies for the alleviation of pain, sleeplessness and thirst.[62]

Apparently, doctors also used the term "palliative" with their patients. Johann Wolfgang von Goethe, for example, gave an account of his experience with the famous doctor Reil, who treated Goethe over the course of a fortnight without giving him a prescription, "except one, which he described as merely palliative."[63] By the late eighteenth century, terms like "palliative" and "palliative cure" had become established to such a degree in everyday language indeed that they could be used and were understood metaphorically. Goethe, for example, declared "Liebeley," that is, flirting with the opposite sex, the "most effective palliative" for his "Teufels Humor," his "devil's mood."[64] Krünitz's voluminous *Encyclopädie* has around 50 entries that use terms such as *"Palliativmittel"* and *"Palliativcur,"* some in a medical context, others referring metaphorically to moral or economic matters.[65] For example, buying-up crops temporarily became an "excellent palliative remedy" to slow a deterioration of crop prices.[66]

The early modern medical conception of a "palliative" approach was in some respects significantly broader than it is today. Insofar as the expression "palliative" focused more than it does today on the difference between it and a radical, causal approach. As can be seen from its metaphoric use in everyday language, the term was very close in meaning to our modern notion of a "symptomatic" treatment. In this sense, illnesses that could be expected to have a fatal outcome in a distant future—illnesses such as scurvy,[67] syphilis, epilepsy, melancholia and leprosy—also would have been addressed with a "palliative" treatment.

The notion of "palliation" was also shaped much more than it is today by the original, literal meaning of the Latin *palliare*. The word derives from *pallium,* meaning "cloak." In the strict sense, *palliare* therefore meant "laying a cloak over

[62] Boerhaave, Institutiones (1721), pp. 386–9.

[63] Johann Wolfgang von Goethe, letter to Carl August, August 10, 1805, repr. in Hans Wahl (ed.), Briefwechsel des Herzogs-Großherzogs Carl August mit Goethe, vol. 1, 1775–1806, Berlin: E. S. Mittler 1915, pp. 334–336, cit. p. 334; my thanks to Christiane Schlaps who pointed this letter out to me.

[64] Johann Wolfgang von Goethe, Goethes Briefe an Frau von Stein. Ed. by Jonas Fränkel, vol. 1, Jena: Diederichs 1908, p. 2 (January 27, 1776).

[65] Krünitz, Oeconomische Encyclopädie (1773–1858).

[66] Ibid., vol. 45 (1789), p. 629.

[67] The early modern notion of "scurvy" differs markedly from that today. The disease was commonly attributed to some acrimonious morbid matter; see Stolberg, Experiencing illness (2011), pp. 110–3; Maximilian Mayer, Verständnis und Darstellung des Skorbuts im 17. Jahrhundert, Mit einer Edition und Übersetzung der Fallgeschichten zu "Skorbut" bei Johannes Frank. Würzburg: med. diss 2012 (URL: https://opus.bibliothek.uni-wuerzburg.de/frontdoor/index/index/docId/6241),

something," "covering something up."[68] As we have seen, the English edition of Vigo's *Chirurgia* of 1563 defined "cure palliative" as a treatment that, for one reason or another, "covered up" ("cloked") the disease.[69] In his widely read medical dictionary of 1709, Johann Jakob Woyt accordingly rendered *palliatio* in German as "Bemäntelung", that is literally "cloaking".[70] Likewise Robert Hooper in his medical dictionary derived the term "palliativus" from "pallio", "to dissemble".[71] In his German translation of Johann Baptist van Helmont's *Opkomst der Geneeskunst*, Christian Knorr von Rosenroth even created the term *"Mantel-Kuren"* ("cloak cures"),[72] which was never widely adopted, however.

Today's proponents of palliative medicine like to refer to the etymological roots of "palliative" to underline the element of caring. According to them, palliative medicine wraps, so to speak, the patient in a protective cloak of medical treatment and empathic caring.[73] This seems a very suitably, heart-warming image but the etymology and original meaning of the word "palliative" are different. In early modern writing, not the patient was wrapped in a cloak but the diseases and defects were "cloaked" or "covered" without actually going away. This explains why originally remedies and procedures such as cosmetics, eyeglasses and prostheses, which no more than covered or compensated external defects, could be counted among the *palliativa* as well. In fact, to some authors, a "cloaking" of such deficiencies that were visible from the outside was the true, basic meaning of *cura palliativa.*[74] Looked at in this way, applying the term "palliative" to the treatment of complaints inside the body was a metaphorical usage. The imagery of cloaking was transferred to symptoms and physical alterations that were not accessible to the senses in the first place and could therefore not be covered up with a "cloak," strictly speaking.

For analogous reasons, failing to pursue a curative treatment could also be seen as a kind of *cura palliativa*. The therapist tried—or pretended—to get hold of the disease at its roots, but at best managed to make the symptoms or external appearance of the illness disappear, while the illness itself continued to make trouble inside the body. Here the "palliative cure" became synonymous with "sham treatment" and "palliative" medicines and healing procedures became "sham remedies."[75] To "palliate" ("palliare"), Georg Handsch noted in one of his notebooks, meant, "to hush

[68] We find the same phenomenon in the Netherlands. It was here that the term *palliatio* first became common on a larger scale with Dutch terms like "manteln" oder "menteln" (cf. Lorenz Diefenbach, Glossarium latino-germanicum mediae et infimae aetatis, Frankfurt: Baer 1857 (repr. Darmstadt 1968), p. 407a); on the history of the term see also Stolberg, "Cura palliativa" (2007b).

[69] Vigo, Chirurgerye (1543), appendix: The interpretation of straunge words, no page numbers.

[70] Woyt, Gazophylacium (1709), p. 673.

[71] Robert Hooper, Lexicon medicum; or medical dictionary, London: Longman et al. 1825, p. 857.

[72] Johann Baptist van Helmont, Aufgang der Artzney-Kunst. Transl. by Christian Knorr von Rosenroth, Sulzbach: J. A. Endters Söhne 1683, p. 6.

[73] D. Morris, Palliation. Shielding the patient from the assault of symptoms, Academy update, in: American Academy of Hospice and Pallliative Medicine 7 (1997), pp. 1–11, cit. by Clark and Seymour, Reflections (1999), pp. 80–1.

[74] Wedel, De cura palliativa (1703), p. 4.

[75] Krünitz, Oeconomische Encyclopädie, vol. 141 (1825), p. 723.

up the disease for a while."[76] Johannes Antonides van der Linden spoke of a *medicatio simulata* in this context, when someone wanted to cure a patient who was unable to pass water due to a bladder stone, for example, by pushing the stone from the internal urethral orifice back into the bladder: Urinary retention would almost inevitably develop again soon. This also applied if someone boasted of having healed someone's fever, when really he had only suffocated the fever without cleansing the blood of its impurities. The morbid matter remained in the body and the illness would come back at the next opportunity.[77]

It was this danger of a premature decision in favor of a "palliative cure" that led medical authors to urge their colleagues to work with the greatest diagnostic and therapeutic care. At the same time, they tended to blame patients for the decision of pursuing "only" palliative treatment when it was not called for. Rosa complained that patients often made it impossible for the doctor to recognize and fight the true cause of a disease. Patients had trouble remembering, came to the doctor with preconceived ideas or underestimated the paramount significance of a person's individual disposition and lifestyle for the development of illnesses. Others were garrulous, never got to the point and the doctor could not break their flow of words. When the doctor did finally succeed in getting to the bottom of things, they rejected the necessary therapy, if only because they happened not to like it. They would also forget or disregard the doctor's advice, not heed the dietary recommendations or even try household remedies.[78]

In large part, doctors were also aiming at their less educated competitors[79] when they criticized inappropriate palliative treatment that merely cloaked the symptoms of a disease that actually stood a chance at being cured. These were in particular the numerous lay healers or *empirici,* who were much sought after and appreciated among the general population and were the target of fierce criticism by doctors at the time.[80] As we have seen, Foreest, who was also the author of one the best-known medical invectives against the "deceitful practices" of the countless traditional uroscopists,[81] had already framed his influential case histories as instructive *exempla* of the *empirici's* "ignorance." The critiquing doctors claimed that the *empirici,* unable to arrive at an adequate diagnosis and therapy or with deceitful intentions, led patients to believe that they were able to cure their illnesses. Yet, they merely made the symptoms disappear or only seemingly removed the morbid matter from the body. Sometimes they were generously rewarded. There is, for example, the

[76] ÖNB, Cod. 11206, fol. 135v.

[77] Van der Linden, Selecta medica (1656), pp. 455–6.

[78] Rosa, De curatione palliativa (1742), pp. 36–40.

[79] Ananius Horer, Artzney-Teuffel, oder kurtzer Discurs, darinn diesem Ertzmörder seine Larve abgezogen. Sine loco 1634; cf. Barbara Elkeles, Medicus und Medikaster: Zum Konflikt zwischen akademischer und "empirischer" Medizin im 17. und frühen 18. Jahrhundert, in: Medizinhistorisches Journal 22 (1987), pp. 197–211.

[80] Küchler, De cura palliativa (1692), p. 21; Wedel, De cura palliativa (1703), pp. 12–19; cf. Rosa, De curatione palliativa (1742), p. 41; still in very similar terms Lund, Palliative medicine (1880).

[81] Pieter van Foreest, De incerto, fallaci urinarum iudicio, Leiden: Raphenlengius 1589.

account by Balthasar Timäus von Güldenklee (1601–1667) about an *empiricus* who had relieved a noble woman from the agonizing itch she had suffered from for years after contracting syphilis from her husband. He earned 500 pieces of gold and, as Timäus wrote, seemed to have snatched the crown from the doctors. However, the *empiricus* had not removed the cause of the disease, the syphilitic *causa morbi,* from the body. The disease spread all the more violently and the woman died soon after.[82]

According to doctors' accounts, *empirici* sometimes even stood in the way of a possible curative treatment by doctors and trained surgeons. In a chapter on *That Death Will Follow When Refraining from Trepanning the Cranium* ("*Daß auf Unterlassung der Durchbohrung der Hirnschal der Tod erfolgt*"), Wilhelm Fabry described his experience with a nobleman who had been hit in the head in battle and had collapsed with a broken skull. Not until 4 days later were Fabry and a colleague called to the patient, who now had a fever. They concluded "that there must be pus hidden under the cranium" and advised enlarging the wound and trepanning the cranium. The local barbers, however, promised they would be able to help the patient without the procedure, "arrogantly rejecting and despising [trepanation] as an unknown and repulsive means, and also making bystanders loathe it." As the barbers fought against the procedure and Fabry and Slotanus recognized that they would "come away dishonorably administering a cure next to men such as these," they stopped their treatment and departed, so that "our name and profession would not unwittingly be endangered because of the barber-surgeons." The patient ultimately lost his speech, became paralyzed on one side and died on the fourteenth day.[83]

2.2 *Cura mortis palliativa* and *Euthanasia medicinalis*

In today's understanding of the term, "palliative" treatment and care principally refers to patients in advanced stages of a terminal chronic disease. However, it has become widely accepted that many of its elements, combined with other therapeutic approaches, may be employed much earlier and not only when death is at the doorstep.[84] The early modern conception of *cura palliativa* embraced from the outset diseases and physical deficiencies that were not immediately life threatening. Alleviating the suffering of the dying, the *cura mortis palliativa,* as Detharding

[82] Balthasar Timaeus von Güldenklee, Casus medicinales praxi triginta sex annorum observati, Leipzig: Impensis Christiani Kirchneri 1667, pp. 277–8.

[83] Fabry, Wund-Artzney (1652), p. 107.

[84] Derek Doyle, Geoffrey Hanks and Nathan I. Cherny, Introduction, in: iidem (eds): Oxford textbook of palliative medicine, 3rd edn, Oxford: Oxford University Press 2005, pp. 3–8, here p. 3; Geoffrey P. Dunn and Robert A. Milch, Introduction and historical background of palliative care: where does the surgeon fit in? in: Journal of the American College of Surgeons 193 (2001), pp. 325–8.

called it in his medical dissertation of 1723,[85] was but an important special type of palliative treatment.

Georg Christoph Detharding, in this vein, also talked about *euthanasia palliativa,* which the dying themselves or those close to them requested so that "they may die a gentle death," as people said, so that they "would not meet a difficult end, fall asleep etc."[86] In this, he resorted to a term that played an increasingly important role in pre-modern literature about medical terminal care: *euthanasia.*

Its roots go back to antiquity. Derived from the Greek word elements for good (*eu*) and death (*thanatos*), "euthanasia" meant a good death.[87] In the medieval and early-modern western Christian world, the term is found predominantly in the religious context of spiritual welfare, in book titles such as *Euthanasia sive de firma spe ac fiducia in Dei misericordia, mortis tempore, collocanda,* meaning more or less: *Good Death, or Of the Firm Belief and Trust One Must Have in God's Mercy when Dying.*[88] In the tradition of the Christian *ars moriendi,* the "art of dying,"[89] such publications were pointed the way to preparation for the afterlife in a way that would be pleasing to God. A considerable number of works dedicated to euthanasia referred to it in this sense. The term "euthanasia" here usually stood for the desired goal, that is, for the good, pious death one wanted to experience; but sometimes it also stood for the actions, the spiritual preparations that would help assure such a pious death.

The English philosopher Francis Bacon (1561–1626) introduced the term "euthanasia" in the medical discourse in the early seventeenth century. Only few years after Pieter Foreest had, with reference to different cases of terminal cancer, established the term and the concept of a "palliative" treatment in the medical discourse once and for all, Bacon voiced his emphatic request that doctors help dying patients die a gentle death: "I esteem it the office of a physician not only to restore health, but to mitigate pain and dolours; and not only when such mitigation may conduce to recovery, but when it may serve to make a fair and easy passage."[90]

---

[85] Detharding, De mortis cura (1723). It is unclear it whether the author was Christoph Friedrich Detharding or his father Georg.

[86] Ibid., pp. 84–9.

[87] Cf. Benzenhöfer, Der gute Tod? (2009), pp. 13–19.

[88] Martin Eisengrein, Euthanasia sive de firma spe ac fiducia in Dei misericordia, mortis tempore, collocanda, Cologne: apud Ludovicum Alectorium & haeredes Iacobi Soteris 1576; Nicolaus Heldwaderus, Omnium mater artium euthanasia [graece], Das ist die beste, nutzlichste und bewerteste Kunst unter allen Künsten dieser Welt, genant Sterbekunst [...], sine loco 1625; Philippus Bebius, Euthanasia seu de praeparatione ad felicem mortem, Cologne: apud Joannem Kinckium 1708.

[89] For the history of the *ars moriendi* see Chartier, Les arts de mourir (1976); on the medieval tradition see Edelgard E. DuBruck and Barbara I. Gusick (eds), Death and dying in the Middle Ages, New York: Lang 1999; Daniel Schäfer, Texte vom Tod. Zur Darstellung und Sinngebung des Todes im Spätmittelalter, Göppingen: Lang 1995; Hiram Kümper (ed.), Tod und Sterben. Lateinische und deutsche Sterbeliteratur des Spätmittelalters, Duisburg–Cologne: WiKu–Verlag 2007.

[90] Francis Bacon, De dignitate et augmentis scientiarum libri IX, Paris: Typis Petri Mettayer 1624, pp. 222–3; cf. Nicolas Aumonier, Bernard Beignier and Philippe Letellier, L'euthanasie, Paris: Presses universitaires de France 2001; Benzenhöfer, Der gute Tod? (2009), pp. 58–62.

Bacon went on to say that it was no small fortune to have a "euthanasia," the death that resembled a friendly, pleasant sleep, which Emperor Augustus had had and wished for, and which Antoninus Pius had written about. About Epicure it was written in an epigram that he drowned his stomach and his senses in a large amount of wine after his illness had been declared hopeless so that he was too drunk to taste the bitterness of the water of the River Styx. Physicians by contrast, Bacon claimed, instead of looking for ways to alleviate pain and the agony of death, were hesitant to stay with an incurable patient. Bacon was therefore using the term "euthanasia" in the classical, ancient meaning of a "good" death. Yet, his phrasing made it possible to understand "euthanasia" also in an active sense, namely as the actions of doctors that accomplished the desired gentle death.

Bacon's use of the term at first created only a faint response in medical writing, but in the second half of the seventeenth century it gradually attracted more attention.[91] Johann D. Horst, in line with the Leiden professor J. A. van der Linden, discussed the "exterior euthanasia," the *euthanasia exterior,* which—in opposition to the religiously connoted "inner" euthanasia—provided an easier and gentler departure from life when there was no longer hope for a recovery. At the same time, both van der Linden and Horst rejected as unchristian a deliberate shortening of life as was practiced in antiquity.[92] Georg H. Welsch also picked up on Bacon's advice, saying that doctors should turn to, among other things, the neglected practice of *euthanasia*, not only with respect to patients' spiritual welfare but also to their physical condition. In 1676, he listed this *euthanasia medicinalis*, as he called it, in his list of 70 desiderata of medicine.[93] Criticizing Horst's somewhat ambiguous phrasing, Welsch, in his commentary on Walaeus's *Methodus Medendi* of 1679, emphasized that euthanasia in this Baconian sense was a far cry from administering poison and shortening life.[94] In 1683, Lucas Schröck, in a commentary on a case history written by the French doctor Guy Patin, praised Patin for granting euthanasia to an 80-year-old patient with a gigantic bladder stone by abstaining from any torturous treatment attempts. This he contrasted with the less praiseworthy doctors who showered their patients with remedies, thus increasing their pain and suffering or even hastening death.[95] Christian Scriver in his work *Gotthold's Siech- und Siegs-*

[91] According to Roelcke, "Ars moriendi" (2006), p. 35, Bacon remained "entirely isolated" in the seventeenth and eighteenth centuries with this call medical euthanasia; however, the passages from the works of Horst, Welsch, Detharding and others that I quote in this chapter are at odds with Roelcke's argument. These authors made Bacon's call their own almost 150 years before for the German physician Reil published his work who according to Roelcke, loc. cit., p. 30 was "one of the very first authors who used the term euthanasia to refer to the practice of physicians."

[92] Johann Daniel Horst, Manuductio ad medicinam, 4th edn, Ulm: Kühnen 1660, p. 215. So far I have not been able to identify the passage in van der Linden's writings.

[93] Georg Hieronymus Welsch, Somnium Vindiciani sive desiderata medicinae, Augsburg: Göbel 1676, p. 36 and appendix with a list of his *desiderata.*

[94] Joannis Walaeus, Methodus medendi brevissima [...] Georg. Hieronymi Welschii [...] animadversionibus illustrata, Augsburg: Göbel 1679, p. 348 (commentary by G. H. Welsch).

[95] Lucas Schröck, Scholion on observation XIX by Guy Patin, in: Miscellanea curiosa sive ephemeridum medico-physicarum Germanicarum Academiae Naturae Curiosorum Decuriae II. Annus primus, anni MDCLXXXII, Nürnberg: Endter 1683, pp. 43–5.

Bette, first published in 1687, referred again to Bacon when he wrote of *euthanasia physica,* which could be used "when someone is nearing his end and has to depart from life to alleviate his pain of dying and to take away his anxiety so he may take his leave without further suffering." With god-fearing people, who were passing away in the knowledge of God's mercy, he had rarely experienced, however, that "these kinds of natural remedies had been necessary."

In medical case histories and similar sources that reflect ordinary practice, the term "euthanasia" in the sense of explicitly seeking to secure the patient a death that was mostly free from physical suffering was came to be used only in the late seventeenth century. The earliest example I have so far been able to identify can be found in the case histories that Ehrenfried Hagendorn published in 1690. Among many other cases, Hagendorn gives a detailed account of a young patient with a breast tumor that, in the care of a healer, developed into a painful cancerous ulcer. In the end, the ulcer seized the entire breast, hardened and gave off an acrid secretion. Hagendorn and his colleague Dr. Ledel saw no other way but to amputate the breast. The patient submitted herself to the procedure and initially improved. However, she then developed pain again and went to a surgeon for treatment. When she was ever more tormented by pain and sleepless nights and began to waste away, she again consulted the doctors. However, they were unable to do anything beyond giving her remedies in an attempt to alleviate the horrible pain and, in Hagendorn's words, to bring about "euthanasia," which came to pass the following month.[96]

Detharding, in his work of 1723, specified this medical meaning of the term "euthanasia" more specific by adding the word "palliativa." However, rather than *euthanasia palliativa* or *euthanasia physica,* another term became established in the time that followed, one that was closer to Welsch's *euthanasia medicinalis* of 1676: *euthanasia medica.* It is first found in 1735 in a dissertation entitled *De euthanasia medica , Vom leichten Todt*, for which Zacharias Philipp Schulz was awarded a medical doctorate from the University of Halle under Professor Michael Alberti (1682–1757).[97] People wished for a gentle, mild and sweet death and feared a difficult, arduous, terrible and hard death, the author explained. This was the subject of their pious prayers as much as of their urgent pleas to the doctor. The text did not refer to *euthanasia medica* as a mode of action, as something that could be done but as an aim. *Euthanasia medica* was used to describe a gentle death in the physical as opposed to the spiritual, sense. The intention of the treatise was to examine more closely the ways in which doctors could contribute to *euthanasia naturalis*, an easy, gentle, short progression of "natural death" ("mortis naturalis") and prevent a death that was miserable physically. This wish, the author held, was absolutely natural and permissible for Christians to have.[98] He discussed the necessary remedies, the suitable nursing and other practical issues only in passing. The focus was on the signs that showed which patients could be expected to die a gentle, mild death

[96] Ehrenfried Hagendorn, Historiae medico-physicae centuriis tribus comprehensae, Rudolstadt: Arnst 1690, pp. 375–9.

[97] Schulz/Alberti, De euthanasia medica (1735).

[98] Ibid., pp. 10–11.

without medical support and which could not. This was of great importance, as the doctor who recognized such a patient was not to disturb the approaching gentle death unnecessarily with his medication and inadvertently turn it into a miserable one. In such cases, the doctor was advised to content himself with wetting the dry tongue and the weary throat of the dying with some liquid. In his congratulatory speech, Alberti underlined the value of this undertaking, stating that man's life on earth was finite after all, so the physician's task was to show people how to live a healthy life but also to give his advice about how to die a "good death."[99]

More explicitly even, another dissertation defended under Alberti in the same year, focused on the need to refrain from therapeutic measures that no longer made sense and caused suffering. Under the title *De dysthanasia medica . Vom schwehren Tod* the author—the doctoral candidate Karl Christian Hennig or Alberti himself[100]—used Quintilian's words as his starting point that not death as such was miserable, but that dying was. Who would not be deeply distressed when faced with the fears, the cries, the torment, the pain, the affliction of the dying? The throes of death, when soul and body had to give up their connection, were bad enough. In addition, all too daring and inexperienced doctors contributed to such a difficult death, a *dysthanasi a*, instead of effecting euthanasia. In cases like these, people said, "the sick man has been held up with so much medication which work in him all the time and make it difficult for him to die."[101] The physician was to facilitate death with means that were permissible and commensurate with his conscience—rather than making it even more bitter.[102]

Thus, to these physicians in Halle, it was more important to exercise restraint when their remedies threatened to increase the agonies of death than to actively try to alleviate the agonies of death. Prior to this there had been a few cases of medical authors urging doctors in a similar fashion, but all in all, this had been a rather marginal phenomenon. In the sixteenth century, Baptista Codronchi , for example, complained about the widespread practice of advising hopeless patients to ingest all manner of food and drink regardless of their appetite.[103] It was no coincidence that the voices cautioning against the dangers of an overly eager medical practice that increased suffering grew considerably louder in Halle during the early eighteenth century. The school of Georg Ernst Stahl in Halle put special emphasis on the

[99] Michael Alberti, Dn. Candidato, appended to Ibid., no page numbers.

[100] Hennig, De dysthanasia medica (1735); again it remains unclear whether Schulz and Hennig were the actual authors or only defended a text written by Alberti. Since both dissertations also contain texts that are explicitly attributed to Alberti himself and since Alberti is also mentioned in the third person in the texts there is considerable evidence that Schulz and Hennig were at least actively involved in writing these dissertations. Both dissertations are of very high quality, however, and quote an unusually wide range of works that only someone like Alberti is likely to have known.

[101] Ibid., pp. 35–6.

[102] Ibid., p. 37.

[103] Codronchi, De christiana ratione (1591), pp. 25–6.

healing powers of nature or the soul within the body.[104] Stahl and his followers recommended caution even in the treatment of curable diseases. When the physician was unable to help, a dissertation defended by another student of Michael Alberti proclaimed, he was at least to make sure that he did not harm the patient with questionable attempts at treatment.[105] "He advised all physicians and surgeons," wrote Stahl's student Carl, "to rather err on the side of fearfulness than audacity and boldness. [...] Our contribution and action in medicine all too often spoil what is best."[106] Michael Alberti even had one doctoral candidate defend the thesis that forgoing medical help and the use of medication may prevent illness and death.[107] Obviously, this attitude also promoted therapeutic restraint with dying patients. As Stahl himself had explained, a gentle death was not to be disturbed with medication if death was inevitable. Consequently, his student Christian Meisner called on doctors to refrain from useless attempts at treating "incurable" diseases. This was a waste of money and, in the worst case, dangerous. He cautioned against the negative effects that might even come from attempts at mere palliative *mitigatio* in the case of paralyses, cancer and anal fistulas, as this only provoked the illness, making it worse.[108] Michael Alberti , too, doubted the usefulness of such healing attempts with patients close to death. They might delay death a little but they also made dying more difficult and could make the patient die a miserable death. "They came to a difficult end," relatives said in such cases. With good reason, thought Alberti, did they object to the thoughtless dispensation of remedies, believing that the patients should not be bothered with further ingestion when it was obvious that nothing helped and that they would die.[109]

In 1759, C.G. Ludwig chose "The doctor's duties to the dying" as the subject of his formal dissertation speech. He came to somewhat different conclusions. He described the doctor as a comforting support, as the expert in judging the patient's ability to leave a will and as the one who guarded against the danger of mistaking

[104] Georg Ernst Stahl, Proempticon inaugurale de synergeia naturae in medendo, [Halle – Magdeburg] 1695; idem, De ministerio naturae salutariter adhibendo. Exp. Johannes Fridericus Siber, Halle – Magdeburg: Henckel 1711; idem, De abstinentia medica. Subm. Gottfried Bateldt, Halle – Magdeburg 1709; Friese, De vehementia (1723), esp. p. 32; on Stahl and Stahlianism see Axel Bauer, Georg Ernst Stahl (1659–1734), in: Dietrich von Engelhardt and Fritz Hartmann (eds), Klassiker der Medizin I. Munich: Beck 1991, pp. 190–201; Johanna Geyer-Kordesch, Pietismus, Medizin und Aufklärung in Preussen im 18. Jahrhundert. Das Leben und Werk Georg Ernst Stahls, Tübingen: Niemeyer 2000; Dietrich von Engelhardt and Alfred Gierer, Georg Ernst Stahl (1659–1734) in wissenschaftshistorischer Sicht, Halle: Deutsche Akademie der Naturforscher Leopoldina 2000.

[105] Alberti, De religione (1722b), p. 37; the author of this dissertation is uncertain but the quality of the writing and the numerous references to other works suggest that it was Alberti himself; in some places, the *praeses*, i.e. Alberti, is mentioned in the third person, however, which may indicate that Broesike wrote at least parts of the text.

[106] Johann Samuel Carl, Medicina aulica, Altona: Gebrüder Korte 1740, p. 363.

[107] Alberti, De abstinentia (1722a), p. 31.

[108] Meisner, De incurabilibus affectibus (1705), pp. 26–7; G. E. Stahl is quoted repeatedly with his works, which suggests that Meisner rather than Stahl was the (principal) author.

[109] Alberti, De abstinentia (1722a), p. 31.

an apparent death for a real one. However, he could, with the means available to him also bring the dying back to life so to speak. This was something the physician was obliged to do, even if this life was now only a sad, unwanted life that would be prolonged a little in this way. Other than that, Ludwig reminded doctors that they had to make use of all resources to relieve patients in the last moments of their lives from the hardship of their symptoms by moistening the patients' tongue, countering cold sweats with heat, alleviating breathing difficulties, strengthening the heart and mitigating pain: in short, by choosing every means available to make the last, burdensome moments of life more bearable.[110]

2.3 Palliative Care in Early Modern Medical Practice

In publications on medical therapy in general as in texts that focused on the treatment of incurable and dying patients in particular, the concept of an alleviating "palliative" treatment was firmly established from the late sixteenth century onward. As we have seen, compared to modern usage, the term "palliative" carried a wider meaning. It could also refer to a literal "cloaking" of disease symptoms and physical defects by means of cosmetics, prostheses and so forth, and it could even include the erroneous abandonment of a curative treatment in curable cases. This wider meaning of the term was limited largely to dissertations and theoretical treatises, however, and in the following, I will refer to "palliative" treatment in the more narrow modern sense as we find it in sources that reflect actual medical practice or indeed describe individual cases. Here, the term *cura palliativa* was often used synonymously with other terms such as *cura mitigativa*, or with dying patients, *euthanasia medica* . The *cura palliativa* was a treatment that (no longer) pursued a radical, curative goal but instead focused on the alleviation of symptoms. It was, as Johann Jakob Woyt (1671–1709) put it, an "interim cure" which, "with desperate and incurable diseases" was used "to alleviate pain, for example, so as not to leave the patient alone in his helplessness, even though the cure has little effect."[111] Krünitz's famous *Encyclopädie* defined it as a "therapy that does not cure a malady but merely alleviates it for some time."[112] This would have included actions taken against the underlying illness, which in itself could no longer be eradicated, in order to slow down its progression and relieve its physical consequences.

The theoretical discourse on the *cura palliativa* or *medicatio palliativa,* as van der Linden referred to it,[113] was commonly coupled with detailed practical advice on the remedies and procedures that worked best for certain complaints and forms of illness. Sometimes medical case histories were used as examples to illustrate how they were applied.

[110] Ludwig, De officio medici (1772), especially p. 178.

[111] Woyt, Gazophylacium (1709), p. 673.

[112] Krünitz, Oeconomische Encyclopädie, vol. 106 (1807), p. 284.

[113] Van der Linden, Selecta medica (1656), pp. 463–466.

The central task in many cases of illness was to relieve pain. Cancer, above all, was feared for the persistent pain, which could be virtually unbearable toward the end. Early modern medicine had a number of remedies available to fight pain. Some of them have been all but forgotten, while others continue to be used today. Prominent among these remedies were the nightshades (*solanum*), the northern water hemlock (*cicuta aquatica*), mandrake root and henbane (*hyoscyamus*).[114] But pride of place was taken by opium in the various forms in which it was administered. Liquid *laudanum* was widespread. Often the term "opiate" stood for a mix of different remedies with similar effects administered along with poppy. Many doctors relied on a specific mix that was reliably effective in their experience. Opium and other narcotics also offered welcome help in combating the sleeplessness of the seriously ill. Further, these remedies sometimes also helped with diarrhea, eased breathing difficulties or reduced the racking cough of patients suffering from consumption.[115]

Otherwise, the three major, most commonly diagnosed fatal diseases—cancer, consumption and dropsy—were each treated in their own way. The palliative treatment of cancer combined medicines against the pain and the sleeplessness with the attempt to counter the carcinoma's growth, its expansion into adjacent areas and its putrid decomposition once an ulcer had formed. In the early modern understanding, the tumor and its ulcerous decomposition were due to an influx of acrimonious, caustic morbid matter, which could eat its way into the surrounding flesh and through the skin. Even when a cure no longer seemed possible, the physicians therefore sought to combat the formation of these acrimonious, "burnt" cancerous substances inside the body[116] and, to the extent that this could not be prevented, to evacuate them from the body as quickly as possible through other pathways than the ulcerating skin. In this manner, it was thought, they might even be able to slow down the progression of the disease.

In many cases, a palliative treatment was considered superior to other options and doctors sometimes explained to patients and their families why they favored a palliative approach over a surgical procedure. In 1634, the Milan doctor Giovanni Battista Sitoni (1605–1660?) advised the brother of a woman who had fallen ill with breast cancer against her having an operation. Surgery was dangerous, he said, and as the patient complained about pain in her back, one could assume that the cancer was already rooted deeply. Explaining that this was called an *indicatio curativa palliativa,* he instead recommended bloodletting to stop any further influx of cancerous substance to the breast, to make the breast firm so it would less likely absorb the substance and, above all, to do everything to prevent the cancer from breaking open

[114] Cf. e.g. Boerhaave, Institutiones (1721), pp. 386–389.

[115] Oberlin, De opio (1752), especially pp. 20–21.

[116] Pierre Darmon. Être cancéreux et mourir 1700–1850, in: Jean-Pierre Bardet and Madeleine Foisil (eds), La vie, la mort, la foi, le temps. Mélanges offerts a Pierre Chaunu, Paris: Presses Universitaires de France 1993, pp. 295–309, here p. 297.

as an ulcer. This was the best way of giving the patient some relief, helping her to live longer and with as little suffering as possible.[117]

In cases of incurable uterine cancer physicians also relied heavily on expelling, evacuating remedies. When, in 1605, Henricus ab Heer treated a 70-year-old woman who suffered from pain in her lower abdomen and in the groin and from a stinking black discharge, he gave up hope for a complete cure ("curam absolutam desperans") and turned to a "palliative" treatment. He attempted to promote urination above all and, among other things, gave borage, dodder and quicksilver preparations.[118] Guillaume Baillou, too, advised a woman suffering from uterine cancer to take purgatives and perform local irrigation. He did not hope to cure the woman in this way, he explained, but to prolong her life a little and to alleviate her pain.[119]

As the *ultima ratio* in advanced cancerous tumors and ulcers a palliative operation could be performed. Even if there was not any hope of a cure, a cancerous breast, for example, could be removed if the pain from the surgery seemed a lesser evil than the intense pain, the secretions and the stench.

With consumptive patients, palliative treatment usually focused on the racking, prolonged cough, on the breathing difficulty and on the loss of appetite, which progressively weakened them and caused them to lose weight. For the increasing respiratory distress of advanced pulmonary consumption, opium and other poppy preparations were the first choice. The persistent cough could be relieved by making the viscous phlegm more fluid and by strengthening the lungs. Franciscus Sylvius, for example, suggested the use of hyssop , lady fern , coltsfoot and horse-heal. If the mucus was acrid or stinging, he recommended medicines against acrimony. Against the weak appetite of consumptive patients, an elixir composed, among others, of myrrh , crocu s, aloe and—Sylvius was an iatrochemist—sulfurous oil was thought to be effective and to improve, at the same time, the digestion—or, as Sylvius explained it the fermentation—of food.[120]

The palliative treatment of dropsy mainly aimed at eliminating the extra water from the body, so the swelling of the abdomen and limbs would recede and breathing would become easier. This was achieved predominantly with diuretics. Specifically with abdominal dropsy, which could cause the belly to distend like a balloon, a paracentesis could bring some relief. This involved opening the abdomen with an incision and inserting a little tube, a *cannula*, to drain the liquid. At times, paracentesis seemed the only option when the bulging abdomen put so much pressure on chest and lungs that it threatened to suffocate the patient. Yet, it was known from experience that more liquid would usually develop quickly—and the

[117] Giovanni Battista Sitoni, Iatrosophiae miscellanea sive sapientia medica, Einsiedeln: Wagenmann 1669, pp. 28–36.

[118] Heer, Observationes (1645), pp. 180–1.

[119] Guillaum Baillou, Consiliorum medicinalium libri II. Ed. by Jacques Thevart, Paris: Quesnel 1635, p. 476.

[120] Sylvius, Praxeos medicae idea (1695), pp. 701–2.

intervention was considered dangerous.[121] The Paduan anatomist and surgeon Gabriele Falloppia, for example, carefully explained to his students in 1553 how a paracentesis was done but cautioned them to perform it only on the patient's request, "because few survive." He himself, he confessed, had performed the operation on three patients and they all had died.[122] The famous surgeon Wilhelm Fabry as well, practicing in the seventeenth century, came to the conclusion that "generally" "opening the patient's navel was of little or no benefit," and he recommended that if the intervention was to be performed at all it should be done at a point in the course of the disease when the patient was not yet severely weakened.[123] Martin Lister's experiences with paracentesis were similarly ambivalent. In the case of a Mrs. Pepper, whose belly became more and more swollen following two miscarriages while the rest of her body became emaciated, he ultimately ordered a paracentesis, which produced five liters of an initially turbid liquid. Subsequent drainage produced sometimes ten, sometimes eight pounds of liquid until no more liquid came out and the patient was able to leave the house again.[124] Yet, he also witnessed a surgeon draining nine pounds of liquid from a man around 50 years in age who had tried all kinds of remedies before. The next day there was almost the same amount again, and on the third day the man was dead.[125] In the late eighteenth century, John Ferriar likewise referred mainly to accounts that pointed out the dangers of paracentesis.[126] Only by the nineteenth century, judging from the writing of Gmelin, had paracentesis become a standard procedure used in cases where the actual causes of dropsy could not be eliminated. "Emptying the water that collects in the abdomen is the most effective means of palliative treatment and is often repeated many times with a beneficial outcome."[127] It is believed that Ludwig van Beethoven, during the last weeks of his life, was drained of several liters of liquid multiple times.[128]

[121] Georg Heinrich Behr, Medicina consultatoria. Oder Sammlung einiger schwehren und seltenen Zufälle, samt denen von ihme darüber verfertigten Berathungen und eingeschickten Beantwortungen, vol. 1, Augsburg: Klaffschenckels sel. Witwe 1751, pp. 96–105, medical consilium by Dr. Bonet, Geneva, October 21, 1750 on the dropsical Mme Bram who was "extremely relieved" after eight pitchers of fluid had been evacuated.

[122] ÖNB, Cod. 11210, student notes of Georg Handsch.

[123] Fabry, Wund-Artzney (1652), pp. 52–3.

[124] Lister, Octo exercitationes (1698), pp. 28–30; when the woman eventually died from an epidemic fever, an autopsy was performed and the whole abdominal cavity was found to be filled with numerous "glands"; from a modern perspective, these descriptions suggest ovarian cysts. In extreme cases such cysts can cause a monstrous swelling of the woman's belly and make her unable to move around.

[125] Ibid., pp. 17–18.

[126] John Ferriar, Neue Bemerkungen über Wassersucht, Wahnsinn, Wasserscheu, ansteckende und andere Krankheiten, nebst Erläuterungen durch Fälle, und Angabe der besten Heilarten, Leipzig: Johann Friedrich Junius 1793.

[127] Gmelin, Allgemeine Therapie (1830), p. 318.

[128] Jörg Zittau, Matt und elend lag er da. Berühmte Kranke und ihre schlechten Ärzte, 2nd edn, Berlin: Ullstein 2009, pp. 173–4.

As Falloppia's writings show, even students of medicine were taught about the palliative treatment of incurable and terminally ill patients. Indeed, contemporary study guides explicitly advised students to learn "the ways in which incurable pain can be alleviated and soothed."[129] At some universities, students were even able to gather practical experience in this area. A manuscript that documents the bedside teaching of Musa Brasavola and other doctors in the town of Ferrara during the first half of the sixteenth century records the fatal case of a 60-year-old man who evacuated lumps of blood along with his urine and ultimately developed seizures. He was given different remedies to strengthen him and his heart, and to prevent further seizures. When he had been ill for 2 weeks, the doctors thought they recognized the signs of death approaching. But they continued their visits, apparently accompanied by students. Four days later, the patient's health declined further; he was weak, threw up and suffered from diarrhea. The doctors ordered that he be given food only bit by bit, with breaks in between. Soon after he was dead.[130] About another patient, a young man who coughed up a lot of blood, the professor said that he would soon die. He prescribed no further medication but merely appropriate food. Nevertheless, the professor went back with his students the next day to see the patient who could now hardly breathe and, as expected, died the following night.[131]

When bedside teaching was introduced more widely also to places outside of Italy, universities there also offered increasing opportunity to gather experience in treating terminally ill and dying patients during their studies. At the famous hospital of Leiden, for example, Franciscus Sylvius taught his students palliative therapy as early as the late seventeenth century. His *Collegium nosocomicum* includes the story of Johannes Toeback, severely weakened and close to death. Treating the disease itself, in Sylvius's judgment, no longer held any promise. Yet, he could not leave him to his own devices and thus prescribed tonic remedies.[132] He cared for another patient suffering from fatal consumption over the course of several weeks, and the prescriptions for this patient included expectorants and sleep-promoting remedies and, in the end, also opiates.[133] Student notes from Edinburgh, another center of clinical teaching in the eighteenth century, also show that palliative care was taught. In his clinical lectures, James Gregory (1753–1821), for example, presented the case of the consumptive Janet Hunter. The diagnosis was very clear, he said, and "consequently the prognosis was very bad, if not certain death." He went on to explain that, "with this kind of clinical picture, in general we can only pretend to

[129] Johannes Brettschneider (aka Placotomus), De ratione discendi ac praecipue medicinam, Leipzig: Bapst 1552, no page numbers.

[130] Biblioteca Comunale Ariostea, Ferrara, Ms. Antonelli 531, fols 10r–15v; on clinical teaching in early sixteenth-century Italy see Michael Stolberg, Bed-side teaching and the acquisition of practical skills in mid-sixteenth-century Padua, in: Journal of the history of medicine and allied sciences 69 (2014), 633–64.

[131] Ibid., fols 160v–161r.

[132] Franciscus Sylvius, Collegium nosocomicum, in: idem, Opera omnia, Geneva: apud Fratres de Tournes 1681, pp. 709–737, hier p. 715.

[133] Ibid., p. 712–3.

palliate the symptoms & avoid occasional causes." His treatment was accordingly cautious: "I gave the mucilaginous mixture, to relieve the tickling cough, and the vitriolic acid, to check the colliquative sweats."[134]

2.4 Medical Care for the Dying—A Professional Dilemma

The physician's duty to alleviate the suffering of incurable and dying patients was, as we have seen, accepted generally and without contradiction in early modern medical writing. Unanimously, authors requested that doctors stand by the side of their moribund patients and offer them support and relief even if there was no hope for a cure. Medical students and doctors in training could consult medical textbooks and medical case histories for concrete, practical advice and some even received hands-on training in working with terminally ill patients.

Whether early modern doctors in their daily practice always and in every situation fulfilled and satisfied their professional obligation to care for the dying is a different question. Without a doubt, many doctors continued to accompany and support their patients even in desperate cases. This is shown by records of medical practice and teaching, such as above-mentioned case histories by Foreest , Sylvius and Lister . It is reflected in students' notes and, occasionally, in accounts of a "last sickness" written by laypeople.[135] In documents about estate settlement, too, we can find notes about fees claimed by the doctors or surgeons who cared for patients until their deaths, or claims by apothecaries, whose bills for the last prescribed medication had not yet been paid. In some cases, it is difficult, of course, to tell in retrospect whether the physician may have hoped for curative success until the very end. The more than 4000 pages of notes on ordinary medical practice that the Bohemian doctor Georg Handsch wrote around 1560 contain various such cases. In the case of a certain Mauricius, for example, who had suffered from progressive cachexia and dropsy over the course of the previous 2 years, Handsch's mentor Andreas Gallus believed that he would still be able to cure the patient, as long as the liver did not become "putrid." Handsch at this point had already described Mauricius as having a very bad color, caved-in cheeks, yellowish eyes and a bloated belly. He coughed, which according to Gallus was a bad sign, as it indicated that the lungs were full of water. Yet, even when Gallus no longer doubted that the patient was approaching death, he prescribed a mild remedy for the liver, which he now indeed found to have putrefied.[136] There are also documented cases of physicians and surgeons taking on

[134] Osler Library, Montreal, Bib.Osl. 7565, notes taken from the clinical lectures of Dr. James Gregory of Edinburgh, 1787, pp. 6–10; James was the son of John Gregory and succeeded him at the Edinburgh Royal Infirmary.

[135] For example, a list of the patients who died in the care of Dr. Jan van Beekhoven de Wind in Haarlem, Netherlands, from September 1 until October 20, 1761, names among others a consumptive patient who had been bedridden for months before her death (Gemeentearchief Haarlem, Collegium medico-pharmaceuticum, 25).

[136] ÖNB, Cod. 11207, fols 65v–66r, fol. 70r and fols 79r–v.

new patients who were clearly already nearing death. Jean-Claude Pancin, for example, wrote in his medical diary about a female patient whose entire body was bloated from dropsy after about 6 weeks of illness, and who had severe difficulty breathing. She died only a few days after Pancin's first visit.[137]

As burdensome as caring for the seriously ill may have been, doctors probably also recognized the positive aspects apart and beyond the fulfillment of a moral duty. As their condition worsened, gravely ill and dying patients needed numerous visits and thus opened the prospect of ample earnings, especially with high-ranking, affluent patients. From April until her death in July 1791, Jean-Claude Pancin, for example, paid 43 visits to a female patient who seems to have suffered from cancer and received 43 *livres* for his services.[138] If a doctor was successful in creating the impression that his treatment significantly alleviated the patient's suffering or even prolonged the patient's life beyond all expectations, he might be met with gratitude by the patient and his family and, as some authors emphasized, he stood to gain "great honor."[139]

Yet, treating seriously ill and dying patients also came with a great risk. The doctor could seriously damage his reputation and even endanger his livelihood, especially with patients of high social status. Patients and their families were convinced that doctors, like other healers, differed greatly in their diagnostic and therapeutic abilities, and a physician's competence and trust were established mainly on the basis of stories about the favorable or unfavorable outcomes under his care. Accordingly, people engaged in a lively exchange with one another about the experiences they had had with different professional healers.[140] Under these circumstances, when a physician treated a hopeless case, he could only hope that the patient and his family would praise his helpful and compassionate support at the deathbed. There was always the danger, however, that the fatal outcome would be attributed to his incompetence and lack of skill, to his flawed, ineffective or indeed harmful treatment.

In his first years as a practicing physician, Georg Handsch learned this lesson the hard way. He repeatedly had to remind himself to exercise more caution in this respect. In one entry in his notebooks, he admonished himself, for example: "Do not take on incurable patients to avoid acquiring a reputation as a bad doctor, as it happened to me Hosska." In another note, he added that a doctor must refrain from giving medication to severely ill patients who were close to death if he wanted to

137 Bibliothèque Municipale, Avignon, Ms. 3997 (Jean-Claude Pancin), "Journal de mes malades principaux", fol. 24v.

138 Ibid., fols 30v–32r.

139 Heurne, Praxis (1590), pp. 343–4.

140 Michael Stolberg, Medizinische Deutungsmacht und die Grenzen ärztlicher Autorität in der Frühen Neuzeit, in: Richard van Dülmen and Sina Rauschenbach (eds), Macht des Wissens. Entstehung der modernen Wissensgesellschaft 1500–1820, Cologne – Weimar: Böhlau 2004, pp. 113–30.

avoid being blamed for their death.[141] His teacher Ulrich Lehner also observed this rule, he remarked.[142] In a similar vein, Johann Jakob Döbeln complained about the excessive expectations of patients who believed that, "if they make use of a doctor, he will cure them and they will not have to die."[143] In 1610, the Breslau doctor Peter Kirsten was outraged about the wrong done to a physician by family and friends when a patient died of a severe, life-threatening disease. Such a doctor deserved gratitude for "the great trouble and inconvenience that a righteous physician necessarily faces in treating a patient such as this, who is burdened with such serious illness, which can also kill him." Instead, his name and honor were damaged.[144]

Great caution was already advised, in this respect, in medieval works on *cautelae medici* with their detailed instructions for the doctor's conduct at the sickbed,[145] and early modern authorities on medical deontology and professional ethics followed suit.[146] The physician was to beware of promising the impossible for the sake of money, cautioned Guy de Chauliac, or else he might acquire a reputation as a bad doctor.[147] Roderigo da Castro, in his *Medicus politicus,* recommended a trick. If the doctor feared the patient would not live much longer, he could play it safe and send a helper who would use a pretext to ask about the patient's condition. And if the doctor went to a patient's home himself, and was surprised to learn of the patient's death, and perhaps sensed that the family might be blaming him, he was to "assume a sad and composed expression and communicate that he had foreseen this death and had come back merely as a friend, to console those left behind and to learn when exactly the patient had died."[148]

A doctor who had talked to family and friends and correctly predicted the imminent death of a patient was not safe from reputational damage either. Even the famous physician Johann Daniel Horst had to endure being "defamed and gossiped about all across town" along with two surgeons after having taken on the terminally ill Anthon Johann Dieffenbach, seeking to grant him at least a gentler death. Ultimately, the bereaved family—presumably upon Horst's request—countered

---

141 ÖNB, Cod. 11240, fol. 42r: "Incurabiles morbos non suscipere, ut est phtisis, apoplexia, asthma in senibus, hydrops inveterata. [... Item extreme affectu propinqum morti non medicatur, ne deinde mortis causam tibi ascribunt."

142 ÖNB, Cod. 11205, fol. 690v.

143 Döbeln, De erroribus (1700), p. 68.

144 Petrus Kirstenius, Trewe Warnung von rechtem Gebrauch und Mißbrauch der Artzney. Breslau: Baumann 1610, p. 99; see also Georg Detharding, Disputatio medica, quae adstruit voluntatem medici habendam esse pro effectu. Resp. Jacobus Battus, Rostock: Typis J. J. Adleri 1732.

145 Gabriele Zerbi, Opus perutile de cautelis medicorum, [Venice] 1495.

146 See e.g. Giovanni Battista da Monte, Consultationum medicarum opus absolutissimum. Basel: per Henricum Petri et Petrum Pernam 1565, p. 458.

147 Guy de Chauliac, Chirurgia, Leiden: apud Sebastianum de Honoratis 1559, fol. a3 verso; see also Augenius, Epistolarum (1602), fol. 87r; Müller, Melemata (1778), p. 29.

148 Castro, Medicus politicus (1662), p. 133.

these "defamations" with a detailed report.[149] They made it known that the consumptive patient had developed a rapidly growing tumor on his back, which the doctors could not operate due to his weak condition. A healer had then treated him locally with a plaster—presumably to pull the morbid matter out—until his entire back was "almost nothing but raw flesh, riddled with large and deep holes." This had caused the sick man "unbearable pain," which he, "had not God given him special extraordinary endurance, would never have been able to bear." At this point treatment with the healer was ceased, so that the sick man approaching his death would at least be freed from the pain caused by the caustic medicines "and his soul might await its farewell breathing calmly and with brief comfort as it were." This was the situation in which Horst and the surgeons had been asked for help, not "in the hope of any reconvalescence (which, with any common sense, could not be hoped for considering the condition)" but "only to alleviate the pain, and so that the patient may breathe a little before his impending death." The doctors and the two surgeons had come to the "very nearly dead" patient and "indicated to those gathered and all friends that nothing but death could be expected here, and that all that should be sought was to relieve the patient of the pain in his back and the flow of blood." They treated his back and were able to take the pain away. The fact that the sick man died in the end could not be held against them. Rather, they were to be praised for the "loyalty, diligence and help they provided, with God's council, as far as was possible in such an extreme situation." Here, the family ultimately stood up for Horst and the surgeons in public, but the case goes to show just how much a respected doctor's reputation and practice could be damaged by accepting to treat a terminal patient.

It is not surprising then that the deontological obligation to assist also the terminally ill and dying was not always respected in actual practice. As we have seen, there are numerous examples in which physicians acted according to this norm. However, in a striking number of medical case histories, contemporary patient letters, accounts of miraculous healing and other sources that reflect the patients' own experience, we also read about patients whom doctors and surgeons had "given up" or "left." In Handsch's notes on other physicians' practice, for example, we not only find descriptions of doctors who accompanied a terminally ill patient all the way to his or her deathbed, or apparently even waited at the deathbed; we also find phrases such as "reliqui ipsam," "I left her" or "relictus est ab illis," "he [the patient] was deserted by them."[150] Patients and their families for their part also wrote about doctors and other medical practitioners who abandoned a sick person as hopeless. Patients and families sometimes used this as an argument in negotiations with authorities, in order to obtain the permission to consult a non-licensed, unauthorized healer. Even the "medici," they would say in the case of a very sick female patient,

---

[149] Stadt- und Universitätsbibliothek Frankfurt, Senckenbergarchiv, letter (February 23, 1671) and detailed history of the disease (March 2, 1671) .

[150] E.g. ÖNB, Cod. 11183, fol. 82v; similarly fol. 80v ("reliqui eum"); Ibid., fol. 136v ("relictus est ab illis"), on a young man who had been sick for months and who recovered, against all expectations.

had "despaired of being able to cure her, and no longer dared to support her with some help or advice."[151]

The danger of doing harm to one's reputation was especially great when it came to surgical interventions, as their success or failure could be recognized readily by anyone. If the patient succumbed during or shortly after the operation, the physician might have to face accusations of having caused the patient's premature death. Thus, a doctor or surgeon, for example, who performed paracentesis on a dropsical patient to drain water from the abdomen, had to fear not only for the patient's life but also for his repute. "Therefore I say thanks to my dear God," wrote Wilhelm Fabry to Abel Roscius in Lausanne concerning such a patient, "that we did not undertake to open his navel or belly." After all, everyone would have blamed the intervention for his death, "although they would have been wrong. For the disease in itself was incurable, because the inner parts such as the liver and the spleen were in a bad condition and weak, I might even say due to their entire destruction."[152]

The doctors' concern about their reputation—rather than their respect for their patients' right of self-determination—was without a doubt also the driving factor for the well-documented willingness of doctors to seek the patient's or at least the family's consent before they undertook a risky intervention. Accordingly, Roderigo da Castro impressed upon the readers of his *Medicus politicus,* as did Falloppia on his students, that, when treating dropsy or empyema (an accumulation of pus in the lungs or in some other cavity), they must never reach for the knife without having explained the uncertain outcome of the intervention to the relatives, the father, mother, children, brothers or sisters, and obtained their consent.[153]

As we can see, the risks associated with the treatment of incurable and dying patients were high. Yet, doctors likewise risked putting their reputation and practice on the line if they abandoned seemingly desperate cases. After all, the course of a disease could rarely be predicted with complete certainty. While there was little doubt of a fatal outcome if a cancerous tumor had already become ulcerated or a consumptive patient hardly stopped coughing up blood and had difficulty breathing, sometimes there was a surprising turn for the better, even in advanced stages of a disease. If the doctor continued his treatment after having predicted a fatal outcome an unexpected positive outcome could be attributed to his excellent treatment. But if he abandoned the patient, another medical practitioner or, even worse, some unlicensed healers, might be consulted—with serious consequences, for the physician and his reputation. If the patient died, as predicted, under the treatment of the competitor the physician who had treated him before might feel validated. Yet, even in this case his reputation could suffer. The competitor could easily attribute the fatal outcome to the ineffective previous treatment: He had only been called in when it was too late for a cure. When the disease took a surprising turn for the better after a physician had abandoned a patient, the consequences were even more dire. Then the

[151] Augsburg, Stadtarchiv, Collegium medicum, Karton 7, supplication by Hieronymus Harder (late sixteenth century).

[152] Fabry, Wund-Artzney (1652), pp. 52–3.

[153] Castro, Medicus politicus (1662), p. 133.

physician was cast as ignorant and the competitor carried off the laurels, even if he had made, in the physician's eyes, the greatest mistakes in his treatment and owed his success only to Nature or God. And the physicians knew from experience that sometimes the most desperate cases improved even under the treatment of an "ignorant" *empiricu s.*[154] In learned medical writing, one explanation for this was what we would call a placebo effects today: The *empiricus* made the patient hopeful of a cure, thus strengthening the patient's spirit, which could often lead to the sick person's nature gathering all its strength against the disease. The patients and their families, however, would inevitably attribute the success to the healer, to the poor prognostic skills of the first physician or to both.

The well-known French surgeon Bartholomé Cabrol had a painful experience of this kind at the beginning of his career. Near Albi, he was called to a man who was suffering from a serious knife injury to the head, which had begun to fester. From his reading of Hippocrates und Galen , he knew of the dangers of treating penetrating head injuries, that is, wounds that were deep enough to reach the brain. He arrived at the conclusion that death was near and inevitable. Against the wishes of the man's wife, who tried to keep him with all kinds of promises, he departed. Another surgeon attempted unsuccessfully to help, and in the end the sick man was, in Cabrol's words, "abandoned by all, robbed of all help." Then came a farmer who cured the sick man within 2 months. Cabrol was not only surprised; he also blamed himself for leaving the patient to his own devices. Thus, he cautioned surgical novices never to declare cases like this incurable. The doctor, he said, was to treat them but first explain to friends and all those present about the dangers associated with wounds of this kind. In this way, it could be prevented, in the case of a fatal outcome, that the doctor would be blamed and that medical means which had been of great benefit to many would be discredited.[155]

No matter whether doctors continued to treat or gave up on people who were incurable or dying: their reputation and their authority were always on the line. From this angle, the growing medical appreciation of palliative treatment may also be seen as the solution for a serious professional dilemma. The palliative approach allowed them to expand their activities to the potentially quite lucrative treatment of hopeless cases, instead of giving up on patients and leaving them to their competitors, who might sometimes be successful in seemingly desperate cases and thus bring shame to the doctors. It also allowed doctors to present themselves as honest healers, guided by Christian compassion, who were not afraid to help ailing patients in their plight and, in contrast to the less educated competitors, did not charge a hefty fee for empty promises. By explicitly forgoing further curative attempts and, at least to the family, expressing their preference for a "merely" palliative treatment, they could at the same time reduce the danger—although not eliminate it altogether—of a fatal outcome being ascribed to their therapy. In this sense, Laurent Joubert, as early as 1580, gave his students the advice of forgoing in hopeless cases

[154] Cardano, De malo medendi usu (1536), p. 9.

[155] Cabrol, Alphabeton (1604), pp. 108–9.

the more powerful, drastic means such as bloodletting or strong laxatives, so that in the end it would not appear that they had killed the patient.[156]

2.5 The Art of Prognosis

In light of all this, it becomes clear why the contemporary medical literature placed great importance on the art of prognosis, especially in chronic and potentially fatal diseases. In the experience of doctors, prognostic skills were invaluable when it came to building a reputation and gaining people's trust.[157] Sick people and their relatives wanted to know what the present disease meant, and what the consequences were for the near future or possibly for the rest of the patient's life. If a doctor was able to predict the course of an illness correctly, he also proved his ability to interpret symptoms well, to identify the mysterious pathological changes within the body and thus he presumably assured his patients and their families of his ability to treat the illness successfully. The stakes were especially high, as we have seen, when it came to treating patients with serious, possibly terminal illnesses.

The study of prognostics, and in particular the study of the symptoms of impending death, goes back to antiquity. The *facies hippocratica*, the typical, sunken face of dying patients, is still a familiar notion today. Basing his work on the Hippocratic tradition, the Paduan doctor Prosper Alpinu s became widely known at the turn of the seventeenth century for his work *De praesagienda vita et morte aegrotantium*,[158] in which he gave a detailed account of the numerous prognostic signs that indicated different kinds of disease processes and allowed the doctor to predict how much longer a patient would live. The book was a great success. It went through numerous editions, was cited frequently until far into the eighteenth century and had various imitators. Changes in breathing, sweat, body odor, physical restlessness, dulled senses, tightness in the chest and similar symptoms were presented to the reader of this book and in many other publications as the signs that allowed the doctor to recognize if death was near.[159] In contemporary treatises on uroscopy—by far the most important diagnostic procedure far into the eighteenth century—readers likewise found many different notes on urinary changes that allowed unfavorable outcomes to be predicted.[160] Vernacular recipe books also offered prognostic tests. One of these tests was said to have been used by a certain Dr. Mannhaber in Leipzig on 74 patients and the resulting prognosis was said to have proven true in all but two cases. One had to boil "crabs eyes" (*oculi cancrorum*), a commonly used medicine

[156] Laurent Joubert, Oratio de praesidiis futuri excellentis medici, Geneva: Stoer 1580, p. 15.

[157] See e.g. Augenius, Epistolarum (1602), fols 86v–87r; Lehmann, De moribundorum regimine (1685), p. 7; since Lehmann mentions a case that he had from his *praeses*, J. D. Major, he rather than Major is the more likely (principal) author.

[158] Prosper Alpinus, De praesagienda vita et morte aegrotantium libri septem, Frankfurt: Rhodius 1601.

[159] Lehmann, De moribundorum regimine (1685), pp. 7–12; Seld, De signis mortis (1747).

[160] Cf. Stolberg, Uroscopy (2009), esp. pp. 55–6 and pp. 154–7.

at the time, and make the patient drink the broth. If the patient vomited, it was a sign that his brain and heart were poisoned and that there was no cure for him.[161]

Learned doctors further saw the art of prognosis as a means of showing themselves in a good light by distancing themselves from the less educated competitors, from the many unskilled empirics and the barber-surgeons. A precise prognosis required, as Hubner emphasized in 1591, great learnedness, a keen ability to discern and prudent circumspection. This would prevent the doctor from daring, out of hubris, to undertake more than God, Nature or the art allowed, as many of the numerous crooks and vagrants did who pretended to be doctors, squeezing money out of gullible people. A trained doctor, C. F. Seld cautioned in 1747, must never risk his reputation by interpreting the signs of a dramatic but ultimately salutary crisis as the signs of death approaching, the way old women mistakenly did.[162] Other authors used similar terms to emphasize the learned doctors' prognostic and therapeutic restraint, dissociating their practice from the empty promises of the "audacious empirics" who promised sick people the world but ultimately only hastened their death.

With patients they considered incurable and doomed to die, physicians had to be particularly careful, however, in communicating their prognosis. The physician, Piper from Riga warned, must never use phrases such as "I no longer know how to help" or "If this is not effective, I don't know what else to do." For if he did, the patient, especially with chronic illnesses, was likely to consult another medical practitioner who might reject the physician's prognosis and promise a cure.[163] The danger that patients and families would ignore the physician's pessimistic prognosis was all the greater due to an attractive offer some of the less learned healers made: They asked to be paid only if their treatment proved successful. It was said about an irregular healer based in Lucerne, for instance, that he "never took money from someone he had not first helped." When the authorities threw him in jail, numerous former patients advocated for his release. As one of them put it, they had "suffered the high costs charged by local barber-surgeons and apothecaries," but without receiving help.[164]

With unconcealed indignation, Pieter van Foreest published cases in which another healer was consulted after he had given an unfavorable prognosis. "To avoid defamation," he had declared in 1563, for example, that the uterine cancer of 50-year-old Adriana Nicolai was incurable and could now be approached merely with "palliation." He told her husband that he could only alleviate her pain and that

[161] Hohenlohe Zentralarchiv, Neuenstein, U5, recipe book of Count Wolfgang von Hohenlohe, late sixteenth century, fol. 174v, "Einen Menschen zu probiren, ob er sterben werde".

[162] Seld, De signis mortis (1747), introduction.

[163] Det Kongelige Bibliotek, Copenhagen, Ms. Thottske S 4689, Dr. Piper (*archiater* in Riga), Collegium pathologicum [...] ut et collegium medico-politicum, fols 257v–258r.

[164] Luzern, Staatsarchiv, Archiv I, Fach 4: Polizeiwesen 740, "Report about a captured doctor and barber", Saturday before Jubilate 1603; for a detailed account of such healing contracts between unlearned healers and patients see Pomata, La promessa di guarigione. Malati e curatori in antico regime. Bologna XVI – XVIII secolo, Bari: Laterza 1994.

she would die. The husband, however, turned to an *empiricus* who relieved him of quite a lot of she would recover.[165] Foreest's account is written with the satisfaction of someone who had been proven right in the end. Nevertheless, he had lost the trust of his patients in these cases.

[165] Pieter van Foreest, Observationum et curationum medicinalium ac chirurgicarum opera omnia, Frankfurt: in officina Paltheniana 1634, pp. 698–9.

Ethical Challenges 3

3.1 The Intentional Shortening of Life

As we have seen, the term "euthanasia" appeared frequently in early modern writings about caring for the terminally ill. Even when they used the term to signify not only the gentle death that medical action would ensure but the medical activities designed to assure such a gentle death, early modern medical writers did not define euthanasia as an active, intentional curtailing of life. However, the widespread assumption according to which it was out of the question for early modern physicians to entertain this possibility of actively shortening life and suffering proves to be wrong when the medical writings of the day are examined more closely. As a possible way to end the agony of the dying person, an intentional acceleration of death was certainly discussed. The physicians could hardly avoid the issue. After all, as the Antwerp city physician Michael Boudewijns (1601–1681) explained, doctors often found themselves faced with patients and their relatives asking them to end the suffering of dying patients.[1] Moreover, the Hippocratic Oath, which was widely translated and commented upon at the time, forbade that a physician hand out deadly poisons, even if explicitly requested to do so, and some commentators took advantage of the opportunity to discuss in more general terms the question of intentionally shortening life.

In their general assessment, medical writers were widely in agreement with one another: Neither the physician nor the patient nor his relatives were allowed to put a premature end to a hopelessly ill patient's life and suffering. Even if the physician was fervently begged for a fatal poison by a patient, as Petrus Memmius explained in 1577, he was not permitted to grant this wish—also for the sake of preserving

[1] Hippocratis iusurandum, in: Alessandro Benedetti, Anatomice, sive de hystoria corporis humani libri quinque, Strasbourg: apud Iohannem Hervagium 1527, fols 111v–112r: "Rogatum mortale venenum nemini daturum, neque id cuiquam consulturum".

M. Stolberg, *A History of Palliative Care, 1500–1970*, Philosophy and Medicine 123,
DOI 10.1007/978-3-319-54178-5_3

people's trust in the physician.[2] In his commentary on the Hippocratic Oath, François Ranchin conceded in 1627 that in antiquity it was allowed in some places to put an end to the suffering of a patient who was ill unto death. But these were barbaric, heathen practices that Christians must not imitate.[3] In 1666, Boudewijns even dedicated a whole chapter of his *Ventilabrum medico-theologicum* to the question "May a Physician Accelerate Death to Free a Desperate Patient from his Agony?" He expressed a certain understanding for the solicitations of the sick people: Disease and death could put the strongest people to the test. Nevertheless, he said, it was a sin even in the worst, most desperate cases to accelerate death, even if only indirectly by forgoing food, water or necessary medication.[4]

For a long time, such issues were discussed only sporadically. However, from the end of the seventeenth century, the debate rapidly intensified. Shortening the agony and accelerating the death of terminally ill patients became a heavily discussed subject, commented upon by countless medical and non-medical authors, especially but not only in Germany. Here, the crucial impetus came from a book, which a Saxon lawyer by the name of Caspar Questel published in 1678. The title appears odd at first glance: *Dissertatio academica de pulvinari morientibus non subtrahendo, von Abziehung der Sterbenden Haupt-Küssen.*[5] The Latin title "de pulvinari morientibus non subtrahendo" like its German translation " von Abziehung der Sterbenden Haupt-Küssen" ("On Removing the Pillows of the Dying") refers to a practice that was widespread at the time, not only according to Questel's observation. Krünitz's popular *Encyclopädie* would later succinctly summarize this practice by saying that in some places sympathetic bystanders would pull away "the pillows of the departing out of mercy, in the opinion that this will provide a quicker and gentler death." As a result, the sick person's upper body would suddenly change from a more or less upright to a horizontal position. It was an act carried out with the declared intention of putting an end to the suffering of the dying person.[6]

Questel and others after him reported a range of other practices as well which, according to their accounts, served to accelerate death.[7] Their depictions may have to be taken with a grain of salt—they were frequently framed by a more general polemical critique of the "backwardness" and "ignorance" of the population as a whole and of the "ignorant" orderlies or relatives providing medical care in particular. So many

[2] Petrus Memmius, Hippocratis Coi iusiurandum commentario recenter illustratum, cui accessit altera pars, qua ratione medicorum vita et ars sancte conservetur declarans, Rostock: typis Augustini Ferberi 1577.

[3] François Ranchin, Opuscula medica. Ed. by Henricus Gras, Lyon: apud Petrum Ravaud 1627, pp. 28–31.

[4] Boudewijns, Ventilabrum (1666), pp. 219–23, chapter on "An medico liceat mortem accelerare, ut desperatus aeger a doloribus liberetur?"; cf. Michael Ernst, Ärztliches Handeln und ethische Fragen am Lebensende im Ventilabrum medico-theologicum von Michael Boudewijns (1666), Cologne: WiKu-Verlag 2012.

[5] Questel, De pulvinari (1678).

[6] Krünitz, Oeconomische Encyclopädie, vol. 73 (1798), p. 175.

[7] For later overviews see Bächtold-Stäubli, Handwörterbuch (1937), pp. 438–450; Falk, Geschichte (1983), pp. 27–9; Cavina, Andarsene (2015).

writers reported these practices, however, across large geographical areas and for centuries, that it cannot be plausibly be reduced to a mere literary topos. The most straightforward way, which only a few authors described, was to smother the dying person. Italian diplomat Giulio Raviglio Rosso in 1560, having first described how relatives would pull on the legs of hanged persons to shorten their death struggle, went on to give an account of a particular form of "mercy" that was practiced above all by the lower classes in the countryside. "The next of kin takes a pillow and places it on the face of the sick person and then sits on it, thus smothering him." According to Raviglio, relatives did not believe that they were doing anything wrong but rather held it a deed that would be pleasing to God.[8] An outraged Johann Peter Frank recounted that still at the end of the eighteenth century one saw how "those who were dying slowly would have their nose and mouth inconspicuously held shut by an officious little gammer eager to do her duty and pretending that she was drying the sick person's face; or that they were rolled over on their face."[9] Dieffenbach in the early nineteenth century recounted that it had happened that "old women in the countryside would put the dying with their faces down and hold their mouths closed, smothering them in this way only to make dying easier!"[10]

Significantly more widespread, according to the writings of early modern physicians and later ethnographers, was the practice of taking dying people from their beds and laying them—naked or very lightly clothed—on either the floor, a bed of straw or a board otherwise used for corpses. An eighteenth-century account from Leipzig describes a husband standing before the court because, together with a maid, had laid his dying wife first on a board, then on straw and then on the cold ground. He made a partial confession but explained that his intentions were not bad. He wanted to liberate his wife from the agony and pain of dying.[11]

As late as 1798, Johann Georg Krünitz's *Encyclopädie* bewailed this "murderous mercy," the fact that if not generally but "among those who would in actuality be called the rabble," it was often claimed that a sick person could not die in his bed and so he was laid on straw.[12] According to John Ferriar's account from the late eighteenth century, this means of accelerating death had been "very common" in Great Britain in the previous 200 years.[13] It also continued to be described in the literature of the nineteenth century, especially for the lower classes.[14]

[8] Giulio Raviglio Rosso, I successi d'Inghilterra dopo la morte di Odoardo sesto fino alla giunta in quel regno del sereniss. Don Filippo d'Austria Principe di Spagna. Scritti volgarmente da Giulio Raviglio Rosso da Ferrara, Ferrara: Francesco di Rossi 1560, fol. 103r; cf. Rodolfo Graziani, Non-utopian euthanasia. An Italian report, c. 1554, in: Renaissance quarterly 22 (1969), pp. 329–333.

[9] Frank, System (1788), pp. 666–7.

[10] Dieffenbach, Anleitung (1832), p. 176.

[11] Georg Andreas Ioachimus, Dissertatio iuridica de vivi sepultura delicto et poena. Submittit Hieron. Wilhelmus Arnold, Leipzig: Langenhemius 1732, pp. 27–8, December 1727.

[12] Krünitz, Oeconomische Encyclopädie, vol. 73 (1798), p. 176.

[13] Ferriar, Treatment (1798), p. 199.

[14] Heinrich Hoops, Sassenart. Niedersächsische Volkssitten und Bräuche, Bremen: Angelsachsen-Verlag 1922, pp. 115–6; further references in Georg Schoppe, Sterbende werden auf die Erde gelegt, in: Archiv für Religionswissenschaft 17 (1914), pp. 341–2.

In retrospect, it cannot be known to what degree this practice actually stemmed from the desire to curtail the life and suffering of the dying person. Laying the dying person on the bare floor could also be understood as a symbolic anticipation of the return of the mortal human shell to the earth.[15] Medieval accounts point in this direction. For example, a dying Caesar von Heisterbach requested to be laid on the floor and for the bells to be rung. About Queen Matilda it was recounted that for her death, in 968, she requested that a rough cloth be spread out on the floor and that ashes be scattered on her head.[16] Alfonso de' Liguori (1696–1787), one of the most influential Catholic moral theologians of his time, explicitly came to the defense of those who, just before their death, asked to be laid on the ground. They did so, he believed, out of humility or to set a good example and not with the intention to shorten their lives.[17] This practice resembles others that in retrospect seem to have had an exclusively symbolic function, some of which continued until well into the twentieth century.[18] In many places, there was a widespread tradition of removing a roof shingle or opening the window in the sickroom so that the soul of the dying person could escape more readily. All these practices were designed, it seems, to help the soul depart from the body at the right time. If the dying had withstood all trials successfully until now, one could also in this way help them enter eternal life, so that they might not at the final moment, with weakened senses and weakened reason, renounce God and God's mercy and thus forfeit eternal salvation.[19]

Excluding some specific conditions such as severe heart failure, we would not today attribute a significant life-shortening effect to these practices or to pulling the pillows from underneath a dying patient, even if they entailed a considerable change of position. For our understanding of the debate at the time, it is crucial, however, that we accept that Questel and generations of physicians and scholars after him were convinced of the very concrete life-shortening effect. They explained to their readers that, especially in several of the most significant and generally terminal illnesses such as dropsy and consumption, morbid humors accumulated in the respiratory tract. If the sick person was suddenly put into a horizontal position, the airflow would be obstructed and the patient would suffocate. According to another explanation, the sudden change of position caused the brain to become flooded with blood.

---

[15] Albrecht Dieterich, Mutter Erde. Ein Versuch über Volksreligion, Leipzig–Berlin: Teubner 1905, pp. 26–7; Ernst Samter, Antike und moderne Totengebräuche, in: Neue Jahrbücher für das klassische Altertum, Geschichte und deutsche Literatur (1905), pp. 34–45, hier p. 36; Bächtold-Stäubli, Handwörterbuch (1937), cols 438–50.

[16] Rudolf Cruel, Geschichte der deutschen Predigt im Mittelalter, Detmold: Meyer 1879, p. 239; Bächtold-Stäubli, Handwörterbuch (1937), col. 446, on St. Benno. Financial considerations may also have been at play. Beds were expensive and the dying might easily soil them with their excretions.

[17] Alfonso de Liguori, Theologia moralis. Ed. by *P. Leonardi* Gaudé, vol. 1, Rome: Typogr. Vaticana 1905, p. 627. My thanks to Isacco Turina for pointing out this passage to me.

[18] See also Arnold van Gennep, Manuel de folklore français contemporain, vol. 1: Introduction générale et première partie: du berceau à la tombe, Paris 1946, pp. 664–7.

[19] Georg Andreas Ioachimus, Dissertatio iuridica de vivi sepultura delicto et poena. Submittit Hieron. Wilhelmus Arnold, Leipzig: Langenhemius 1732, pp. 27–8, December 1727.

This interrupted the flow of the "nerve juices" to the heart and thereby the activity of the heart, or it led to a sudden stroke or apoplexy.

Questel' s book gave new meaning and significance to the question of the "jus abbreviandae vitae et accelerandae mortis," that is, to the right to shorten life and accelerate death, as Schilter put it in his preface to Questel's work in 1678. Questel's treatise found a powerful resonance, considering that it was learned treatise written in Latin. By 1718, it had gone through at least five editions or reprints and countless authors cited it until well into the nineteenth century.

Questel presented his own position clearly and unequivocally. Life and death for him lay in the hands of God alone. Even if the patient begged the doctor for a hastened death, one could not justify such an immoral act.[20] Other contemporaneous lawyers saw it in much the same way. One expert's report from the faculty of law at the University of Tübingen in 1699 expressed the opinion that one must not approve of "killing before the day that is determined by God a person who lies ill unto death."[21] With a typically charged polemic against the female bedside attendants or "old women," who called medical authority into question at the sickbed, Questel went on to warn against the danger of abuse. The female attendants, he wrote, would occasionally remove the pillow willfully, under some pretext, so as to shorten the travails of caring for the sick person or to secure their modest pay or a mourning dress more quickly.[22]

Other learned writers also unanimously rejected the shortening of life. "This kind of love goes too far," wrote Karl Christian Hennig succinctly in 1735.[23] Krünitz's *Encyclopädie* warned emphatically:

> O, you loveless faithful! You religious murderers! [...] Be warned; and if such a treatment has taken place until now out of innocence, or good intentions, you are nevertheless murderers! From now on, do not sin so cruelly against mankind and the holy law of nature![24]

Until well into the nineteenth century, medical literature regularly made reference to—and simultaneously denounced—the practice described by Questel. There was all the more reason for doing so because in many cases this practice was regarded a typical example of popular "superstition," which doctors in those days were determined to fight.

The arguments invoked to reject the abrupt removal of pillows applied all the more to the purposeful shortening of life in medical practice. It was rejected across the board until the end of the eighteenth century. Georg Ernst Stahl, for example, argued that a physician could and should in hopeless cases forgo further attempts at treatment, but he must not administer deadly medication so as to "take all of the

---

[20] Questel, De pulvinari (1678), p. 13.

[21] Hauptstaatsarchiv Stuttgart A 209, Bü. 558, expertise by the Faculty of Law in Tübingen, 1699.

[22] Questel, De pulvinari (1678), p. 8.

[23] Hennig, De dysthanasia medica (1735), p. 40; deliberately shortening a patient's life was alien to the physician's identity ("character medici") we read in another dissertation with the same praeses, Michael Alberti (Alberti, De religione (1722b), p. 36).

[24] Krünitz, Oeconomische Encyclopädie, vol. 73 (1798), p. 175.

patient's fear away." That was also not even necessary, Stahl continued, because the doctor could use opium to give the suffering patient comfortable sleep, which was commonly known as death's brother. A true, happy *euthanasia* at the right time could only be asked of the true Lord of life and death.[25] No one, according to Hennig in 1735—and especially no Christian doctor—was permitted to give a desperate patient a remedy to hasten death, even if death was clearly at the doorstep.[26]

3.2 The Unintentional Shortening of Life

Even when the doctor did not mean to end the patient's life but administered remedies to alleviate the dying person's agony, he was of course risking that he might thereby shorten the patient's life. Today, this frequently discussed ethical dilemma is sometimes known as "indirect euthanasia." Even leading Catholic moral theologians such as Juan de Lugo (1583–1660) and Alfonso de' Liguori (1696–1787) did not see it as a categorical obligation to avoid everything that might result in shortening life.[27] According to Alfonso, it was forbidden to kill oneself or another "directly" and with intention. But to bring death to oneself or others "indirectly" by doing something with fatal consequences or by forgoing something was sometimes permitted. He was referring to the ascetic penitential practices of some clergy, however, which could have consequences for their health, and pointed to the blacksmiths who through their constant work in the heat of flames consumed their life-sustaining radical moisture prematurely.[28] It remained an open question as to whether the "mere" alleviation of pain, shortness of breath, a tormenting cough or ulcerous, decaying tumors was enough to warrant the risk of shortening life, especially since the agony of illness and death was widely understood as a divinely ordained test.

Yet, the question arose quite frequently in the case of the terminally ill. For example, Wedel explained that the remedies for the tormenting cough could in some circumstances make a consumptive patient get worse and hasten death if the causes of the illness were not treated at the same time. The patient, he wrote, would be glad to be relieved of his cough, but without the coughing the phlegm could accumulate in the airways with grave consequences.[29] The debate became more heated—as it also does today—when it came to the dangers of an unintentional hastening of death by giving strong pain medication. Opium's lethal potential had long been known. Early modern doctors were well aware of the accounts of ancient authors according to which people died after having taken opium or intentionally killed themselves by

[25] Stahl, Mortis theoria (1702), p. 39.

[26] Hennig, De dysthanasia medica (1735), pp. 38–9.

[27] Overview in Bonifacio Honings, L'eutanasia attiva e passiva secondo i manuali classici. Dal XVI al XX secolo, in: Lateranum N. S. 44 (1978), pp. 515–34.

[28] Ibid., especially pp. 521–526; cf. Alfonso de Liguori, Theologia moralis. Ed. by *P. Leonardi* Gaudé, vol. 1, Rome: Typogr. Vaticana 1905, p. 627.

[29] Wedel, De cura palliativa (1703), pp. 24–31.

taking an overdose.[30] At the same time the dosing of opium, which was also considered a remedy for many an illness,[31] was notoriously difficult because of the great variation in its effectiveness. The dangers were widely known among the lay public as well. In fact, according to Wedel in the seventeenth century, common women considered opium a poison, a "viaticum," a messenger of death.[32]

Many physicians urged medical professionals to use opium only with the greatest caution. In careless hands, wrote Severinus Hee in 1734, opium was like a double-edged sword in the hands of a madman.[33] George Young in his *Treatise on opium* (1753) warned that opium shortened the lives of cancer sufferers in particular.[34] But there were other views. Oberlin cautioned against an overly prudent approach. According to him, one should, with appropriate care, be more liberal in giving opium than many doctors were, their hands trembling every time they prescribed it.[35]

The possibility of palliative operations for the terminally ill posed the question with particular urgency as to whether or not the effort to alleviate suffering justified the risk of curtailing the patient's life, indeed perhaps bringing it to an abrupt end. Some of Henry Fearon's patients at the end of the eighteenth century seem to have consciously accepted the risk of a fatal outcome. For example, 40-year-old Mary Smith explained that she had such intense and nearly constant pain that she was willing to "risk everything."[36] Another patient, 46 years of age, had not wanted to hear anything, at first, about an operation in spite of the favorable prospects but then wanted to have her breast removed and have "everything possible done" to relieve her from her intense pain.[37] Forty-year-old Elisabeth Auger suffered from such intense and constant pain that she even asked Fearon to operate on her a second time, after her breast tumor had again grown extensively. Fearon declared the patient's condition hopeless, but granted her request.[38]

---

[30] Georg Wolffgang Wedel, Opiologia, Jena: Sumptibus Johannis Bielkii 1682, pp. 153–4.

[31] Cf. Philippe Hecquet, Reflexions sur l'usage de l'opium, des calmants, et des narcotiques pour la guerison des maladies, Paris: Guillaume Cavelier 1726.

[32] Wedel, Opiologia (1682), p. 155.

[33] Severinus Hee, De methodis medendi in medicina et chirurgia suspectis. Praes. Georg Detharding, Copenhagen: Höpffner 1734, p. 17.

[34] George Young, A treatise on opium founded upon practical observation, London: Millar 1753, pp. 124–9.

[35] Oberlin, De opio (1752), preface.

[36] Fearon, Abhandlung (1790), pp. 83–5.

[37] Ibid., pp. 80–3.

[38] Ibid., pp. 88–91. The patient survived the operation but he died 5 months later, after his pain and the resulting insomnia had become refractory to opium; Siena, Suicide (2009), p. 59, mentions similar cases of patients who declared that they would rather suffer the torments of medical treatment.

3.3 Forgoing Treatment

Doctors also could become complicit in the death of terminal patient, however, if they no longer attempted a radical cure. Today we would call this "passive euthanasia." This was not always by deliberate choice. Sometimes patients refused to accept their advice, especially when the physicians came to the conclusion that an operation was needed. Work on the history of "informed consent" has sometimes given a different impression but the consent of patients for more significant surgical interventions was, for obvious reasons, generally indispensable at the time. If a patient was not prepared to undergo an operation whilst entirely conscious, without anesthesia and effective pain relief—neither existed at the time—the doctor or surgeon could hardly force him.[39] Cancer patients above all were reluctant—and with good reason—to go under the knife. Operations were generally associated with horrendous pain, the healing process could extend over a long period of time, the outcome was uncertain and the risks were high.[40] In the early nineteenth century, the memoirs of Margarete Milow, a burgher's wife from Hamburg, still give graphic testimony to this. When the tumor in her breast became harder after various very painful treatment attempts, her doctors presented her, in her own words, with the agonizing choice of

> [either] living another year and then dying in the most terrible pain, or undergoing an operation. Both were ghastly. The operation, cutting off an entire breast, it all appeared dreadful to me. I went to a woman who had been operated on and who told me the most dreadful things about it. My knees shook and I was in a deeply saddened and anxious state.

Nevertheless she agreed to have the operation performed. Immediately before the intervention, she wrote "my fear began to increase every quarter of an hour. I paced to and fro; my knees shook." She survived the painful operation, but in the end succumbed to her cancer.[41]

The deep fear that preceded a surgical intervention in such conditions found vivid expression in a prayer that was published in the eighteenth century. The author faced an operation to remove stones. As he put it, he was "offering his damaged body, martyred with daily pain, as a sacrifice to the Lord, my God, and to his tool, the physician, no different from how Isaac lay down on the sacrificial wood ready to be butchered." He asked that God bless "the hand, the tools and the cutting of my

---

[39] On the history of informed consent Martin S. Pernick, The patient's role in medical decision-making. A social history of informed consent in medical therapy, in: The ethical and legal implications of informed consent in the patient-practitioner relationship, vol. 3, Washington: U.S. Government Publishing Office 1982, pp. 1–35; Ruth R. Faden and Tom L. Beauchamp, A history and theory of informed consent, New York: Oxford University Press 1986; Elkeles, Schweigsame Welt (1989).

[40] For a detailed account of the surgical treatment of cancerous breasts see Lorenz Heister, Chirurgie, Nürnberg: Johann Hoffmanns sel. Erben 1724, pp. 612–8; on the negotiation of surgical interventions between Heister and his patients see Marion Maria Ruisinger, Patientenwege. Die Konsiliarkorrespondenz Lorenz Heisters (1683–1758) in der Trew-Sammlung Erlangen, Stuttgart: Steiner 2008.

[41] Margarethe E. Milow, Ich will aber nicht murren. Ed. by Rita Bake and Birgit Kiupel, Hamburg: Dölling und Galitz 1993, pp. 298–9.

doctor," so that "this great work may go tolerably and favorably, without excessive bodily pain, and bring healing and well-being." May God strengthen him, he went on, "so that I may be able to withstand chivalrously and confidently the painful wounding and opening of my body, and powerfully overcome it. Strengthen and protect my heart against immoderate fear and agonizing trepidation."[42]

It is not surprising then that medical case histories repeatedly describe patients who, at least initially, rejected undergoing a recommended operation, even more so if they already knew from personal experience what they had to expect. Bartholomé Cabrol at the end of the sixteenth century wrote about a woman who had been successfully operated on to remove her breast cancer. When, following menopause, she developed a cancer of the lip, she refused any new surgical procedure "because of the great and agonizing pain of the earlier treatment." She died after suffering more than 2 years of agonizing illness.[43] Henry Fearon also described a number of such cases at the end of the eighteenth century. When Ellis of Camberwell's doctors diagnosed her with breast cancer in 1783 she could

> not make up her mind whether to follow the advice of her doctors and submit herself to such a terrible and painful operation, one that in the end might not even go well. And if I may make use of her own words, this opinion had grown deeper roots in her soul ever since she had seen the suffering of her neighbor who had been operated on under the supervision of one of the most distinguished surgeons in the city and who had described to her the pains of the operation, and what it was like to stay at home and have your wounds dressed every day for a number of months.[44]

Another female patient rejected the doctor's recommendation to undergo surgery "because she did not experience any discomfort except for the weight of the lump and at times a dull pain."[45] For one of Henry Fearon's patients, even the intense pain and the occasionally bloody and generally malodorous, festering discharge of his testicular tumor were initially not enough to move him to submit to the recommended surgery.[46]

In many cases, it was the physician who came to the conclusion that it would be better to forgo further attempts at a radical, curative therapy in favor of a "mere" palliative treatment. This decision not only raised issues of professional politics but also some serious ethical problems. In the case of many incurably sick and dying patients—here, early modern authors were in unanimous agreement—a palliative

---

[42] Johann Friderich Schwalb, Andächtiges Gebet vor und nach der schmertzhaften Operation weiland Marx Albrecht Sturm, wohlverdienten Handelsbedienten, welcher Dienstags den 28. Januarii 1772. in dem 43. Jahr seines christrühmlich geführten Alters Vormitag an einem Stein glücklich geschnitten worden, verrichtet von M. Johann Friderich Schwalb, Diac. II. Minorit., Augsburg: [N.N.] 1772, fols 4r–v.

[43] Cabrol, Alphabeton (1604), pp. 108–9.

[44] Fearon, Abhandlung (1790), pp. 95–7; in the end, when it was already too late according to Fearon, she did ask for an operation. On her urgent request, he sent her to a surgeon who performed an operation, which initially yielded good results.

[45] Ibid., pp. 85–7.

[46] Ibid., pp. 77–80.

treatment made sense and was necessary. After all, no reasonable person could expect even the best medical art to wipe out a disease if the body was already in a very weakened state or if the disease or morbid matter had become too powerful or too deeply rooted in the body. In such cases, the treatment had to follow symptomatic indications.[47]

The problem was again the uncertainty of the prognosis. With any given case of illness, the doctor ran the risk of making a mistake.[48] Should he be wrong, should it actually have been possible against all expectations to halt the progress of the disease by carrying out a rigorous treatment, then the physician was partly responsible for the premature death of the patient. Critics did not hesitate to hit upon this sore spot. As Helcher in the early eighteenth century wrote, "when signs of death begin to show, many, indeed most, give no medicine or only medicine that is too weak and serves [to sooth] the throat more than [to combat] the disease." Insofar as the doctor, for a fine penny, was addressing "the symptoms alone" such as pain, coughing or a poor appetite, he was treating "in only a palliative manner, not attacking the main work […]." But Helcher held that the prognosis was always uncertain. If, unlike himself, a doctor did not, "until the soul left the body, administer everything that was possible and strong enough, even if [the patient] was already in the throes of agony," he burdened his conscience heavily and carried great responsibility on Judgment Day.[49] "So, praised be he who attempts all possible cures and leaves nothing untried that might help, even with those who are already dying."[50]

Helcher, judged by the standards of the day, was a somewhat dubious character. He sought to win new patients by boasting the success of his treatment with gold tinctures that supposedly cured patients who had been deemed lost causes by other doctors. Yet, some highly respected physicians came to quite similar conclusions. Johannes Bohn, for example, quoting Galen and Celsus in his support, declared that unless the condition was completely hopeless, it was better to give a medicine of uncertain effectiveness than to give none at all. There were enough examples, he wrote, of seemingly desperate cases turning out for the better. If a doctor was reluctant to give powerful medicines, he might accelerate the patient's death in such cases.[51] Friedrich Hildebrandt in 1795 wrote that although one should leave the disease to nature rather than give remedies on the off-chance that they will work, in

[47] For a detailed analysis of the differences between a "symptomatic indication" and therapeutic approaches that targeted the very essence of the disease see Gmelin, Allgemeine Therapie (1830), pp. 64–71.

[48] Cf. e.g. the case histories in Augenius, Epistolarum (1602), fol. 86v, and in Henricus Casparus Abelius, Dissertatio inauguralis medica in casu practico complicatissimo, exponens aegram phthisicam, diu quidem pro desperata habitam, ast per Dei gratiam feliciter curatam. Praes. Heinrich Christoph Alberti, Erfurt: Groschius 1692.

[49] Hanß Heinrich Helcher, Cur incurabler Kranckheiten beweiset durch Gottes Seegen und mit Goldes Hülffe, Leipzig: Tietzen [around 1723], pp. 240–1 and p. 259.

[50] Ibid., p. 259.

[51] Johannes Bohn, De officio medici duplici clinici nimirum ac forensis, Leipzig: Gleditsch 1704, pp. 67–8.

the case of severe complaints or in the face of great danger, it was better to give a questionable medication with an uncertain chance at success than nothing at all.[52]

However, here doctors were not in agreement. There were opposing voices, medical authors for whom it seemed more important not to increase the suffering of the dying than to do everything within one's power to extend their lives. For these critics, it was the physician who persevered in attempting to combat the disease itself and not its symptoms until the patient's hour of death who risked shortening the dying person's life. This was because any futile treatment attempts meant an additional strain on the weakened body. For example Girolamo Cardano in the sixteenth century emphatically opposed the "not few" physicians who attempted a radical, causal cure in incurable diseases and thereby only shortened the patients' lives. Some of these physicians, he felt, truly believed that they could still cure or at least improve the illness; others were driven by glory or greed.[53] Along these lines, a dissertation defended under the direction of Michael Alberti in the early eighteenth century argued that the physician was under the obligation, through his faith and his conscience, to preserve the life of the patient as long as possible. The *religio medici* did not, it went on, allow questionable and dangerous remedies to be used, especially in the case of delicate or weakened patients such as infants, pregnant women, or those suffering from dropsy, consumption or other chronic illnesses.[54]

The question of surgical treatment in the case of breast cancer offered a particularly illustrative example—one that was corroborated by the testimony of ancient authorities—of why it was sometimes better not to try out every remedy. Wilhelm Fabry, for example, writing about cancer patients, distinguished between, "the actually true cure (which requires the complete elimination of the tumor, be it by burning, cutting or cauterization)" and the "ostensive" or *Schein-Cur* which was limited to "alleviating pain and preventing the disease from further settling in." While it did not help permanently, he for one would "rather choose the ostensive cure than putting the patient in a certain and inevitable mortal danger."[55]

The proponents of therapeutic reserve also argued that a palliative treatment could sometimes not only alleviate the symptoms but could even indirectly work in a curative manner or at least serve to prolong life.[56] The "palliation" of incurable consumption for example aimed, according to Sylvius, not only at alleviating the

[52] Friedrich Hildebrandt, Ueber die Arzneikunde, Erlangen: bei Johann Jacob Palm 1795, pp. 99–100.

[53] Cardano, De malo medendi usu (1536), pp. 8–9.

[54] Alberti, De religione, p. 37.

[55] Fabry, Wund-Artzney (1652), pp. 1269f, letter to the physicians and surgeons in Geneva, September 15, 1596.

[56] Heurne, Praxis (1590), pp. 343f; Guy de Chauliac, Chirurgia magna, 1585 (repr. Darmstadt: Olms 1976), pp. 398–400; Guido Guidi, De curatione generatim, in idem: Opera omnia sive ars medicinalis (separate pagination), Frankfurt: typis et sumptibus Wechelianorum 1626, p. 121; Wedel, De cura palliativa (1703), p. 33; similarly idem, Opiologia, Jena: Sumptibus Johannis Bielkii 1682, p. 157.

complaints, but also at restoring and strengthening the patient's failing vigor.[57] The treatment of pain, too—a central element of palliation—could indirectly delay death. For Wedel, it was "stupid" to aim at the elimination of the disease itself while neglecting urgent complaints. Pain weakened nature and made it difficult for nature to free itself from the burden of the illness. When the pain subsided, nature was in a better position to fight the disease of its own accord. In this way, opiates were useful not only in treating the complaints but often indirectly in fighting the cause of these complaints as well.[58]

These arguments took some of the bite out of the ethical dilemma of possibly shortening a patient's life due to abstaining from treatment. But they could not eliminate it altogether. While we may not share this belief today, early modern physicians were convinced that they could, in principle, cure many diseases. Doctors who decided in favor of a palliative treatment, in what appeared to be desperate cases, were inevitably taking a risk: by not attempting a possible curative treatment they were, at least in some cases, failing to save a life that could otherwise have been saved.

In cases where the choice was between further pursuing a radical, curative treatment and refraining from this in favor of alleviating pain, doctors were confronted with an analogous moral dilemma if a patient was clearly in the final stages of dying. There was no hope of a cure, but the physician could at least try to keep the patient alive for as long as possible with strengthening, invigorating remedies. As we will see, this was common practice. However, there were some, above all Georg Ernst Stahl and his followers, who clearly opposed attempts to prolong life at all costs. In their eyes, what took priority was to allow for a death that was as gentle and painless as possible. For Stahl, remedies that served only to delay death a little were unworthy of the art of medicine.[59] Along the same lines, Z. P. Schulz in his *Euthanasia medica* spoke out against the apparently common contemporary practice of giving dying people generous doses of strengthening remedies and nerve tonics. They were not able to turn the situation around, and they made those close to the dying person call out, "[He should] not be held back so fruitlessly, his end made difficult still." In Schulz's perspective, this kind of medication required special justification: Sometimes, due to spiritual or worldly reasons, the attempt to delay death might be indicated, but that was something the doctor could only do if he achieved it with mild and safe remedies and not with dubious and daredevil attempts.[60]

---

[57] Sylvius, Praxeos medicae idea (1695), p. 701 ("Incurabilis ergo phthiseos palliatio consistet in symptomatum molestorum alleviatione vel alteratione, viriumque collabentium convenienti reparatione ac sustentatione").

[58] Wedel, Opiologia, Jena: Sumptibus Johannis Bielkii 1682, p. 157.

[59] Stahl, Mortis theoria (1702), p. 39; Alberti, De abstinentia (1722a), p. 31.

[60] Michael Alberti, Nobilissimo et clarissimo Dn. Candidato, in: Schulz, De euthanasia medica (1735), appendix (no page numbers).

3.4 Medical Morality and Lay Culture

In retrospect it is difficult to judge what the majority of physicians thought about such matters. To all appearances those doctors who adhered to Stahlianism were a minority, and even this minority, to the degree they put particular trust into the healing powers of nature, may have been in favor of refraining from further curative measures not because they wanted to reduce suffering but based on the belief that more energetic interventions risked having a life-shortening effect insofar as they disturbed the natural power to heal. For all we know, the majority of physicians felt that they must not do anything that could contribute to shortening a patient's life or neglect means that could help prolong it. As physicians' polemical medical stance against popular practices such as removing pillows quoted above already suggested, however, there are signs of a certain gap between the deontological norms, the medical morality of learned physicians and the views of the population at large when it came to the question of whether to prolong the life of a dying person as much as possible.

Many contemporaries, it seems, believed that there was a "right" time to die, one that was determined by Nature or God. The effort to preserve a person's life beyond this time, to "delay" death, was from this point of view senseless; indeed, it counteracted God's plans.[61] It is therefore completely imaginable that relatives and caregivers, all scholarly polemics aside, truly believed they were acting most piously ("optime religionem suam moribundo probari"), as I. Zach reported, when they refrained from giving tonic remedies as soon as they heard that the person was dying.[62] And if the death throes were severe because the soul found it difficult to separate from the body at the time that God had ordained—this battle was, according to a widespread view, the cause of death agony—then promoting this separation was indeed entirely in line with Christian faith.

We do not know precisely how widespread the popular practices of curtailing life described above actually were. In their indignation, the physicians and scholars may well have exaggerated their scale and significance. What we do know is that ethnographic surveys and personal testimonies continued to describe these practices as common until the end of the nineteenth century. Many people, it seems, were at least familiar with such practices that aimed at shortening the sufferings of a dying patients, even if they did not resort to them personally. We must assume all the more that many ordinary people rejected attempts to keep dying people alive with heroic measures or to bring those who seemed dead already back to life for a limited time. Peter Kennedy, for example, wrote from personal experience at the end of the eighteenth century that if symptoms appeared that were usually considered harbingers of death, bedside attendants and other helpers would neglect giving the remedies that had been prescribed by doctors to preserve the fading life that remained. They declared it pointless in such cases to prolong the agony of death.[63]

[61] Cf. Johannes Upmarck, De euthanasia (1760), pp. 60–4.

[62] Zach, De cura (1792), p. 28.

[63] Peter Kennedy, An account of a contagious fever, which prevailed lately at Aylesbury, and in some of the adjacent parts of Buckinghamshire, Aylesbury: printed by W. Nicholls 1785, pp. 33–4, footnote; my thanks to Kevin Siena for pointing out this passage to me.

3.5 Truth at the Sickbed

Another question that was determined in the border zone between questions of medical ethics on the one hand and physicians' concern for their reputation and practice on the other was, whether the physician ought to inform patients and relatives when death was imminent or not. If we believe Philippe Ariès, telling the truth was the norm in early modern Europe and it became common practice only since the mid-nineteenth century to conceal from the dying their unfavorable prognosis and impending death. The centuries-old familiarity with "tamed death" and the naturalness with which one had until then encountered it became lost according to Ariès. It was omitted with abashment and became a forbidden thing.[64] But Aries's account does not stand up to closer examination. As we will see, it was precisely in the nineteenth century—a time that according to Ariès was characterized by concealment—that the demand was voiced increasingly to secure the patient's right to be informed about his unfavorable prognosis. Conversely, for the early modern period, a significantly more complex picture emerges than the one implied by Ariès. In the sixteenth century, we find contradictory statements. Leonardo Botallo demanded that the physician should give his dying patients hope but should not hide an unfavorable prognosis from them.[65] Baptista Codronchi, by contrast, held that doctors were justified to hide an unfavorable prognosis from him if revealing it risked causing great damage.[66]

From the seventeenth century, as numerous sources indicate, this was the mainstream position.[67] Early modern writings about medical ethics or the duties of a physician routinely recommended concealing the truth. Ideally, the physician was to confront the patient with his fatal diagnosis only when death was imminent, when it was time to call the clergyman and give the last rites. When patients exhibited strength of character and asked directly and bluntly for the prognosis, some physicians saw the possibility of being more open about the truth. According to Roderigo da Castro' *Medicus politicus*, one of the most influential early modern texts on the professional duties of the physicians, if a patient's mental state indicated that he would not be terrified, then the doctor could indicate the true state of the disease. Some patients had, especially thanks to their religious faith, the necessary spiritual strength. Even with the most philosophical and mentally firm patient, the doctor had to be very careful, however, and to avoid everything that could put the patient in a state of distress and thus cause damage to his body and life. With a cheerful face, he

---

64 Ariès, Western attitudes (1974), pp. 85–6.

65 Leonardo Botallo, I doveri del medico e del malato. Ed. by Leonardo Careri and Anita Bogetti Fassone, Turin: Unione tipografico-editrice torinese 1981 (orig.: Commentarioli duo, alter de medici, alter de aegroti munere, Lyon: Gryphius 1565).

66 Codronchi, De christiana ratione (1591), pp. 57–9.

67 On the controversial contemporary debates about telling patients the truth see Schleiner, Medical ethics (1995), pp. 5–48; on communicating a fatal prognosis, in particular, ibid., pp. 27–9; see also Bergdolt, Gewissen (2004), pp. 145–7. By contrast, Roy Porter, Death (1998), p. 82, possibly relying on Ariès's work, has claimed erroneously that traditional medical etiquette demanded that patients be informed about their poor prognosis without any reservations.

was to give the patient hope, console him, strengthen his trust in the Savior, and take away his fear of death, which, after all, lasted but a brief moment.[68] And when patients were fearful—as most were, Castro thought—the truth should be concealed and cloaked.[69]

This position was based on widely accepted notions about the role affects in the body.[70] Negative emotions were believed to have a powerful impact on the body and the course of diseases. In early modern medicine, the affects were closely associated or even largely identified with the movements of the vital spirits and of the blood, which were thought to move toward the pleasant and to retreat from the negative to the interior of the body. Causing a withdrawal towards the heart, negative emotions like grief, fright or anger, in particular, interfered with the natural movement of spirits and blood from the center to the periphery. As numerous medical case histories illustrated at the time, affects could bring on illness and sudden death, and in those who were sick already they were likely to make the disease worse. From this perspective, the revelation of a fatal prognosis was bound to have extremely negative effects. After all, according to contemporary accounts, nothing was considered as more frightening than death. As soon as people heard tell of death, Guazzus stated, for example, in the early seventeenth century, their blood would become "ice cold," their faces would turn pale, their hearts would be "robbed of all liveliness," which was why "one thought it improper and impolite if death were recalled during meals."[71] The doctor who shattered the hopes of a moribund patient by informing him of his unfavorable prognosis might just as well have administered a poison since fear and desperation would kill the patient just as effectively. Conversely, if he was able to preserve the person's hope, the vital spirits and thus also the body's healing power would continue to fight the illness with full force and in some cases might even still gain the upper hand, defeating the illness against all expectations. In the eighteenth century, the old ideas about the effects of emotions on the movement of the blood and the spirits gave way to knew theories that focused on the brain and the nerves. The belief in the potentially harmful and sometimes indeed fatal effects of negative emotions remained very much alive, however. The physicians had to be all the more careful not to shatter their patients' hopes, because they could always be wrong in their prognostic judgments. Experience taught that sometimes even "the most desperate illnesses" could be survived.[72] In the worst case, the physician might cause a patient's death by giving a false prognosis.

---

[68] Castro, Medicus politicus (1662), p. 145.

[69] Ibid.; see also Zacchia, Quaestiones (1651), pp. 392–3; Seidel, Liber morborum incurabilium (1662), p. 133.

[70] Michael Stolberg, "Zorn, Wein und Weiber verderben unsere Leiber." Krankheit und Affekt in der frühneuzeitlichen Medizin, in: Johann Anselm Steiger (ed.), Passion, Affekt und Leidenschaft in der Frühen Neuzeit, Wiesbaden: Harrassowitz 2005, pp. 1033–59.

[71] Stephanus Guazzus, Euthanasia, Das ist: Ein lehrreich, nütz- und sehr tröstliches Gespräche, wie man nemlich christlich leben und seliglich sterben soll. Transl. by Melchior Wisaeus, Leipzig: Bey Abraham Lamberg 1625, p. 6.

[72] Döbeln, De erroribus (1700), p. 65; similarly Rosa, De curatione palliativa (1742), p. 5.

Against this background, the medical practice of concealment must not be interpreted as simply the expression of a predominant paternalistic attitude. Regarding many other questions, early modern physicians were quite respectful of the wishes and ideas of their patients. When it came to prescribing medication or a "regimen"—the recommendations for a health-promoting lifestyle and diet—they frequently took patients' personal preferences into account.[73]

Works on medical ethics and terminal care in the eighteenth century continued to demand that the physicians should withhold the truth as long as possible. The doctor, as succinctly explained by Ignatius Zach in his 1792 work on treating the dying, was to give the patient hope until the end because this made a critical difference to his physical constitution.[74] Occasionally only, there is now a sense of moral dilemma. According to John Gregory, the author of one the most influential works on medical ethics in the eighteenth century, the physician was often "in a loss in speaking to his patients of their real situation when it is dangerous. A deviation from truth is sometimes in this case both justifiable and necessary. It often happens that a person is extremely ill; but yet may recover, if he is not informed of his danger."[75]

Sources that reflect ordinary medical practice confirm that withholding a fatal prognosis remained common. A very weak Mme de Graffigny, who had coughed up blood and lost consciousness at various times, reported on 8 December 1758 that the doctor explained to her that she was not fully cured and that her complaints would periodically return. On 11 December, she was dead.[76] Even Albrecht von Haller, one of the most famous European doctors, who had been severely ill for months, was told only 10 days before his death that he was going to die.[77]

The patient's families or friends, by contrast, were to be put in the picture early on in the opinion of most authors. According to John Gregory, this was also a matter a fairness because it allowed for the possibility "of calling for further assistance, if they think it necessary."[78] Informing relatives was also very much in the doctor's own interest. He could not be blamed later for the inevitably unfavorable course of a disease or even be accused of having concealed an unfavorable prognosis out of personal economic interest. It appears that the patient's relatives usually played along in this game. They too saw it as their duty to spare the sick person as long as possible. All it took was seeing his mother's weight loss, cough and glowing cheeks, and Jean-François Marmontel (1723–1799) understood that his mother was suffer-

[73] Michael Stolberg, La négociation de la thérapie dans la pratique médicale du XVIIIe siècle, in: Olivier Faure (ed.), Les thérapeutiques: savoirs et usages, Lyon: Fondation Marciel Mérieux 1999, pp. 357–68.

[74] Zach, De cura (1792), p. 18.

[75] Gregory, Lectures (1772), p. 34.

[76] Beinecke Library, Yale University, New Haven, Gen. Mss. 353 60, letters from Mme de Graffigny, here letter, December 8, 1758, the handwriting is probably that of Mme de Graffigny's daughter.

[77] Haller, Briefe (1923), pp. 545–6, December 3, 1777.

[78] Gregory, Lectures (1772), pp. 34–5; a similar approach can be found with Lorenz Heister; see Rüdiger Korff, Das Berufsethos in der Chirurgie Lorenz Heisters 1683–1758, Zürich: typescript med. diss. 1975, p. 37.

ing from the same contagious, fatal lung disease that had killed his father. Yet he did everything to conceal his mother's true condition from her.[79]

Some authors recommended that the physician not even inform the relatives because the patient might learn the truth from them. Along these lines, J. J. Döbeln argued, for example, that one must not reproach a doctor who was reluctant to share the prognosis in the case of some illnesses. The patient would, "upon hearing a sad message become intensely worried and would therefore also, whilst suffering from his bodily illness, slip into the greatest sadness." Relatives and attendants as well became "agitated to no small manner by this. They start to scream and cry so that the doctor becomes afraid of being near them." The patient became saddened "often more for his friends, and he enters a state of melancholy and constant wakefulness, gives up everything."[80] In the surviving sources, we very rarely find evidence, however, that relatives and attendants were really less cautious in this respect. Belzer is a rare exception, when he recounts, in 1738, that his "dear wife" said to him that she was unable "to feign as the doctor did, but rather had to tell me that a recovery was out of the question."[81]

Authors whose primary concern was the spiritual welfare were likely to put more stress on the need to inform dying patients about their fatal prognosis. Writing "On the duties of physicians", the Anglican priest and poet Thomas Gisborne, for example, underlined the physician's duty to support the patient's drooping spirits but held that "truth and conscience forbid the physician to cheer him by giving promises, or raising expectations, which are known or intended to be delusive". The physician was "at liberty to say little; but let that little be true." However, "the state of the malady, when critical or hazardous, ought to be plainly declared without delay to some at least of the patient's near relations" and on "many occasions it may be the duty of the physicians spontaneously to reveal it to the patient himmself." Moreover, "conscience will frequently prompt him discreetly to turn the thoughs of the former towards religion."[82]

Some medical authors, too, conceded that physicians were depriving terminally ill patients of the possibility of preparing for the end, in both a worldly and a spiritual sense, as long as they withheld their unfavorable prognoses. Knowing about their close and inevitable end, some patients might still want to prepare a will, distribute their wealth and secure a future for their wives and children. John Gregory advised the physician to adapt his approach accordingly. If a sick person had "made

[79] Jean-François Marmontel, Mémoires. Ed. by John Renwick, Clermont-Ferrand: G. de Bussac 1972, pp. 56–7.

[80] Döbeln, De erroribus (1700), p. 65.

[81] Stadt- und Universitätsbibliothek Frankfurt, Senckenbergarchiv, letter from Belzer to Senckenberg, January 13, 1738.

[82] Thomas Gisborne, An enquiry into the duties of men in the higher and middle classes of society in Great Britain, resulting from their respective stations, professions, and employments, London: printed by J. Davis for B. and J. White 1794, pp. 383–426 (chapter "On the duties of physicians"), cit. pp. 401–2; Gisborne explicitly drew on Gregory's "Lectures" and on parts of Percival's "Medical ethics" that Percival had already composed and communicated to Gisborne (ibid., note on p. 383).

no settlement of his affairs, and yet perhaps the future happiness of his family may depend on his making such a settlement," then it was proper for a physician "in the most prudent and gentle manner, to give a hint to the patient of his real danger, and even solicit him to set about this necessary duty."[83] Along similar lines, Thomas Percival declared it the physician's duty to give the patient's friends "timely notice of danger, when it really occurs" and "even to the patient himself, if absolutely necessary." Since the disclosure of a poor prognosis was particularly alarming when it came from a physician, the task was preferably assigned "to any other person of sufficient judgment and delicacy", however.[84] Bruno Seidel, in the late seventeenth century, had even preferred to leave this task entirely to the relatives or to the clergy, adding that people were generally best advised to make their wills early, in healthy times.[85]

Particularly in Catholic regions, difficult questions arose when it came to deciding on when to call the priest to perform the last rites. Church authorities insisted that physicians must make their severely ill patients go to confession early and must fetch the priest in time so that the last rites could be performed while patients were still of clear mind. While asking a patient to receive confession might have appeared relatively harmless, calling the priest to give of the last rites would have unmistakably brought home to severely ill patients just how bad their prognosis was.

It is difficult to ascertain how often early modern physicians in their practice actually called for a clergymen in a timely manner. Insofar as a call to perform the last rites amounted to an admission of defeat, the physician had good reason to delay it, unless the relatives demanded it of their own accord. After all, the doctor risked that the patient would seek medical help elsewhere if he declared him a lost cause. As a result, secular and ecclesiastical authorities repeatedly found themselves compelled to reinforce the relevant ordinances. For example, the government of Anterior Austria in 1779 pointed once again to previous, identically worded ordinances, stating that physicians must

> urge their patients to receive the holy sacraments at even the slightest sign of danger, and to do so upon the third visit at the latest, but further, should the sick person refuse to do this, to take their responsibility seriously and actually lay down their work and not visit [the patient] again.

Apparently this could not be taken for granted. The reminder was prompted by several sad cases "in which the sick person died without a minimum of spiritual preparation."[86]

---

[83] Gregory, Lectures (1772), p. 34.

[84] Percival, Medical ethics (1803), p. 31.

[85] Seidel, Liber morborum incurabilium (1662), pp. 131–3.

[86] Freiburg, Stadtarchiv, C1 Medizinalwesen 1, N. 44, ordinance of the government of Vorderösterreich, October 9, 1779; similar ordinances can still be found in the nineteenth century; see Joseph Müller, Systematische Darstellung der Krankenpflege nach den im österreichischen Kaiserstaate geltenden Normen bearbeitet, Vienna 1844, note on p. 70, referring amongst others to a *Hofdekret* (Imperial ordinance) of 1812.

4 The Experience of Death and Terminal Care in Everyday Life

4.1 Hopes for the Afterlife and the "Final Hour"

Much more than today, the way death was perceived and dealt with in the early modern period was profoundly shaped by religious belief. The hope for a bodily resurrection in the hereafter—and conversely the fear of eternal damnation—also had a major impact on the experience of dying and terminal care. Death was far less the endpoint, the border to nothingness, that it is for many people today. When the process of dying began, this did not spell the beginning of the end, but rather the beginning of the transition to a new life, from one physical, social and metaphysical state to another.

As Philippe Ariès has shown, the more images of a universal last judgment on doomsday receded into the background, the more the hour of death gained importance in the Middle Ages. Whether a deceased person would be granted eternal salvation, or whether the soul would first have to be cleansed in purgatory or might even be condemned to eternal damnation, all this, it now was widely believed, was decided at the time of her or his death. The sick person's spiritual state and behavior in the hour of death became crucially important to his fate in the hereafter: Like an uprooted tree, the soul remained in precisely the state that it was in at the moment of death.[1] If the person died sinful, without repentance, without forgiveness, the soul at the moment of death was sullied and the person was not granted eternal salvation. One last sinful thought just before death or a weakening in resistance against the temptations of the devil could obliterate the rewards of a God-fearing life. On the other hand, if a person found his way back to his faith during the hour of death and repented his sinful life, he could, in spite of his sinful past, be granted eternal salvation. The death room became the place where eternal salvation was decided. "His attitude during this fleeting moment will erase all at once all the sins of his life if he wards off temptation, or, on the contrary, will cancel out all his good deeds if he

[1] Favre, La mort (1978), p. 83.

M. Stolberg, *A History of Palliative Care, 1500–1970*, Philosophy and Medicine 123,
DOI 10.1007/978-3-319-54178-5_4

gives way. The final test has replaced the Last Judgment."[2] This idea took hold more and more. Wollgast with a view to the seventeenth century summarizes that increasing importance became attached over time to "the moment of death" because "on the deathbed—so it was said—the devil and his helpers fought desperately one final time to obtain the person's soul."[3]

For these reasons, it was widely believed, over the entire course of the early modern period and across the different denominations, that religious, pastoral presence at the deathbed was indispensable.[4] The clergyman had an established, largely uncontested place at the deathbed, in the early modern period. As stated in the statutes of the Brotherhood of the Birth of Christ in Rome (whose telling epithet was *delli Agonizzanti*), at that most extreme moment in life, on which eternal happiness depended, one was—more than ever—in need of help and prayer, because the fight between the dying person and the devil was extremely fierce.[5] For clergy and relatives this meant that they were to do more than stand at the dying person's side and console him. They had to do everything in their power to prevent the dying from wavering in their belief at the last moment. The concern arose especially when the dying person was no longer able to speak or became unconscious. In an effort to reach the dying, it seems to have been a widespread practice to yell ever louder prayers or warnings into their ears. When the former mayor of Sitta appeared to be close to death in 1580, the pastor yelled the psalm verse "Into your hand I commit my spirit" into his ear and the deep sigh that followed was interpreted by those in the room as an affirmation.[6] According to his funeral sermon, 55-year-old Michael Jeger even explicitly requested that, when he lay dying, the priest would "scream into his ears, so that his Lord Christ may not leave his heart again."[7]

There were, however, important differences between the denominations, at least at the theological level.[8] Since the Middle Ages, Catholic doctrine had opened the prospect of purgatory, which was both frightening and in some respects comforting. What awaited the dead in some circumstances was tortuous pain, but in the end they would enter eternal life. Further, God was willing, as it were, to negotiate. Those left behind could, through prayers and indulgences, help ensure that the tortured soul would not suffer as long in purgatory, and before his death, the dying person could

[2] Ariès, Western attitudes (1974), p. 36.

[3] Siegfried Wollgast, Zum Tod im späten Mittelalter und in der Frühen Neuzeit, Berlin: Akademie-Verlag 1993, p. 22.

[4] For a brief overview see Jésus Conde Herranz, Les soins palliatifs: les origines, les antécédents et l'histoire vus à partir d'une perspective chrétienne, in: Dolentium hominum 20 (2005), pp. 54–63.

[5] Bayerische Staatsbibliothek, Munich, Cgm 44, Statuti della Venerabile Archiconfraternità della Santissima Natività di Nostro Signor Gesù Christo delli Agonizzanti di Roma [1690].

[6] Funeral sermon by Bruno Quinos for Nicolaus Dornßpach zu Poritsch, 1580, Herzog August Bibliothek Wolfenbüttel, I 1. 4° Helmst. (3), cit. in Kümmel, Leichenpredigten (1984), p. 210.

[7] Funeral sermon by Hartmannus Creidius on Marx Hueber, 1652, Staats- und Stadtbibliothek Augsburg, 4° Aug. Leichenpredigten 394 (3), cit. in Kümmel, Leichenpredigten (1984), p. 210.

[8] Michael Fischer and Rebecca Schmidt, "Mein Testament soll seyn am End". Sterbe- und Begräbnislieder zwischen 1500 und 2000, Münster: Waxmann 2005, introduction; Kümmel, Leichenpredigten (1984).

take precautions by buying indulgences.[9] The Catholic priest also played an indispensable role at the deathbed as a mediator, lighting the way. In 1615, Pope Paul V gave the Catholic death ritual its enduring form, with a confession, viaticum (Eucharist for a dying person) and final anointment. Above all, the viaticum, that is spiritual "provisions for the journey," which was brought to the house of the dying person and presented in an elaborate ceremony, was considered an essential prerequisite for a good death in the seventeenth century.[10] Other elements were a number of different prayers, an invocation of Christ, Mary and the Saints and kissing the crucifix. Consecrated candles were lit and the dying person was sprinkled with holy water.[11]

Lutheranism made a clearer distinction between the world of the living and the world of the dead and left little room for the mediating role of clergy. The idea of purgatory was rejected. Indulgences and requiem masses had no influence on salvation in the afterlife. It was a person's faith in God in his life and death as well as divine grace that determined whether he would have eternal life.[12] This made the hour of death more significant in some respects, as those in the room considered the circumstances of the dying person as signs that could be read. Although there were clear exceptions that called for explanations, in general a peaceful or even joyful death was the mark of a good, pious person. A "good death" thus brought consolation to relatives and friends. It indicated that the dead person had found divine grace. On the other hand, a "bad," agonizing death or even despair on the part of the dying person could give rise to doubts about God's grace and therefore about the dead person's eternal salvation, unless these physical and spiritual trials could be interpreted as a final divine test which the dying person would master by ultimately putting his fate in the hands of God, with humility and composure.[13]

In the course of the early modern period, the perception and evaluation of the hour of death began to change in humanist circles and gradually among the educated classes in general as well. When the question was whether a dying person had a prospect of a blessed life after death, the focus shifted from direct physical signs of a "bad" death, such as twitching and expressions of pain, to the state of the soul.[14] An agonizing death, as Johann Christoph Kemme (1738–1815) put it, was as little the sign of an evildoer as a gentle and painless death was of a saint.[15] The question

[9] Margaret Aston, Death, in: Rosemary Horrox (ed.), Fifteenth-century attitudes. Perceptions of society in late medieval England, Cambridge: Cambridge University Press 1994, pp. 220–2; cf. Chaunu, La mort (1978), p. 464.

[10] Ibid., pp. 348–9.

[11] Georg Handsch's notes suggest, in particular, that making the dying patient hold candles in his or her hand was an essential feature of this *rite the passage.* A candle was put even into the hands of dying infants and adult patients might ask for a candle when they felt the moment of death approaching (e.g. ÖNB, Cod. 137v).

[12] Koslofsky, Reformation (2000).

[13] Favre, La mort (1978), pp. 117–8; Gleixner, Pietismus (2005), pp. 198–9.

[14] Kümmel, Leichenpredigten (1984), pp. 224–5.

[15] Johann Christlieb Kemme, Von der Heiterkeit des Geistes bei einigen Sterbenden, Halle: Hendels Verlag 1818, p. 4.

of how piously one had led one's life gained significance as the basis of hope for eternal salvation, while the question of one's spiritual state in the hour of death lost significance. In Pietist eulogies, depictions of final trials that were mastered by the dying person took a back seat to images of a silent and serene trust in one's own chosenness.[16] In everyday practice, however, what remained essential across all denominations into the eighteenth century and beyond was a perception of the central significance of the hour of death and, for Catholics, the faith in the last rites as the key to Heaven's gate.

4.2 Subjective Experience

How did terminally-ill and dying patients experience their condition and approaching death? What physical and spiritual pain were they subject to in the final weeks and days of their lives? How did they wish to die when death was inevitable and imminent? What did they expect from medical care and nursing, and what significance did they attach to this, for example in comparison to pastoral care? To these and similar questions, historians can so far only give rather vague and general answers. The ethical norms and therapeutic methods of doctors and the theological views about the significance of the hour of death can be reconstructed quite well. The same is true of contemporary ideas of a dignified death that was pleasing to God, as illustrated in the extensive literature on the *ars moriendi*, and in death reports and eulogies. But what dying was like for those affected, how they perceived the medical care and nursing and what status it had compared to pious faith and hope for an afterlife, has by and large remained in the dark.[17] For obvious reasons, personal testimonies give only limited information. Most dying people no longer had the energy or the desire to record their spiritual and physical condition in a letter or diary. Thus, we must largely rely on what we know of the external circumstances of death and of the dominant religious and cultural norms and convictions to arrive at a rough answer to the question of how sick people and their relatives experienced the "final illness" and death and how they perceived the role of physicians in their situation. The accounts and published case histories written by doctors provide important information in this regard.

In the wake of Philippe Ariès's groundbreaking work, historical studies, using the extensive literature about the *ars moriendi* as a basis, have painted quite a positive, at times almost romantic, picture of death in the early modern period: the image of an authentic death at home in contrast to the anonymous and alienated death in the modern hospital today. People in former times, they have claimed, died in the company of their friends, family and community members. They were able to bid farewell in a dignified manner and to prepare themselves for the afterlife, finding

[16] Gleixner, Pietismus (2005), p. 203.

[17] Cf. Chartier, Les arts de mourir (1976), p. 70.

support in the helpful rituals of the traditional art of dying.[18] In this account, death and dying were not hidden taboo subjects, pushed into concealed corners, but rather an integral part of daily life in villages and towns.

It is true that, before 1800, only a very small minority of people died in in-patient institutions such as hospitals or the *Pfründnerhaus* (an old folks- or almshouse). For most, life came to an end at home, in the company of family members and friends. And, unlike today, the hope for a better life after death was, without a doubt, very important in helping people deal with death and dying. The rituals that accompanied dying and death had an established, visible place in everyday life. In rural parts of Germany, it remained common custom even after W orld War II that the village community would bid farewell to the deceased in their houses and later, after the funeral, would celebrate the return to normality with a hearty funeral feast. Yet, the image of dying in pre-modern times that we find with Ariès and his adherents is in some respects all too one-sided in emphasizing the positive aspects, engaging in romantic nostalgia. According to his critics, Ariès "confused rites and memories, terms, myths and norms with the reality of dying itself," reconstructing in this way a history "which had little to do with the historical experiences of people, with their life and death."[19] As we will see in the following, it is indeed rather questionable, for various reasons, whether this image of a conscious, peaceful death—a death that people entered willingly given their hope of a better life after death, a death that was in harmony with God and those left behind—does justice to the subjective perception and experience of the dying and their relatives.

4.3 The Horror of Death

In order to arrive at a realistic and nunaced picture of the subjective experience of dying, we must first of all spotlight once again the often terrible, utterly unbearable physical pain of dying, which could not be fought nearly as effectively as today. Dying in a hospital bed today may appear very anonymous, mechanized, even inhuman. However, it would be historically naïve to assume that dying is much more horrifying today than it was in the past when we consider the agonizing, often months-long suffering of many patients in previous centuries. Even in funeral sermons, a genre that tended to emphasize the peaceful circumstances of a composed death, the sheer, unbearable pain of some patients makes itself felt. About the princely Württemberg councilor Johann Cunrad Miller, for example, it was said in 1655 that, over a long period of time before his death, he had "endured terrible pains and agony in his body, as he certainly whimpered like a crane and a swallow, having

[18] Cf. Arthur E. Imhof, Ars moriendi. Die Kunst des Sterbens einst und heute, Vienna–Cologne: Böhlau 1991.

[19] Elias, Einsamkeit (1982), pp. 23–8; Mischke, Umgang (1996), pp. 5–6.

to yell out overloudly and so pitifully that it would have aroused pity in a hard rock."[20]

For relatives as well, the sight of their suffering, moribund family member was often a difficult burden psychologically and emotionally. One unnamed author in 1761 wrote that he had often seen people near the dying become dismayed, watching "the struggle that came to pass with trepidation of the soul, trembling limbs, paling of the face and a quick movement of the heart before life ceased to be."[21] Mme de Graffigny explained in 1739 why her friend Devaux was feeling worse and worse. It was making him positively ill to keep watch over his uncle who lay in death agony, whose legs were being cut open every day and who was vomiting every minute.[22] When we look back, it is indeed almost impossible to imagine what it meant to accompany a sick person as they approached death, with pain and cramps that could hardly be controlled with the existing medication, who screamed almost uninterruptedly day and night, writhing with cramps or whose body literally appeared to be dissolving into foul, sanious excretions.[23]

Rich families sometimes also hired paid bedside attendants but even in circles who could afford such services it was often a young unmarried daughter, granddaughter or niece who cared for the terminally ill in the final weeks and months. Their personal testimonies give vivid and times dramatic expression to their emotional burden. Julie Verdier's account of her last months with her cousin, the author Sophie Cottin (1770–1807), is a good example.[24] Verdier cared for the sick woman until the end of her life. Her account is complemented by a letter of farewell written by Cottin herself and by various other letters from friends and acquaintances. The diagnosis that was made at the time is not known, but the symptoms—particularly vaginal bleeding—suggest that the young woman had uterine cancer, a disease that was well known already at the time. According to her cousin, Mme Cottin did not die of weakness but of an excess of pain and, in her agony, was not able to find the peace that unconsciousness could grant. With dramatic words, she described what followed for her psychologically and physically: "And I saw it all! Heard it all! Felt it all! And I'm still alive!" She had this terrible image constantly before her eyes, she wrote. "In vain do I try to escape it; it burns my heart; consumes my body, controls my imagination, my thoughts." She did not cry about the loss, she wrote, about

[20] Funeral sermon by Johannes Georgius Esenwein on Johann Cunrad Miller, 1655, UB Tübingen, 4° L XVI 138 ang., cit. in Kümmel, Leichenpredigten (1984), p. 217.

[21] Anonymus, Die guten Wirkungen des Kranken-Bettes bey dem merkwürdigen Ende eines Sterbenden, 3rd edn, Dresden–Leipzig: Richter 1761, p. 5.

[22] Letters from A. Devaux, March 24 and April 1, 1739, in Graffigny, Correspondance, vol. 1 (1985), letters n° 108 and 109. Graffigny writes of the "vapeurs" that virtually killed Devaux. His uncle died 5 days later in Devaux's arms.

[23] Contemporary physicians were well aware of the emotional repercussions on the families; see e.g. Kortum, Kleine Aufsätze (1800), pp. 38–9.

[24] On Cotting see David-Paul Bianciardi, Sophie Cottin, une romancière oubliée à l'orée du Romantisme, une vie, une œuvre, contribution à l'étude de la réception, doctorat de lettres, Metz: http://dabianc.free.fr/these.html 1995; this doctoral thesis comprises about 1.400 pages but these documents on S. Cottin's dying and death seem to have escaped the author's attention.

the emptiness left behind. She cried about her cousin's pain and had only her "unbearable torture" on her mind. In addition, she felt exhausted physically, suffered from cramps and complained of "inner hemorrhoids," which were completely new for her and which she traced to her great unrest, which, locked entirely within her, had burned her blood.[25]

In the eighteenth century, some patients, even a long time after the event, traced their own disease to the great burden of caring for parents, husbands, children or other relatives. Mme de Merande, for example, had devoted herself to her consumptive aunt for 4 years, from the age of 15 to the age of 19, and eventually developed a chest ailment herself.[26] Another factor was the widespread fear of contagion, which existed long before the discoveries of modern bacteriology.[27] For the Comtesse de Mouroux, the hardship of lending support, her worry and fear for herself and her children, whom her husband suffering from a lung disease had wanted to see until the end, had ruined her emotionally.[28]

4.4 Dying at Home

Not only was death in earlier centuries often extremely painful. The external circumstances were not necessarily as favorable either as the romantic images of death in the familiar home setting lead us to believe. For one thing, we must not be too quick in drawing general conclusion from sources that reflect primarily the situation of upper-class patients. They were a small minority. Most people who died came from humble backgrounds. Many of them slept on straw and even people who were terminally ill might have to share their bed with others. Among the less affluent, dying was also frequently linked to economic concerns, especially where the dying person had provided for the family. For some it was barely feasible to put aside their work to take care of a dying family member and funeral costs were a considerable burden.[29]

Some dying patients had no one at all. They died alone or, at best, in the care of a hired nurse. In Nuremberg, according to a 1769 report of the town's alms office, those who suffered from a protracted, non-contagious illness were "taken in and fed" by "specially hired bedside attendants." Yet, their watch and care was, as the report (which called for the founding of a hospital) stated, often bad, the rooms often hardly suitable and poorly heated and the food inferior.[30] There seems to have

[25] Bibliothèque Nationale, Paris, NAF 15985, letter (draft) September 1807.

[26] Bibliothèque Cantonale et Universitaire, Lausanne-Dorigny, IS 3784, Fonds Tissot, letter from Mme de Merande to Tissot, October 4, 1783.

[27] Lachmund and Stollberg, Patientenwelten (1995), pp. 43–5; Stolberg, Experiencing illness (2011), pp. 118–20.

[28] Bibliothèque Cantonale et Universitaire, Lausanne-Dorigny, IS 3784, Fonds Tissot, letter from the Chevalier d'Alberey, with a report about the countess, February 13, 1790.

[29] Cf. Houlbrooke, Death (1998), p. 192; Nolte, Wege (2006b), p. 45.

[30] Stadtarchiv Nürnberg D1 209, report from the Stadtalmosenamt, July 22, 1769.

been a similar arrangement in Augsburg, at least around 1800, judging from an account about Carolina Bachin, who was suffering from uterine cancer. Her hired bedside attendant Barbara Rosengardtin no longer wanted to stay with her. The attendant's account, in turn, highlights just how burdensome caring for such a patient could be. She explained that the patient's condition had gotten so much worse that she "would not keep anything in and that the sick woman was not able to hold anything back and there was such a foul smell that one could hardly stand being in the same room with her." The rags which the attendant laid under her and which she tried to keep as clean as possible smelled so strongly that everyone had to hold their nose when she took them to the brook to wash, which she had to do "so as to prevent the sick woman from rotting."[31]

Even when there was company, the question arises whether dying patients always experienced the presence of others as helpful and beneficial. Our current ideas about death in pre-modern society—our notions of death in the familiar, private circle of one's own family—accord with the actual circumstances of the time to a limited extent. Much more than is the case today, dying was a public event. It was very common for friends, acquaintances, relatives and even passersby to come pouring into the dying person's room.[32] In some circles, these visits seem to have been viewed as an imperative. This is well documented in particular for the Pietists, who considered visiting and giving spiritual support to the sick and dying an obligation.[33]

According to the dominant conception, a death was successful for nobles and other high-ranking individuals if one died surrounded by one's servants. For example, according to his chronicler, Friedrich Karl, Bishop of Bamberg and Würzburg explained some days prior his death in 1746: "You folks, I am much more ill than you believe; I can feel it." Yet, the doctors played down the issue and so everyone went to bed on the evening before his death. It was not until the bishop was in the throes of death that the doctors, clergy and other employees were called to his bedside. "And so it was decided *in fatis,*" wrote the chronicler, "that this great bishop and powerful prince of the empire", in spite of his many servants, was to die "in circumstances of abandonment and misery."[34]

Medical writers in the Enlightenment increasingly took offence at the lively visits to the sickbed and deathbed. In their opinion, the dying patients needed peace and quiet and were not to be pestered by the sight of numerous spectators, not to be exposed to the clamor of their mourning.[35] There are accounts from as late as 1860 in rural Bavaria that describe loud, public lamentations on the part of relatives

[31] Stadtarchiv Augsburg, Bestand St. Servatius Akt 26, Num 328, Bl. 2 (um 1806); I owe this source to Hannes Langrieger.

[32] Chaunu, La mort (1978), pp. 347–8.

[33] Gleixner, Pietismus (2005), p. 81 and p. 90.

[34] Stadtarchiv Augsburg, Evangelisches Wesensarchiv 115, account of the last hours of bishop Friedrich Karl of Bamberg and Würzburg, August 8, 1746.

[35] Zach, De cura (1792), p. 31; Collner, Specimen (1799), p. 12; Baltes, De euthanasia (1842), p. 14.

and friends.[36] Doctors also cautioned about health risks. Visitors, they said, were putting their own health in jeopardy when they spent time in the polluted air of the sickroom, and they were spoiling the air in the room even more with their candles.[37]

Whether the doctors were successful with their cautioning is a different matter. In the rural Bavaria of the nineteenth century, physicians continued to complain that when someone was dying, "quite a number of people from the neighborhood come together" to "pray and to keep watch, but mainly to eat and drink, and quite often things become less than proper."[38] Another doctor wrote that, "When the throes of death begin, certainly to the great vexation of the dying person and not always without danger for those in the room, the sickroom fills up with people around the bed who are waiting for the dying person's last breath."[39] As late as the mid-nineteenth century, Pierre Chaunu found a similar situation in the rural regions of France.[40]

For the upper classes by contrast, the first indications that dying was becoming more private emerge in the eighteenth century. There were no longer countless people standing around the sickbed, at least not until the actual moment of death.[41] However, we can hardly trace this change to the physicians' cautioning. It reflected a much wider cultural development, in which greater value came to be assigned to the private, the familiar, the intimate.

For most of us today, the desire for privacy goes without saying. This makes it difficult for us when we look back to judge what the numerous everyday visits to the deathbed meant to the dying people themselves and to what degree the visits corresponded to the dying people's desires and needs. After all, those present inevitably included not only close relatives and friends but also people with whom the dying person was less familiar. Karoline Sulzer, the wife of a doctor from Weimar, wrote very evocatively in her diary about how she viewed it as her duty, in the summer of 1821, to stand by at the deathbed of the Duchess of Kurland "with many others." She and the duchess were not very close, and when she later cried by the coffin of the deceased it was not, as she admitted, because of the loss she had suffered but out of pity for the farmers and poor people who depended on the duchess's support. At the bed of the dying woman she had been very aware that the sick woman had "only tolerated" her during the four nights she kept watch at her side. In the end, she could not comfort herself with the idea that she "had done something useful for her—or that she had been anything."[42]

[36] Bayerische Staatsbibliothek, Munich, Cgm 6874/123, Dr. Geith, Neustadt an der Waldnaab.

[37] Collner, Specimen (1799), p. 12.

[38] Bayerische Staatsbibliothek, Munich, Cgm 6874.

[39] Ibid., Cgm 6874/136, Ottobeuern, 1860.

[40] Chaunu, La mort (1978), p. 348.

[41] Jalland, Death (1996), pp. 26–7; McManners, Death (1981), pp. 255–8; Chaunu, La mort (1978), pp. 347–8; see also Kümmel, Leichenpredigten (1984), p. 225.

[42] Zentralbibliothek Zürich, Ms. ZII 665, diary of Karoline Sulzer 1815–1821, fols 51r–53r.

4.5 The Normative Constraints of the Art of Dying

The way in which pre-modern people dealt with death and dying has frequently been described as a positive model. It is seen to have offered the support and meaning that modern death often lacks. Some authors have even called for a revival of the old, pre-modern art of dying.[43] As we have seen, a closer look at sources which reflect the experience of the dying and those around them, leads to a much more shaded picture, however. Undoubtedly, the practices and rituals that characterized the old art of dying could provide some security and support—but they came with a price. The *ars moriendi* was not only an art. It was also and above all a set of norms and expectations, which the dying person and his relatives had to meet, no matter how pained, weak or sad they were. The dying person was to stage the final drama of his life, his departure from Earth. His "audience" could expect to hear some dignified and pious last words that would be eagerly noted down for posterity[44] and that would allow the death—and with it the deceased—to be characterized as good and devout, indeed as exemplary.[45] The bereaved were to give expression to their grief in the predetermined manner. If they were Pietists, they might even have to keep it entirely to themselves. Pietists were meant to be happy that the person was now in a better place beyond this world and if they manifested their grief this could be taken as a sign that they had some doubts whether the dead had lived and died in a way that ensured that he would be among the elected.[46]

Werner F. Kümmel has given a vivid summary of the "the ideal-typical process of dying" as it was reenacted again and again in funeral sermons and eulogies as in personal correspondences. If the patient's condition kept getting worse in spite of thorough medical treatment,

> he has no difficulty, no matter what his age, to prepare for death, because he has been long familiar with it. He puts his house in order, turns away from all earthly things, asks to receive Holy Communion and sends for the minister. He confesses his sins, receives absolution, professes his faith and receives Holy Communion. He forgives all those who have committed any offense against him, bids farewell to his relatives and friends and comforts those who seek to comfort him. He spends most of his time in prayer and song, in spiritual reading and uplifting conversation. All pains and complaints, as intense and disturbing as they might be, he bears with the greatest patience and reiterates with confidence that he longs to leave this world and to come to his Lord Jesus Christ, that he holds to his faith unswervingly and has not the slightest fear of death but rather is full of joy because through it he will enter heavenly life. As long as he is able, he prays and sings with the minister and those present, who are usually many, and he lets himself be prayed to, sung to and read to, and he sometimes chooses himself the words to be read during his eulogy. Day and night he

---

[43] Arthur E. Imhof, Ars moriendi. Die Kunst des Sterbens einst und heute, Vienna–Cologne: Böhlau 1991; Ziegler, Les vivants (1975).

[44] Cf. Karl S. Guthke, Letzte Worte. Variationen über ein Thema der Kulturgeschichte des Westens, Bern–Munich: Beck 1990.

[45] This culture of exemplary dying was particularly influential among Pietists; see Gleixner, Pietismus (2005), pp. 195–208.

[46] Eadem, Enduring death in pietism: Regulating mourning and the new intimacy, in: Lynne Tatlock (ed.), Enduring loss in early modern Germany, Leiden–Boston: Brill 2010, pp. 215–29.

> is surrounded by passages from the Bible, prayers and song, until he finally dies without so much as making a face or moving a finger, almost without those present noticing.[47]

One may rightly wonder if this kind of public death with its pressures to comply with the ideals and norms of the traditional art of dying was "more authentic" or better suited to meeting the emotional and spiritual needs of the dying person. As Rolf Winau has pointed out, death was celebrated with ceremony, but emotions were not part of this ceremony.[48] This was because a level of self-control, which, from today's perspective, seems almost inhuman, was demanded of dying people, and even dying children.[49] Physically weakened, often plagued by horrific pain and awaiting their approaching death in fear, they were supposed to appear calm and composed. There was no room for expressions of fear, of desperation and of pain because the "death that is awaited in faith and patience" was considered "the true euthanasia of just Christians."[50]

Some, inevitably, failed. Medical authors warned against rash conclusions in this respect. They pointed to the influence of the person's respective illness, temperament and age on the dying process. For example, phlegmatic people were said to generally have an easier death.[51] But a widely accepted view was that a person's painful, agonizing death, visible to everyone, posed the question whether his life had been perhaps only ostensibly virtuous and God-fearing. Apparently, God wanted to punish him.[52] The "choreography of correct dying," as Ulrike Gleixner has put it, demanded that "shortly before death a certain calm would come over the dying person, which stemmed from the certainty of attaining the desired nearness to God."[53] Accordingly, funeral sermons tended to underline that the deceased had passed away "without twitching and jerking," "without moving and snorting," "without any sort of bustling and rollicking," indeed "without any sign of fearing death, with a laughing mouth."[54] And the bereaved sometimes might feel the need to counter rumors by "evil, envious people who make malicious remarks." The former mayor of Sitta, for example, was said had died "in great impatience, with a lot of screaming and poor conduct." In another case, "papists" were said to have spread the rumor that a deceased minister had clamored loudly "for his blessed end."[55]

---

[47] Kümmel, Leichenpredigten (1984), p. 202.

[48] Rolf Winau, Einstellungen zu Tod und Sterben in der europäischen Geschichte, in: idem and Hans Peter Rosemeier (eds), Tod und Sterben, Berlin–New York: De Gruyter 1984, pp. 15–26.

[49] Gleixner, Pietismus (2005), p. 199.

[50] Immanuel Friedrich Gregorius, Sendschreiben an Sr. hochedlen Herrn M. Samuel Seidelns, des Laubanischen Lycei hochverdienten Rektorn, bey dem Absterben dessen herzlich geliebten andern Sohnes Carl Samuels, Lauban: Gedruckt mit Schillischen Schriften 1751; the term "euthanasia" is written in Greek letters.

[51] See e.g. Detharding, De mortis cura (1723), p. 86.

[52] Kümmel, Leichenpredigten (1984), pp. 206–7.

[53] Gleixner, Pietismus (2005), p. 199.

[54] Kümmel, Leichenpredigten (1984), pp. 203–4 and p. 207, with further references.

[55] Funeral sermon by Bruno Quinos on Nicolaus Dornspach zu Poritsch, 1580, Herzog August Bibliothek Wolfenbüttel, I 1. 4° Helmst. (3); funeral sermon by David Pistorius on Caspar Sautter, 1604, Stadt- und Kirchenbibliothek St. Mang, Kempten, 4° V.3a.52f (18), both quoted in Kümmel, Leichenpredigten (1984), p. 205.

4.6 Dying with a Clear Mind

In the light of all these expectations, it becomes obvious why for many contemporaries an essential prerequisite to a dignified, devout death was the person's being clear minded until the very end, in a state, that is, in which he or she could bid farewell, receive the last rites, make a confession and pray and could be on the guard against demonic temptations.[56] As Johann Valentin Andreae put it in his *Christianopolis*: "When they enter sleep, which is what they call death, they make an effort to stay completely conscious."[57] Accordingly, funeral sermons and deathbed-accounts regularly emphasized that the deceased person had indeed remained clear minded until the very end. The preservation of mental capabilities conversely served as evidence that God was well-disposed, doubtlessly with good reason, toward the deceased. Sulzer wrote about his deceased father that "such a calm and gentle death [is] granted to only few and certainly only to upright men." He had been "of sound mind until the end."[58]

Of course, this ideal of death in a state of consciousness was at odds to some degree with efforts to reduce pain. As early an author as Aretaeus advised in his widely known work about chronic diseases that the dying person should be put in a state of numbness if nothing more could be done to counter the illness itself.[59] In the early modern period, the choice between pain relief and preserving a clear mind arose above all with opiates. Detharding in 1723 questioned whether the doctor could administer opiates at all in good conscience as they had a soporific effect that adversely affected the mind. After all, a dying person in particular needed presence and strength of mind.[60] Along those lines, it is said that when Samuel Johnson was near death he consciously stopped taking opium so as to die in full possession of his mental capacities.[61] As late as the early nineteenth century, some medical authors championed a cautious approach: With reference to Cicero, Marx stated, "The best end to life is when a person dies fully conscious and with unperturbed senses."[62] Wilhelm Schriever accordingly considered it a major goal of medical treatment to preserve the consciousness of the dying person or to bring it back, and he presented a number of alternatives to opium, which he said had a soporific effect in high

[56] Piller, Private Körper (2007), pp. 230–4.

[57] Johann Valentin Andreae, Christianopolis (orig. title: Reipublicae christianopolitanae descriptio, Strasbourg: Zetzner 1619), Stuttgart: Reclam 1975, pp. 137–8.

[58] Stadtbibliothek Winterthur, NSW3/2 (type-written copy), Sulzer to Johann Jakob Tiger, cit. in Piller, Private Körper (2007), p. 230.

[59] Aretaeus, De morborum acutorum curatione liber II, in: Aretaei Cappadocis medici lib. VIII. Ruffi Ephesii de hominis partib. li. III, Paris: apud Guilielmum Morelium, & Iacobum Puteanum 1554, pp. 280–336, here pp. 313–4.

[60] Detharding, De mortis cura (1723), pp. 86–7.

[61] Porter, Death (1998), p. 93.

[62] Marx, Ueber Euthanasie (1827), p. 17; Marx is referring here to Marcus Tullius Cicero, Cato maior de senectute, paragraph 72: "sed vivendi est finis optimus, cum integra mente certisque sensibus opus ipsa suum eadem quae coagmentavit, natura dissolvit."

doses.[63] According to Schalle, a physician worked contrary to his conscience when he deliberately administered "sleep-inducing" remedies "just to be absolutely sure that [the body] did not suffer pain." If death was inevitable, then the aim should be to "keep [the soul] free" while "neglecting the physical well-being." If pain impaired the abilities of the soul, one could treat it, but only as long as the pain medication did not befog the soul.[64]

It remains the question, however, whether this attitude accorded with the desires and beliefs of the wider population. Schalle was presumably right when he saw himself as contrary to the "general opinion" which held that the soul should be put into a state of "dizziness" to "save the body from pain and fear and the soul from battle and fright."[65] Although many people could not access expensive opiates simply for financial reasons, medical accounts show that it was very common in the early modern period to give dying people plentiful alcoholic beverages. Even dying children were given wine to drink, according to Detharding, so as to comfort their hearts and ease their death, as it was put.[66]

4.7 Sudden Death

The central significance accorded to a person's spiritual state and to pastoral support in the hour of death also had a profound influence on which form of death was considered desirable, which form was feared and what contribution the doctor might be able to make. For most people today, a quick death without pain and free from trauma, is the epitome of a "good" death. An enviable death is when someone goes to bed at night in good spirits and does not wake up in the morning. The desirability of such a sudden death without pain is lessened only by the traumatic consequences for the bereaved. Historically speaking, this widespread the desire for a quick death is a relatively recent phenomenon, however.[67] In the early modern period, quite to the contrary, a quick, surprising death was greatly feared, such as death from apoplexy or stroke. "A subitanea et improvisa morte, libera nos Domine!", a well-known prayer asked, meaning "Deliver us Lord, from a sudden and unforeseen death." The dying person needed enough time to prepare for death, to make peace with God, to receive the last rites and thereby to ensure his happy existence in the afterlife.[68] Some authors even defined a concrete, most desirable time span. In this

[63] Schriever, De euthanasia (1836), pp. 24–5.

[64] Schalle, Zur Psychologie (1832), cit. p. 293 and p. 295; this stance was criticized by Hellwag, De euthanasia (1841), p. 19.

[65] Schalle, Zur Psychologie (1832), p. 292.

[66] Detharding, De mortis cura (1723), pp. 86–7.

[67] Favre, La mort (1978), p. 83; Siegfried Wollgast, Zum Tod im späten Mittelalter und in der Frühen Neuzeit, Berlin: Akademie-Verlag 1993, p. 22.

[68] Kümmel, Leichenpredigten (1984), pp. 213f; Rudolf Mohr, Der unverhoffte Tod. Theologie- und kulturgeschichtliche Untersuchungen zu außergewöhnlichen Todesfällen in Leichenpredigten, Marburg: Schwarz-Verlag 1982; McManners, Death (1981), pp. 253–4.

sense, Le Maître de Claville (ca. 1670–1740) felt that a terminal illness that lasted one to 3 weeks was most desirable.[69]

This ideal of a somewhat more protracted death lost significance as eternal life came to be determined not so much by a person's spiritual constitution in the hour of death but by his or her entire life, and it lost some more of its power as the belief in an afterlife declined in general. For some, a quick and unexpected end became desirable because it did away with unnecessary suffering. Accordingly, when Mme de Sabran in 1787 related the fate of M. de Tingry, who had collapsed, motionless, at his wife's feet after having just called his horses, she wrote that he "died the most desirable death, namely a sudden one."[70] However, according to John McManners's summary of the situation in eighteenth-century France, even in those circles in which the deathbed was losing its religious significance, the desire for a sudden death remained an exception. Apart from religious considerations, a very quick death was at odds with the traditional worldly rites and the ideal of relatives being given the chance to bid farewell.[71]

4.8 Doctors and Clergy at the Deathbed

Historical studies have repeatedly emphasized that one of the most important changes in how dying and death is dealt with has been a shift toward a more central role of the physician at the deathbed. It has been said that for a long time medical care for the dying hardly played a role because of the enormous significance of faith and the religious art of dying. Pierre Chaunu speaks of the "much more discrete presence" of the doctor in comparison with that of the clergyman even with regard to the upper classes. As to the poor, he continues, the doctor stayed away from their beds into the early nineteenth century, and it was only later that the doctor became recognized for his special role and function: His task had long consisted not in prolonging the life of a dying person and easing his agony, but rather in announcing that death was approaching and calling the clergyman.[72] "The decisive final service that was to be performed for dying people," as Katharina Ernst ascertains in regard to the Pietist culture was, as late as the eighteenth century, "not of a medical but of a religious nature, words of comfort and encouragement."[73] Cornelia F. Falk summarizes her findings with the words "Until the Enlightenment, doctors minded the dying only little or not at all, as this was the task of the priests, the point where the medical art reached its limit."[74] For England, Roy and Dorothy Porter date the beginnings of medicalized dying, that was no longer centered on the hereafter but

[69] McManners, Death (1981), p. 253.

[70] Mme la comtesse de Sabran, Correspondance inédite de la comtesse Sabran et du chevalier de Boufflers, 1778–88. Ed. by E. de Magnieu and Henri Prat, Paris: Plon 1875, p. 217.

[71] McManners, Death (1981), pp. 253–5.

[72] Chaunu, La mort (1978), p. 348.

[73] Ernst, Krankheit (2003), p. 217.

[74] Falk, Geschichte (1983), p. 22.

on the alleviation of physical suffering with medicines, to the second half of the eighteenth century.[75]

As Werner Kümmel in his studies on early modern funeral sermons has shown, however, the historical caesura was not nearly as sharply defined.[76] The transition from spiritual to medical care at the deathbed can at best be described as a gradual shift in emphasis. On the one hand, the belief in an afterlife and the desire for pastoral care in the hour of death remained central for the great majority of the population well into the nineteenth century. On the other hand, a valuing of spiritual support at the deathbed did not necessarily stand in contradiction to the desire for intensive and comprehensive medical care.[77] In general, the opposition between religion and medicine was far less pronounced in previous centuries than is often assumed. Even medieval and early modern monks and clergymen did not simply rely on God's care when they fell ill; rather it was obvious to them that they would avail themselves of medical aid. In many places, monasteries could even be considered the most important "employers" of physicians. Especially from a protestant perspective, it seemed simply imperative that the worldly remedies God had provided be used to preserve the divine gift of health and life. It was only when death was unquestionably near that the dying could feel free in good conscience to turn away from medical care and medication.[78] Thus, it was generally the case that the medical practitioner took center stage. Even when death seemed inevitable and a clergyman was called, this in no way meant that the doctor would vacate his chair for him. After all, there still might remain a glimmer of hope that medical treatment could save the sick person yet. Further, it was the doctors' undisputed duty—albeit one that was not always applied in practice—to at least alleviate the symptoms when there was no more hope of a cure. The idea that a calm, composed death was a sign of a God-fearing life on Earth and of a coming salvation in the afterlife even gave the palliative efforts of doctors a central, religious significance. With their remedies, they could contribute significantly to a death without screams of pain and lamentations and could keep the patients from being so weakened that they could no longer resist the temptations of the devil.

The thorough descriptions of the death of famous contemporaries show just how intensive medical care given by doctors at the deathbed was as early as the sixteenth and seventeenth centuries. Philipp Melanchthon's final days, for instance, are described in a very detailed account, which was composed by his personal physicians, in large part presumably by his son-in-law Caspar Peucer.[79] His death offers

[75] Porter and Porter, Sickness (1988), pp. 245–57.

[76] Kümmel, Leichenpredigten (1984), pp. 218–21.

[77] A special case are the medieval Cathars in southern France who regarded the body as a contemptible casing from which the soul had to escape, thus leaving little room and justification for any medical activities; see Peter Biller, Medicine and heresy, in: idem and Jean Ziegler (eds), Religion and medicine in the Middle Ages, York: York Medieval Press 2001, pp. 155–74.

[78] Kümmel, Leichenpredigten (1984), pp. 218–9.

[79] Nikolaus Müller, Philipp Melanchthons letzte Lebenstage, Heimgang und Bestattung nach den gleichzeitigen Berichten der Wittenberger Professoren. Zum 350. Todestage Melanchthons, Leipzig: Verlag von M. Heinsius Nachfolger 1910; I am quoting from the German "Kurtzer Bericht", ibid. pp. 47–87.

an illustrative example of a patient whom doctors did not—likely to some extent in view of his renown and significance—relinquish, taking all available therapeutic steps until the end and striving, even when the situation was hopeless, to maintain his life as long as possible. The 63-year-old was clearly close to death. His pulse was becoming weaker, his extremities were becoming colder, and his vital forces seemed to be leaving him. He briefly lost consciousness and explained when he came to, "I entered death, but God mercifully pulled me out again."[80] Then he lost consciousness again. Those around him "rubbed and anointed" him and he came to his senses again, asking, "Ah, what are you doing?"[81] When they tried to sit him up in bed shortly after, he lost consciousness once more, whereupon the physicians "refreshed [him] (as one tries to do in these circumstances)." This is to say they revived him from unconsciousness once more with their stimulants. When he came to this time, he said, "Ah, what are you doing, why do you hinder my gentle peace? Just give me peace until the end, it won't be long now."[82] He died shortly thereafter.

From the early seventeenth century, a detailed description of the death of the 45-year-old duchess Anna von Sachsen has come down to us, written by the deacon Johann Altenburger.[83] They called the deacon to her in January 1613, 8 days before her death, due to her "great weakness." Along with the physician, Dr. Schön, he set off on his way to her. "I've never been this ill before," the patient was quoted saying. Schön, who needed to go to a wedding, agreed with the patient that remedies would be sent to her, "with instructions on how to use them." But an hour after the sick woman had taken the remedies in the absence of the doctor, the color of her face changed. She felt she was suffocating, "was in great fear, lost the ability to speak, and there was nothing to do with her but pray, yet God was merciful and she recovered." She asked the deacon if she should take the remaining medication. He advised her to wait until the following day, "considering her great weariness and the fear she had suffered, and since she had experienced nausea due to the angel's wort that was mixed in." The next day the doctor returned and prescribed different remedies, "which she praised highly, as they did her well." She said, according to the account, that she had told the deacon many times that "she did not want to scorn proper remedies, so people could not say she was stubborn." They spoke of it again and she stood firm: "If it helps I have God to thank, if doesn't help, I have hope of something better." Toward evening things improved, and "all [that was prescribed] were supportive remedies." Nevertheless, the sick woman thought that she could not be helped anymore and asked if it were already time for confession and communion. The deacon did not want to deprive her of this source of solace, even if one would "make slow progress with the communion due to the cough, vomiting etc. that befalls her from time to time." In no way did the attending physician give up his spot at the sickbed for the clergyman. He continued to be present until the patient turned

[80] Ibid., p. 79.

[81] Ibid., p. 80.

[82] Ibid., p. 81.

[83] Thüringer Universitäts- und Landesbibliothek, Jena, Ms. Prov. fol. 26 (16), fols 375v–392v.

down his help at the very end. When she was offered a liquid to give her relief, she would not take it, saying, "but the throat will have to become swollen and the windpipe blocked at some point." Then things quickly worsened. She developed a strong sensation of pressure in her chest and had convulsive seizures. According to the account, she repeatedly said, "I wish I were dead" and, "Now, dear God, come and get me." When the doctor and the deacon spoke in Latin in her presence, she bid them to speak openly, saying, "I will not live long." She died the following night.

This account is illuminating in several ways. It describes the clergyman as an important figure, while at the same time calling deeper into question—as did the account of Melanchthon's death—the idea that doctors only began to play an important role at deathbed in the eighteenth or even nineteenth centuries. The physician had his own uncontested place at the deathbed. Although obviously close to death, the sick woman was still taking the prescribed remedies a week before she died. Moreover, direct reference is made to "alleviating" remedies which the doctor wanted to give the dying woman and which she only rejected shortly before her death. The clergyman, in turn, was involved in some measure in the medical treatment: When the doctor was absent, the dying woman asked for his advice. The deacon also recalled how he and the doctor had conversed in Latin in the sickroom, apparently—and this is how the patient understood it as well—about the woman's condition and her imminent death.

One essential reason why a medical presence at the deathbed played an important role was that it was difficult for relatives and even doctors in cases of serious, chronic and by all indications terminal illnesses to be entirely sure that a sudden deterioration in the patient's condition truly signaled the beginning of the dying process. Mme de Graffigny, for example, had suffered for a long time, had brought up blood and had temporarily lost consciousness. But when she, on the night before her death, began to utter only incomprehensible words and finally collapsed, her daughter immediately fetched the doctors. They gave the very ill woman emetics and for 2 or 3 h she returned to consciousness.[84]

In the case of Honoré-Gabriel-Victor Riquetti Comte de Mirabeau (1749–1791) we have the renowned P. J. G. Cabani s, one of the attending physicians, to thank for the detailed description of his final weeks and his hour of death.[85] Cabanis made no secret of his subjective, emotional involvement in the case. He cried, he wrote, when the man, seriously ill from a disease that remains unknown, disclosed that he believed he would die that very same day. But his account also goes to show just what torments the doctors allowed their patients to suffer out of fear of prematurely ending their lives, and in this case out of a lack of agreement among themselves. As we see in retrospect, the man's high social status, which allowed him to call several physicians at once, and which made them work with great caution, contributed to his especially painful death. Cabanis described the doctors' failure in remarkably plain terms. The dying man begged for medical aid to allow for the most gentle

[84] Beinecke Library, Yale University, New Haven, Gen. Mss. 353 60, letter from the daughter, December 23, 1758, responding to a letter of condolence.

[85] Cabanis, Journal (1791).

death possible: "Give me your word that you will not let me suffer any unnecessary pain. I want to enjoy unreservedly the presence of all that is dear to me." That evening, his condition worsened and the pain returned. The count was no longer able to speak and requested a piece of paper on which he wrote just one word: "dormir" ("sleep"). Cabanis knew what the count wanted—opium—but he acted as if he did not understand. Thereupon the sick man, who seems to have been medically knowledgeable, expanded on his wish: As long as administering opium harbored the danger of hindering the evacuation of the morbid matter, it was good to forgo it. But now that nothing more could help, he wanted it. Was it right to let one's friend die like someone woven onto the wheel, over the course of several days even?, he asked. The pain became more and more intense, and now that it threatened to accelerate death, it was his obligation—here Cabanis justified his actions—to alleviate it. With this, he implied that the desire to spare the patient pain was not enough of a justification in his eyes in view of the risks of opium. But valuable time slipped away. Cabanis, at first, was not able to come to an agreement with the second doctor, the equally famous Marc Antoine Petit, about the correct medication, and then, once agreed, it took more time before the remedy could be prepared and delivered. Meanwhile, the sick man's pain intensified further. In his agony he said, "I'm being cheated." He was placated and told that the remedy would soon arrive. Yet, the doctors had hesitated too long. Not with pious words but with desperation about the doctors who would not help him in the end, the sick man departed this world. "Oh, the doctors, the doctors!" he said to Cabanis, with a mixture of "rage and tenderness": "Were you not my doctor and my friend? Did you not promise me you would spare me the pain of such a death? Do you want me to take with me my regret that I trusted you?" These were his last words and, as Cabanis wrote, they rang unceasingly in his ears.[86]

[86] Ibid., pp. 59–62.

Part II

Modern Times (1800–1970)

The time period ranging from the nineteenth to the early twentieth century brought with it dramatic and far-reaching demographic, cultural, social and political changes in the Western world. These changes also had a profound impact on the way palliative care was perceived and given shape. Some developments led to increased attention given to questions of palliative medicine and helped establish structures for palliative care. Others led the perception of death and of medical terminal care in new directions. Others still could be said to have rather stood in the way of an increased recognition and advancement of palliative care.

The shift in demographics and epidemiology should be named first of all. The average age of the population in European states rose. Acute illnesses were less and less the cause of death in adults. Instead, the percentage of people dying from chronic and incurable diseases increased. Consumption, that is tuberculosis, became the most important cause of prolonged and frequently fatal illness in adults. Although the mortality rates for tuberculosis decreased significantly in the second half of the nineteenth century—in England for instance from 0.30% (1875) to 0.14% (1910), and in Prussia from 0.32% (1875) to 0.15% (1910), both calculated for the total population—the disease nevertheless remained the most important of the chronic terminal illnesses.[1] As life expectancy increased, however, cancer gradually gained more significance than ever as it principally affects higher age groups. Already in 1938, there were 140,000 estimated cancer deaths in Germany.[2] Much more so than in the past, doctors—especially those working in urban practices and hospitals—were now confronted with the prolonged and often agonizing suffering of patients with advanced tuberculosis, cancer, dropsy and other long-term, terminal chronic illnesses.

In addition to this came cultural changes. The erstwhile rootedness in religious belief lost significance for larger and larger segments of the population. And, to the extent that the physical agony of death was no longer interpreted as a divine test but

[1] Hermann von Hayek, Das Tuberkuloseproblem, Berlin: Springer 1920, p. 53.

[2] M. Kirschner, Zur Bekämpfung der Krebskrankheit, in: Der Chirurg 12 (1940), pp. 177–92, here p. 177.

as meaningless pain, medical terminal care gained importance. This development had its beginning in the early modern period, as did the slowly disappearing role of clergymen at the deathbed. In the different countries, it took its course differently from class to class, from region to region and from denomination to denomination, and usually it was slower in the countryside than in urban areas. But over the long term, the deathbed was by and large becoming increasingly secularized.

Alongside and in the place of religious norms emerged worldly ideals. The "culture of sensibility"[3] nascent in the eighteenth century rendered the ability to feel compassion for others the sign a cultivated, sophisticated character. Physical suffering was now not only described as hard to bear for the suffering person herself, but as an experience that heavily burdened those around her as well. The ideal of the humane, concerned and committed doctor found its way into the medical literature. Medical authors described with dramatic turns of phrase the physical suffering of the pauperized lower classes, wanting to stir the consciences of their fellow citizens.[4] The sensibility of doctors also expressed itself at the sickbed when they showed themselves as brimming with compassion for their suffering patients, perhaps literally shedding tears of lamentation over their dying and death.[5] According to Fanny Burney, tears welled up in the eyes of "the good Dr. Larrey" when her cancer was diagnosed.[6] Even Michel-Philippe Bouvart, whom some contemporaries described as sarcastic, is said to have cried when the child of Jean-François Marmontel died in his care.[7]

---

[3] Cf. G. J. Barker-Benfield, The culture of sensibility. Sex and society in eighteenth-century Britain, Chicago-London: University of Chicago Press 1992; Anne C. Vila, Enlightenment and pathology. Sensibility in the literature and medicine of eighteenth-century France, Baltimore-London: Johns Hopkins University Press 1998.

[4] Laqueur, Bodies (1989), pp. 176–204.

[5] McManners, Death (1981), pp. 53–8.

[6] Burney, Journals and letters (1975), p. 603.

[7] Jean-François Marmontel, Mémoires. Ed. by John Renwick, Clermont-Ferrand: G. de Bussac 1972, p. 304.

The Rise and Fall of *Euthanasia Medica* 5

In the field of medical science itself, a growing interest emerged in the bodily changes that marked process of dying. The origins of this can be traced back significantly further. Authors such as Theophilus Müller had addressed this subject as early as the seventeenth century,[1] moved in part by a practical interest in the signs of an approaching death.[2] But around 1800 the "physiology" of death became a central subject of contemporary medicine.[3] Vitalist views had become widespread in the eighteenth century, and according to vitalism, the living organism is endowed with particular characteristics and powers, which it then loses in the dying process. Attracting a great deal of attention, Xavier Bichat's *Recherches physiologiques sur la vie et la mort*[4] offered the first comprehensive survey of the topic in 1800. Other physiologists took up the subject.[5] The medical interest in the physiology of the dying process was nourished further still by the fear—very widespread around 1800—of apparent death and being buried alive.[6] Having a precise knowledge of the different forms and stages of dying promised to contribute significantly to preventing erroneous proclamations of death.

One thing that is striking in this period is the tendency of doctors to play down the horrors of death. Some early modern authors already, understanding death in the traditional way as a moment of separation of the soul from the body, had sought to reassure their readers. Plempius, in the seventeenth century, wrote that this loosening of soul from body was only a moment. It happened without pain and usually

[1] Müller, De aegro agonizante (1675).

[2] Prosper Alpinus, De praesagienda vita et morte aegrotantium libri septem, Frankfurt: Rhodius 1601.

[3] Cf. Ackerknecht, Death (1968).

[4] Bichat, Recherches (1800).

[5] E.g., Karl Friedrich Burdach, Die Physiologie als Erfahrungswissenschaft, vol. 3, Leipzig: Voß 1830, pp. 557–746 (= book 10: Vom Tode); see also Carol, Médecins (2004), pp. 128–40.

[6] See Gerlind Rüve, Scheintod. Zur kulturellen Bedeutung der Schwelle zwischen Leben und Tod um 1800, Bielefeld: Transcript 2008.

M. Stolberg, *A History of Palliative Care, 1500–1970*, Philosophy and Medicine 123,
DOI 10.1007/978-3-319-54178-5_5

without sensation, and could sometimes even be exciting. It was not death that was wretched but the way to it.[7] Some Enlightenment philosophers and physicians in the eighteenth century already described natural death as a peaceful transition to the beyond, accusing the church and clergymen of being the ones who made death difficult and bitter.[8] In the nineteenth and early twentieth centuries, however, this became the central message of numerous medical treatises. Doctors were seeking not just to "tame" death by promising to alleviate physical torment through medical means. Backed by their scientific authority, they also rejected people's fear of death as unfounded. Certainly, the disease that would ultimately lead to death could be accompanied by many agonizing symptoms. Here medical palliation showed itself to be valuable and necessary.[9] But death itself was usually far less agonizing than generally assumed.[10] Indeed, it was often the case that when death approached after a painful disease, "the sick person would enter a comfortable state."[11] Thus, most people's fear of an agonizing death was founded on a misunderstanding. "The majority of deaths," Richter explained in 1841, were "terrible to external appearances more than agonizing and irritating to the dying person himself."[12] C. A. Ewald too thought that "signs pointing to pain and agony, the so-called death throes, [...] the terrifying rattling sound over the lungs which can go on for days," all this seemed horrifying to the bystander only. The diseased themselves usually perceived it only in a minimal way or not at all. He had witnessed hundreds of people die, and experienced the same thing each time without exception: "without consciousness or pain they drift into eternal sleep."[13] Further proof was offered by the accounts of people who had seemed dead after a fall or a choking fit, but who regained consciousness—today we would speak of near-death experiences.[14] Some told how their entire lives passed before them, sometimes with long-forgotten details.[15]

The doctors were largely in agreement that with most illnesses, nervous functions and the brain in the dying process were so impaired that no thinking or sensation was possible. There came shortness of breath and for the bystanders the sight of the unconscious patient could be hard to take: the convulsions, the relaxing of the sphincter muscles and the sound of a loud rasping and rattling from the sick person's chest. However, the dying themselves were not aware of much of this.[16] Only

[7] Vopiscus Fortunatus Plempius, De togatorum valetudine tuenda commentatio, Brussels: Typis Francisci Foppens 1670, p. 26.

[8] McManners, Death (1981), pp. 251–3.

[9] Munk, Euthanasia (1887), p. 20; numerous further references can be found in Steingießer, Sterben (1938), pp. 29–44.

[10] Hornemann, Vom Zustande (1881), pp. 13–4; Munk, Euthanasia (1887), pp. 7–8.

[11] Capellmann, Pastoral-Medicin (1895), p. 212.

[12] Richter, Euthanasia (1841), pp. 363–4.

[13] C[arl] A[nton] Ewald, Über Alter und Sterben, Vienna: Hölder 1913, p. 30.

[14] Richter, Euthanasia (1841), pp. 363–4; Putz, De euthanasia (1843), p. 7; in very similar terms: Mendelsohn, Ueber die Euthanasie (1897), p. 3.

[15] Hornemann, Vom Zustande (1881), p. 37, footnote.

[16] Cf. Watson, Grundgesetze (1851), p. 76.

a few—so it was said—died a truly agonizing death, in particular people with tetanus or rabies, who suffered massive convulsions while in a fully conscious state.[17]

In their own way, changes in the healthcare marketplace led to heightened medical attention given to terminal care. As we have seen, medical care for terminally ill and dying patients was a potentially remunerative field for physicians already in earlier times. But as long as doctors' professional and economic success depended above all on the reputation they were able to gain with a relatively small upper class clientele, and as long as this reputation was largely based on how a doctor's therapeutic outcomes were perceived, accepting to treat patients with unfavorable prognoses was very risky. When a patient died in a doctor's care this almost inevitably cast a negative light on his skills. The treatment of different kinds of diseases was not yet standardized in the same manner it is today. Even if the doctor had predicted the patient's death, there always remained the suspicion that a more capable doctor might nevertheless have prevented it, or even that the present doctor had hastened it with his treatment.

The fear that the physician's reputation might suffer if he accepted incurable patients continued in the nineteenth century. But in the course of a successful professionalization process, physicians were able to secure a much more prominent place in the health market in many countries and to push to the sidelines the unwanted competition from lay healers and those who were "only" trained as artisans, the barbers and barber-surgeons.[18] The more the doctors secured a near monopoly for themselves in healthcare, at least in urban areas, and won the trust of ever wider parts of the population, the more they were in a position to take terminal and dying patients without risking their reputation and their practice. They could trust that their patients and the patients' families would understand that an illness against which a true professional, a learned, well-trained doctor, could do nothing was one for which there was simply no effective curative treatment.

For those physicians who did accept incurable and dying patients, acquiring the specific knowledge and skills in the face of dying patients brought welcome psychological relief. After all, as Klohss put it, the physician was "witness to indescribable pain, to unspeakable fear and anxiety in the final hour of life, witness to some difficult departures from life, to some heart-rending scenes, to some long and hard throes of death," and to "the agonizing suffering of the preceding days and weeks."[19] The doctor who knew how to provide medical care to the dying could remain true—even with terminal patients—to his positive self-image as an active helper, providing effective care for patients thanks to his special experience and competence. He was not condemned to witness as "a passive spectator," as Joseph Bullar put it, or,

[17] Munk, Euthanasia (1887), p. 21.

[18] Claudia Huerkamp, Der Aufstieg der Ärzte. Der Aufstieg der Ärzte im 19. Jahrhundert. Vom gelehrten Stand zum professionellen Experten. Das Beispiel Preußens, Göttingen: Vandenhoeck & Ruprecht 1985; Michael Stolberg, Heilkundige. Professionalisierung und Medikalisierung, in: Norbert Paul and Thomas Schlich (eds), Medizingeschichte. Aufgaben, Probleme, Perspektiven, Frankfurt: Campus 1998, pp. 69–85.

[19] Klohss, Euthanasie (1835), p. XI.

in Klohss's words "simply an observer at the deathbed."[20] Rather, with his growing experience "in the difficult art of euthanasia" Klohss's courage had grown, in the conviction that he had "alleviated many death throes, made drifting off easier, made many homecomings milder."[21]

Medical knowledge alone was not enough in this situation. Patience and sympathy were as important, and the ability to keep patients' trust. Only few doctors, "and if they were as medically skillful as could be," claimed Vogel, were "through nature, education and art, equipped with all the characteristics necessary to fully satisfy those requirements in all circumstances."[22] Taking care of dying patients was no easy task, Baltes acknowledged as well. More than the general practice of medicine, it required qualities such as strength of character, humanity, erudition as well as experience and a good knowledge of human nature. But carried out successfully, it was a source of joy for the physician.[23]

From the end of the eighteenth century onward, the medical discussion of the possibilities and limits of palliative treatment became more animated than ever. Terms like "to palliate" or "palliative cure" appeared in innumerable medical treatises, handbooks and encyclopedias.[24] Hospital records and admissions statistics indicate patients who were released from treatment as "palliatively cured."[25] Some also spoke of "palliative medicine", long before Balfour Mount, who has been widely credited with having coined it, made the term popular in the 1970s.[26] The *Encyclopédie méthodique* already dedicated a separate entry to *médecine palliative* in 1819.[27]

Alongside terms like "palliative cure", another old term gained increasing prominence: "euthanasia" or "medical" euthanasia, meaning the palliative treatment of the dying. The Leiden professor Nicolaas Paradys (1740–1812) drew great attention far beyond the borders of the Netherlands in 1794 with his *Oratio de euthanasia naturali*. Paradys understood *euthanasia naturalis* to be "the art of making death as

---

[20] Bullar, Opium (1856), p. 268.

[21] Klohss, Euthanasie (1835), pp. XI–XII.

[22] Vogel, Euthanasia (1834), p. 602.

[23] Baltes, De euthanasia (1842), pp. 7–8.

[24] E.g., Gmelin, Allgemeine Therapie (1830), pp. 342–3.

[25] I. N. Thomann, Annales instituti medico-clinici Wirceburgensis, vol. 1, Würzburg: apud A. M. Köl 1799, list of patients from April to December 1798; Salzburg Museum, Salzburg, Hs 1896/1, surgical case histories written by students.

[26] Clark, From margins (2007), p. 434; W. U. Eckart even claimed that Balfour Mount "coined the term 'palliative'" (Wolfgang U. Eckart, Auch Sterben ist Leben. Hospiz- und Palliativmedizin damals und heute, in: Michael Anderheiden, Hubert J. Bardenheuer and Wolfgang U. Eckart (eds), Ambulante Palliativmedizin als Bedingung einer ars moriendi, Tübingen: Siebeck 2008, pp. 43–52, cit. p. 44).

[27] Dictionnaire des sciences médicales, vol. 39, Paris: Panckoucke 1819, p. 123; Encyclopédie méthodique. Médecine, vol. NOY-PHT, Paris: Panckoucke 1824, pp. 283–4; the earliest use of the term "palliative medicine" in the English language is not known but the term was already used in the nineteenth century and occurs in book titles such as Lund's "Palliative medicine and palliative treatment" of 1880.

easy, as bearable, as is within our power and to the extent that it depends on natural causes."[28] The task of medicine was "not only to restore health but also to reduce the suffering of the sick," and when there was no longer any hope of a cure, "to make death itself less felt by the sick."[29] "Go to the beds of the dying [...]", he urged his listeners. "It is a sad but beautiful duty. [...] Learn humanity there!" Especially in the case of diseases against which the body defended itself powerfully, the doctor through a skillful use of weakening remedies could "contain the intense effects of the vital forces" and thus "ease death" and possibly even prolong life by facilitating the orderly work of Nature. Conversely, the doctor could gently strengthen weakened patients with invigorating remedies.[30]

Paradys stood at the outset of a movement that would rapidly gain strength. In England, William Heberden (1710–1801) called on physicians to at least reduce the terror of inescapable death and to ensure that it took place in the most merciful way.[31] John Ferriar (1761–1815), as early as 1798, wrote a whole chapter *On the treatment of the dying*.[32] When all hope had been lost and the organism was already breaking down, the physician was not permitted, according to Ferriar, to torment the patient with useless therapeutic attempts. He had to distance himself from the widespread practice of imposing liquors on the dying, forcing them into their mouths when they could no longer swallow.[33] Henry Halford (1766–1844), royal physician and president of the Royal College of Physicians—one of the most prominent members of the medical profession in the country—took up the topic of dying in various works. A *bon mot* circulated about him, allegedly made by a high-ranking lady in English society, who said that she would rather die under Halford's care than recover under the care of any other physician.[34] While he dealt with specifics of practical medical terminal care only in a marginal way, he gave a further major impetus to medical interest in the topic of dying thanks to his influential position.[35]

In German-speaking areas, the palliative treatment of terminal and dying patients garnered particular attention in the early nineteenth century. In 1806, an anonymous author complained that the "advancement of euthanasia" was unfortunately [still] "not enough of a subject in medicine." As a reason for this he saw the physicians'

---

[28] Nicolaas Paradys, Oratio de euthanasia naturali et quid ad eam conciliandam medicina valeat, Leiden: H. Mostert 1794; in the same year, a Dutch edition of this oration appeared under the title "Rede over het natuurlijk wel-sterven en den invloed der geneeskunde op hetzelve" (Leiden: N.N. 1794); I will quote from the more easily accessible German translation (Paradys, Rede 1796).

[29] Paradys, Rede (1796), p. 561.

[30] Ibid., p. 567.

[31] Heberden, Commentaries (1802), p. 272; a Latin edition made Heberden's text accessible also to physicians whose knowledge of English was limited (Commentarii de morborum historia et curatione, Frankfurt: apud Varrentrapp et Wenner 1804); certainly in Germany, good Latin skills were still standard among physicians, however.

[32] Ferriar, Treatment (1798).

[33] Ibid., pp. 192f and p. 204.

[34] William Munk, The life of Sir Henry Halford, London: Longmans, Green & Co. 1895, p. 265.

[35] Halford, On the deaths (1842), pp. 159–89; idem, On the climacteric disease, in: Medical transactions of the College of Physicians in London 4 (1813), pp. 316–32.

self-serving ambition for reputation and esteem, which caused them to avoid patients whose "healing offers little or no prospect of honor." Further, the incurably ill were usually "morose, stubborn, moody" and were "a great burden [to physicians] with their gloomy thoughts."[36] Soon, however, leading medical authors such as Johann Christian Reil, Ludwig Choulant, Ferdinand Gmelin and Friedrich Puchelt were discussing *euthanasia medica* in their manuals.[37] Practitioners such as Karl F. H. Marx and the Zerbst physician Karl Ludwig Klohss explored the topic in monographic treatises.[38] At German universities, terminal care became a popular topic of medical dissertations.[39] Between 1820 and 1850, almost two dozen dissertations, mostly still composed in Latin, appeared on the subject of *euthanasia medica*.[40]

These writings described *euthanasia medica* as the art "that suppresses all forceful symptoms, controls painful attacks and prepares to make the hour of death that cannot be averted as easy as possible."[41] The line between a *cura palliativa* and *euthanasia medica* was thus blurred in this conception. *Euthanasia medica* for many authors was a special form of palliative cure,[42] and some writings about *euthanasia medica* characterized it expressly as "palliative"[43] or as a "special modification" of "symptomatic" indications.[44] In the long run, the particular attention medical writers paid to the alleviation of dying patients' pain also had an effect on the dominant understanding of "palliative" treatment. The term now increasingly referred more specifically to the care of terminally ill and dying patients rather than,

[36] Anonymus, Vom Verhalten (1806), cols 537–8 and 540.

[37] Vgl Reil, Entwurf (1816), pp. 560–82 (on "Euthanasia, oder von den Hülfen erträglich zu sterben"); Puchelt, Umriss (1826), pp. 522–3 (on "Euthanasie. Verfahren des Arztes am Sterbebette"); Gmelin, Allgemeine Therapie (1830), esp. pp. 14–16; Choulant, Anleitung (1836), pp. 183–9.

[38] Marx, Euthanasie (1827); Klohss, Euthanasie (1835); see also idem, Ueber Euthanasie oder über die vom Arzte ausgehenden Hülfen, den Tod zu erleichtern. Bruchstück einer größern Schrift, in: Journal der practischen Heilkunde 67 (1832), n. 1, pp. 67–108.

[39] Cf. Hoffmann, Inhalt (1969); Falk, Geschichte (1983).

[40] Kessler, De euthanasia medica (1828); Scheidhauer, De cura (1831); Beschuetz, De euthanasia medica (1832); Salzmann, De euthanasia medica (1835); Schriever, De euthanasia (1836); Stubendorff, De euthanasia medica (1836); Jahn, De euthanasia (1839); Schalle, De euthanasia (1839); Pfeiffer, De euthanasia medica (1839); Jäger, De euthanasia (1840); Goetz, De euthanasia (1841); Hellwag, De euthanasia (1841); Baltes, De euthanasia (1842); Hauffe, De euthanasia (1843); Putz, De euthanasia (1843); Brockerhoff, De euthanasia medica (1843); Heinzelmann, De euthanasia medica (1845); Ziemssen, De euthanasia medica (1845). Outside of Germany: Johann Schönbauer, De euthanasia, Budapest 1820; Jentink, De promovenda euthanasia (1840), F. É. F. Billon, Essai médical sur la dysthanasie, med. diss., Paris: Didot jeune 1820 (I have not been able to see the works by Schönbauer and Billon). The only dissertation of this kind, which I am aware of, that appeared after 1850 is Schaffrath, Euthanasie (1869) and it is telling that, according to author, it was his father, an experienced physician himself, who encouraged him to choose this topic and who provided him with accounts from his own practice.

[41] Marx, Euthanasie (1827), p. 3.

[42] Richter, Euthanasia (1841), p. 364.

[43] Putz, De euthanasia (1843), p. 8.

[44] Gmelin, Allgemeine Therapie (1830), pp. 15–6.

in a general sense, to forgoing a curative, causal treatment in favor of a "merely" symptomatic one. For example, in Hooper's medical dictionary of 1825, "palliative medicine" is defined as "medicine given only with an intent to palliate or relieve pains in a fatal disease."[45]

Those who wrote about *euthanasia medica* usually linked two concerns. For one thing, they urged their readers, as Hennig had done in the early eighteenth century, to give up on further therapeutic attempts early enough in hopeless cases, or else they might cause a *dysthanasia*[46] or *kakothanasia*, as W. Hennemann in 1830 termed a "bad" death for which the doctor was to blame.[47] Hennemann bewailed the "busy-ness, which although well-intentioned is therefore not less objectionable," practiced by colleagues who "will not leave any means untried to save patients, and if it is the most torturous and forbidding," even "if the hope for success lacks any inherent probability."[48]

The term *kakothanasia* found its way into contemporary lexicons and encyclopedias. As suggested by Hennemann's complaint, it aimed at a practice that seems to have been widespread at the time. The mesmerist K. Chr. Wolfart, in an article on *Behavior at the Deathbed*, asserted that "the usual way of treating those for whom one must give up all hope" is to heap "agony upon agony." Is it not agony, he asked, if you give the dying patient revolting remedies every quarter or half an hour, administer all too strong wines, "in the foolish opinion that his vital force must still be stimulated," or apply vesicating plasters? Could one imagine "how burdensome and painful the poor suffering person's final hour can become through all this bombarding?" A physician who acted like this was "unfortunately often nothing but an experimenting executioner who just doesn't know that he is one."[49] Anecdotal accounts such as Alfred Meissner's report of the treatment of the terminally ill poet and author Heinrich Heine suggest that there were good reasons for such concerns:

> They tested on him the effect of strychnine as a remedy for palsies, drilled fontanelles in his neck, lit moxa on him and worked on his back in the lumbar vertebrae area with cauterizing irons. I had never seen the likes of it in my whole life.[50]

Combined with the admonition to refrain from painful and aggressive treatment procedures, the medical writers wanted to impress upon their readers that caring for

---

[45] Robert Hooper, Lexicon medicum; or medical dictionary, London: Longmans et al. 1825, p. 857.

[46] Hennig, De dysthanasia medica (1735); Jahn, De euthanasia (1839), p. 10; Baltes, De euthanasia (1842), p. 17.

[47] Hennemann, Kakothanasie (1830).

[48] Ibid., p. 175.

[49] Wolfart, Betragen am Sterbebette (1819), cit. pp. 60–1; Putz, De euthanasia (1843), p. 10 also criticized those who experimented on dying patients.

[50] Alfred Meissner, Die Matratzengruft. Meissners Besuche bei Heine im Wortlaut, Baden-Baden: Keppler 1947, p. 64; see also Wilhelm Kühlmann. Abschied von der "Sterbekunst". Heinrich Heines Briefe und Gedichte aus der "Matratzengruft", in: Hans Helmut Jansen (ed.), Der Tod in Dichtung, Philosophie und Kunst, 2nd edn, Darmstadt: Steinkopff 1989, pp. 327–36.

dying patients was to be understood as the "highest duty,"[51] one that remained neglected all too often.[52] One anonymous author complained in 1838 that there were doctors who had cared for families over the course of decades, but when it came to dying, they unfortunately believed all too often that they were released from their duty and withdrew, "when it was time to take the hardest step a person can take [...], medical help and love." Of course, he went on, it is difficult "to stand by until the end." But "the concern for people" belonged to the duties of the doctor "until the walk to the grave [...] The heart of the dying person yearns for the physician more than does the heart of the sick person." As the reason for the widespread neglect of duty on the part of physicians, the author recognized not so much a lack of feeling among doctors as a "nagging awareness of being powerless, the realization that one is helpless," as well as "mental fatigue."[53]

The critique targeted in particular those physicians who in Baltes's words believed "that they have only to concern themselves with the illness and not with the patient; those who want to treat the body but not at the same time the soul."[54] Along these lines Franz Xaver Putz in Vienna turned against those doctors who held that they were responsible for the illness only, not the human person and neglected making an effort when their remedies were no longer effective against a deadly illness.[55]

The palliative care of severely ill and dying patients also remained present in medical literature at the turn of the twentieth century. Encyclopedia entries declared the "concern for euthanasia" to be one of "most noble tasks of the physician."[56] In 1887, William Munk went public with what was the most comprehensive English language depiction of medical terminal care so far: *Euthanasia: or, Medical Treatment in Aid of an Easy Death*.[57] In comparison with other subject areas covered in the medical literature of the time, however, the interest in terminal care declined significantly in the late nineteenth and early twentieth centuries. By all appearances, this was due to a marked change in the perception of the powers and limits of medicine. Many doctors at the time felt that medicine was finally becoming a real natural science that was gaining increasingly precise knowledge about the human body and its diseases through microscopic examination and chemical analysis. The discoveries of bacteriology revolutionized the understanding of some of the most important and widely feared diseases, and with X-ray technology, physicians were now able to almost literally shed light on the innermost secrets of the sick body. In hindsight, the hope that all this would lead to new, effective therapies proved deceptive until after World War II. However, epochal discoveries and developments such as radiotherapy,

[51] Marx, Euthanasie (1827), p. 4.

[52] Hauffe, De euthanasia (1843), p. 20.

[53] Anonymus, Arzt (1838), p. 229.

[54] Baltes, De euthanasia (1842), p. 7.

[55] Putz, De euthanasia (1843), p. 7.

[56] Mendelsohn, Euthanasie (1898), p. 245.

[57] Munk, Euthanasia (1887); on Munk see also Hughes and Clark, "A thoughtful and experienced physician" (2004).

Salvarsan as a "magic bullet" against syphilis and the successful treatment of diphtheria kept alive the hope of new, unanticipated therapeutic possibilities, even if many other new pharmaceutical preparations were proving to be ineffective or even harmful in the short or long term.

In such a time of overwhelming therapeutic optimism with its keen propensity for medical action at the sickbed there was little room, it seems, for "mere" palliative treatment. Fatal outcomes were perceived as a "failure" rather than as an inevitable fate, and physicians found it difficult to accept that their capacity of even just easing the suffering of dying patients were also severely limited. It was likely due in part to the "hopelessness of all interventions," to the "difficulty of making possible even a tolerable existence for the unlucky sick person," Gessner wrote in 1899 that the palliative treatment of uterine cancer was "still largely treated like a stepchild,"[58] even though most cases were treated so late in the disease that a curative therapy was no longer thinkable. No one, he said, wanted "to undertake the difficult and most of the time seemingly unrewarding task."[59]

Students were no longer forcefully encouraged to take an interest in this field either. In the training of doctors, terminal care played only a modest role. "The treatment of the dying is not made a subject of systematic instruction," complained Joseph Bullar in 1866.[60] And William Munk in 1887 found that there was little about dealing with the dying, or the "management of the dying" as he put it, in the medical literature, or about therapies that would be most suited to alleviating the suffering of the dying. Medical students, he went on, were not specially trained in these matters; the young physician who was just beginning to practice had to teach himself what to do and not do in this difficult situation.[61]

[58] This complaint was repeated by Albert Plathner, Zur palliativen Behandlung des Uteruscarcinoms, med. diss., Jena: Frommann 1904.

[59] A. Gessner, Palliative Behandlung des inoperablen Carcinoms, in: J. Veit (ed.), Handbuch der Gynäkologie, vol. 2, part 2, Wiesbaden: Bergmann 1899, pp. 461–87, p. 464 (cit.) and p. 466.

[60] Bullar, Chloroform (1866), pp. 10–12.

[61] Munk, Euthanasia (1887), pp. 3–4.

The Practice of Palliative Treatment

6

The concrete instructions for dealing with the dying, as we find them in the numerous works on *euthanasia medica* prior to 1850, are similar in many respects to the recommendations for a symptomatic, palliative treatment of illnesses in general that were passed on from the previous generations. The decision in favor of a "euthanatic" method, as Richter and Putz called it,[1] did not entail a fundamental change in the therapeutic process. But with dying patients, certain complaints and problems were often more prominent, and doctors had to adapt their treatment to the reduced strength of the dying body and its limited ability to react. In their work on the medical treatment of terminal and dying patients, Karen Nolte and Katharina Schilling have shown, drawing on extensive case histories, that doctors did precisely this in their practice.[2]

The most important task in most cases was the alleviation of pain and shortness of breath. Here opium was the medicine of choice. There was, however, a good measure of reserve in this regard, especially in Germany. Doctors were aware of the potential side effects and of the danger of an overdose, and they were wary of the body's habituation to the drug, which meant that higher and higher doses would be required the longer the illness went on.[3] In the 1830s, the influential Christoph Wilhelm Hufeland (1762–1836) passionately condemned doctors' "too great fear" of opium. Certainly, he said, like every powerful weapon, opium did harbor dangers, including "opium addiction" which was "analogous to alcoholism and its effects."[4] However, the excessive fear robbed "medicine of one of its most superb remedies and some sick people of the help that is possible through it alone." Its ability to "alleviate suffering and pain, to calm and lift the spirits and to make dying

[1] Richter, Euthanasia (1841), in German "euthanatisch"; Putz, De euthanasia (1843), p. 9.

[2] Nolte, Ärztliche Praxis (2010a), esp. pp. 46–55; eadem, Todkrank (2016); Schilling, "Ach gib mir doch nur etwas Luft" (2011).

[3] Th. A. R. Figulus, De opio, ejusque in quibusdam morbis abusu, Berlin: Nietack 1837 ("quum per periodos alia interponenda sint, ne consuetudine dosium opii mediocrium vis frangatur.")

[4] Hufeland, Enchiridion medicum (1837), p. 854.

M. Stolberg, *A History of Palliative Care, 1500–1970*, Philosophy and Medicine 123,
DOI 10.1007/978-3-319-54178-5_6

easier,"[5] made opium one of the greatest gifts of God.[6] No other remedy, he said, was able "to alleviate pain and fear to such a degree, indeed to magically dispel them for a time." "Not a hundred but a thousand times," had he seen his patients "completely transformed the next day, in the look on their faces, their language and in their entire expression, having taken opium the previous night." Who, he asked, would want to be a doctor without opium, considering the desperate situation of the "incurable consumptive who is slowly dying under fear and a lack of air" or in the face of "the horrific, torturous pain throughout the day and night of the cancer patient for whom there is no rescue," or the "mortal fear of the patient with hydrothorax." The soothing power of opium was at its "most glorious," however, in the "easing of death in severe cases, in the effecting of euthanasia." Here it could "not only [take away] the pain of death"; it also gave "the courage and the power to die; indeed it physically encourages that disposition that makes the spirit adept at lifting into heavenly realms."[7]

In this sense, medical aid even secured, through the administering of opium, the very composure, or even cheerfulness that was demanded by the centuries-old tradition of the art of dying. Hufeland described the case of a man that illustrates this point well. The man had suffered from chest complaints and vomiting for a long time and finally lay dying: "The most terrifying fear of death with the constant danger of suffocation took hold of him; he fell into a state of true desperation and his condition was unbearably painful even to bystanders." He was given a grain of opium every hour, and after the fourth grain he fell asleep, awakening the next day as if transformed: "Very cheerful, free from all pain and fear and so strengthened and calmed in his soul that he bid farewell to his family with the best composure and joyfulness, giving them his blessing and some good counsel as well, and then he fell asleep again, and in sleep ceased to be."[8]

Physicians in England heaped similar praise on opium and there are indications that they were less reluctant to use it than their colleagues on the Continent.[9] In the case of the severely ill Albrecht von Haller, it was his English physicians who advised him to take opium.[10] Leading English authors extolled the effects of opium in particular with dying patients. For example, William Heberden (1710–1801) stated that with intestinal obstruction, it did not hasten death but it made it less

[5] On the curative uses of opium see Samuel Crumpe, An inquiry into the nature and properties of opium, wherein its component principles, mode of operation, and use or abuse in particular diseases are experimentally investigated, London: Robinson 1793.

[6] Similarly Ziemssen, De euthanasia medica (1845), pp. 45–6.

[7] Hufeland, Enchiridion medicum (1837), p. 853.

[8] Ibid.

[9] Albrecht von Haller, Commentatio de opii in corpus humanum efficacia, in: Novi commentarii Societatis Regiae Scientiarum Gottingensis 7 (1777), pp. 1–16, here p. 10; see also Jalland, Death (1996), pp. 86–7.

[10] Haller, Briefe (1923), pp. 490–1 (December 12, 1773).

agonizing by lulling the dying person to sleep.[11] And John Kent Spender emphasized that one of opium's blessings was its ability to allow for a comparatively painless death. Without snuffing out consciousness, it took the sharpness out of the pain with many diseases and made the departure from this world less dreadful.[12] In Joseph Bullar's words, opium in the case of consumption in particular, "changed a scene of hopeless and distressing agony into one of calmness and peace." It could alleviate "not only this last distress of the dying, but also of the relatives around."[13] Herbert Snow at the end of the nineteenth century, based on his own experience as a physician at the London Cancer Hospital, even strongly advocated in favor of accepting the development of an "opium or morphia habit." With incurable cancer patients, the habitual consumption of opium or morphine was "the most powerful and useful weapon we possess, not only for the relief of pain, but for the prolongation of life, and even for checking the development of the disease." This was because "these drugs (and they alone) render life endurable, and even pleasurable, under so heavy a burden."[14]

As indicated above, opium derivatives increasingly came to be used alongside opium, especially morphine, which was identified by F. W. Sertürner at the beginning of the nineteenth century as one of the most important active ingredients of opium, as well as Pantopon, a purified opium preparation.[15] In the second half of the nineteenth century, the development of subcutaneous injections of morphine permitted a more rapid and powerful pain relief.[16] This, however—much more even than the conventional treatment with opium—stirred fears of the dangers of overdose and addiction.[17] Morphinism with its devastating consequences became common and was widely discussed. It became strongly associated with artists and—because they had easy access to it—with physicians. But contemporary authors usually identified the true beginning of morphinism in the treatment of chronic, incurable illnesses.[18] "The very small pain of the needle prick," wrote Capellmann, a medical officer of health, "the prompt and certain effect is all too tempting," yet soon the sick person becomes "increasingly defenseless against the pain" and asks for the injection more and more frequently.[19] Many authors advised

[11] William Heberden, Commentarii de morborum historia et curatione, Frankfurt: apud Varrentrapp et Wenner 1804, pp. 200–1.

[12] Spender, Therapeutic means (1874), p. 62.

[13] Bullar, Opium (1856), pp. 268–9.

[14] Snow, Palliative treatment (1890), pp. 46–7; in addition, Snow assumed a direct positive effect on the cancer.

[15] Berridge and Edwards, Opium (1987), pp. 135–41.

[16] John Kent Spender, The hypodermic action of morphia, in: British medical journal (1860), pp. 436–7.

[17] Eduard Levinstein, Die Morphiumsucht. Eine Monographie nach eigenen Beobachtungen, Berlin: Hirschwald 1877, p. 3.

[18] Albrecht Erlenmeyer, Die Morphiumsucht und ihre Behandlung, Neuwied–Leipzig: Heuser's Verlag 1883; on the French situation see Szabo, Incurable (2009), pp. 142–51.

[19] Capellmann, Pastoral-Medicin (1895), p. 41.

the use of great caution especially when death was not yet knocking at the door: One should administer morphine as late as possible, if not wait until the pain became entirely unbearable, and even then limit the use to once or twice a day. Only in urgent cases should patients or their relatives be allowed to make decisions about the administration of pain medication, and preferably they should not make them at all.[20] Agnes Karl, who worked in private care, wrote in 1894 that a doctor had at least left the decision to her discretion as a nurse working with a patient dying of intestinal cancer, but only, as she angrily noted, after the patient had suffered the worst agony.[21]

In spite of the new possibilities of treating pain more effectively, the situation for many patients suffering from pain and shortness of breath thus seems to have actually become worse again around the turn of the twentieth century because medical professionals had become more wary of the addictive qualities and side effects of pain treatments. The present generation of physicians, complained Oscar C. Young in 1920 "has been so thoroughly warned, both by teaching at college and by observation that now they are in many instances so very afraid to give it, even for the worst pain, that the patient suffers agonies worse than any hell for want of one-eighth of a grain of morphine."[22] Other authors also felt compelled to admonish their readers that with cases of cancer or consumption, one should not be "too sparing with morphine and similar preparations." The danger of morphinism, they argued, "does not enter the picture in terminal cases."[23]

Alongside opium and morphine, other pain suppressants and/or antispasmodic medications could be used, such as henbane, hemlock, jimson weed and cherry laurel.[24] Some of these remedies were attributed with particular effectiveness for certain illnesses: hemlock for malignant bone and nerve diseases for example, and cherry laurel for uterine and breast cancer.[25] Cannabis, which has experienced a remarkable renaissance as an analgesic in recent times, was used as well. Ada Lovelace, one of Lord Byron's daughters, who suffered from cancer, took cannabis among other medications.[26] In addition to these remedies, new substances were being produced in the laboratory. Granville, for example, praised the alleviating

[20] The same warning was already voiced by Jentink, De promovenda euthanasia (1840), p. 24.

[21] Nolte, Pflege (2010b), p. 102.

[22] Oscar C. Young, On the use of opiates, especially morphine, in: Medical news 80 (1902), pp. 154–7, cit. in David T. Courtwright, Dark paradise. Opiate addiction in America before 1940, Cambridge, Mass.: Harvard University Press 1982, p. 54.

[23] Franck, Moderne Therapie (1926), p. 530, on cancer treatment; B. Bandelier and O. Roepke, Die Klinik der Tuberkulose. Handbuch der gesamten Tuberkulose, 2nd edn, Würzburg: Kabitzsch 1912 (orig. 1910), p. 183.

[24] For a useful contemporary survey see Spender, Therapeutic means (1874); on pain relief in cancer of the uterus see Wilhelm Schrader, De carcinomate uteri, med. diss., Berlin: Nietack 1842, pp. 29–30.

[25] Putz, De euthanasia (1843), p. 15.

[26] Jalland, Death (1996), p. 89; on the history of the medicinal uses of cannabis in Western medicine in general see Manfred Fankhauser, Haschisch als Medikament. Zur Bedeutung von Cannabis sativa in der westlichen Medizin, Liebefeld: SGGP/SSHP 2002.

effects of hydrocyanic acid in the face of the "horrible suffering" of the consumptive patient. It had, in his words, "even at the approach of death" proved "a most advantageous palliative." He had, for example, treated the son of a tradesman with it, who whose "grateful acknowledgements" proved "how much more supportable the last days of his existence had been rendered, by the action of this powerful sedative."[27]

Revolutionary possibilities of rapid pain relief emerged in the form of new anesthetics, which, from the mid-nineteenth century onward, made their way into surgical practice. As early as 1834, Vogel praised the beneficial effects of sulfuric ether, which, inhaled from a bowl, calmed the "agonizing [person]."[28] Ether, confirmed Schaffrath, was able to "significantly reduce the constriction of the breath that came with approaching death in some cases."[29] Spender in 1874 enthusiastically recommended chloroform, alongside ether, against "the restlessness and misery of slowly dying." The physician was to always have a small supply of it on his person. He would "joyfully discover many opportunities which he did not expect for his benevolent intervention." Looking back on his professional life, nothing gave him "more satisfaction than the quantity of positive suffering which I have been able to alleviate through the mercies of that 'sweet oblivious antidote,' chloroform."[30]

At the end of the nineteenth century, there were several new, chemically produced drugs that added to the palliative care arsenal. While most products of the young pharmaceutical industry proved to be ineffective or even harmful in the short or long term, the development of new analgesic and sedative medication such as aspirin, pyramidone, sulfonal and chloral hydrate ranks among the few real pharmacological success stories of the time, and these medications became highly valued in the palliative treatment of cancer.[31]

With time, doctors also learned that the different painkillers and narcotics could be combined, meaning that the individual substances could be administered in smaller doses. John Harley reported his good experiences with a mixture of opium and henbane that both relieved pain and acted as a sedative. Herbert Snow recommended the combined use of opium and cocaine.[32] From this followed the so-called Brompton cocktail, a combination of morphine, cocaine and alcohol, which remained a cornerstone of palliative pain treatment until the late twentieth century.

In addition to this, some doctors treating concrete cases of illness began to give opium and other pain medications consistently at regular intervals, rather than

---

[27] Augustus B. Granville, An historical and practical treatise on the internal use of the hydrocyanic (prussic) acid in pulmonary consumption and other diseases of the chest, London: Longman et alii 1820, pp. 60–1.

[28] Vogel, Euthanasia (1834), p. 601.

[29] Schaffrath, Euthanasie (1869), p. 15.

[30] Spender, Therapeutic means (1874), pp. 147–52.

[31] J. Heitzmann, Die palliative Behandlung der inoperablen Uteruscarcinome, in: Centralblatt für die gesammte Therapie 17 (1899), pp. 705–18; Max Berl, Zur palliativen Behandlung des inoperablen Uteruscarcinoms, med. diss., Munich: Gerstenberg [1910], p. 8.

[32] Spender, Therapeutic means (1874), p. 62 and pp. 71–2; Snow, Palliative treatment (1890), p. 34.

waiting until the patient could no longer tolerate the pain.[33] Around 1935, this became standard practice at St. Luke's Home for the Dying in London and was later adopted by Cicely Saunders at St. Christopher's.[34]

The most frequent symptom of advanced consumption or tuberculosis of the lung was, alongside shortness of breath and weakness, a racking cough, which exhausted the patients and robbed them of their sleep. Again, opium was the drug of choice in such cases. Other possibilities were codeine derivatives such as dihydrocodeine or oxycodone.[35] Cocaine was used and even heroin was marketed as an excellent medication for cough and lung diseases around the turn of the century. It was tried, for example, with the consumptive Habsburg Archduke Franz Ferdinand in 1912.[36]

Alongside opium, bloodletting was occasionally recommended for the massive shortness of breath that frequently accompanied pulmonary consumption and some heart diseases.[37] At the end of the nineteenth century, inhalations of highly concentrated oxygen mixtures from steel cylinders offered a welcome alternative.[38] Sometimes it was given in the hope to prolong the patient's life but even if the patients' physical condition did not improve, oxygen offered, at least, in Ortner's words "shortly before the exitus, often enough subjective relief from the feeling of sickness."[39] In Thomas Mann's novel *The Magic Mountain,* Joachim Ziemssen explained accordingly to his cousin the purpose of those "great-bellied vessels" which were standing before certain doors. It was "pure oxygen, six francs the container. The reviving gas was given to the dying in a last effort to kindle or reinforce their strength. They drew it up through a tube."[40] One figure in this novel, the "gentleman rider," survived "only by the aid of enormous quantities of oxygen." In a single day, he used 40 containers. Mann's rather critical attitude toward this practice shines through in these paragraphs. Mann has a nurse comment that "mounted up, the gentlemen could reckon the cost themselves, [...] and his wife, in whose arms he had died, was left wholly penniless." "Why delay by these torturing and costly artificial expedients a death absolutely certain to supervene," Mann has Joachim respond. "One could not blame the man for blindly consuming the precious gas they urged upon him. But those in charge should have behaved with more reason. They

[33] Snow, Palliative treatment (1890), pp. 34–5, on the case of a patient with breast cancer.

[34] Goldin, A protohospice (1981), p. 384; Saunders, Evolution (1988), p. 170.

[35] See the contemporary survey in Franck, Moderne Therapie (1926), pp. 419–26; see also Hans Auler, Über die Wartung und Behandlung Krebskranker (offprint from Monatsschrift für Krebsbekämpfung), Munich: Lehmann 1933.

[36] Ibid., p. 424; F. G. Chandler, Cocaine for euthanasia (letter to the editor), in: Lancet 207 (1924), p. 629; Sabine Fellner and Katrin Unterreiner, Morphium, Cannabis und Cocain. Medizin und Rezepte des Kaiserhauses, Vienna: Amalthea Signum 2008, pp. 142–3.

[37] Callegari, Cura palliativa (1828), pp. 4–5.

[38] Historical survey in Christina Koßobutzki, Die Geschichte der inhalativen Sauerstofftherapie in Deutschland, med. diss., Lübeck: urn:nbn:de:gbv:841-20090420356 2009.

[39] Norbert Ortner, Die Sauerstofftherapie in der inneren Medizin, in: Max Michaelis (ed.), Handbuch der Sauerstofftherapie, Berlin: Hirschwald 1906, pp. 535–41, cit. p. 539.

[40] Mann, Magic mountain (1929), p. 137.

should have let him go his way, in God's name, quite aside from the circumstances, more so when taking them into consideration. The living, after all, had their rights—and so on."[41]

6.1 Palliative Surgery

In spite of various innovations, as outlined above, the number of scientific articles on palliative care remained very modest in the late 19th and early 20th centuries, compared with a flood of articles on other topics. There was, however, an important exception: Numerous articles and a whole series of medical dissertations, especially in France and Germany, were dedicated to "palliative" surgical operations. The term "palliative" was used here in the traditional sense of a "merely" symptom-alleviating, non-curative treatment. Palliative surgery aimed at pathological changes in a specific organ, which were identified as the major source of serious symptoms and which could be improved with a local, surgical intervention.

As we have seen, the history of surgical palliation can be traced far back into the early modern period. Beginning in the late eighteenth century, the readiness to perform surgical interventions on the curable and incurable alike grew. Even if a radical surgical cure was no longer possible, explained Brodie with regard to breast cancer in particular, the operation could be worthwhile to "give [the patient] some peace and quiet through an alleviation of the pain and to make life tolerable for her or to prolong it."[42] According to Brodie, an amputation of the breast was in some cases advisable to at least spare the patient the torturous stage of "extremely painful exulceration [...] during which a plague-like stink spreads and very frequent bleedings take place, which makes the sick person's existence extremely miserable."[43] As an example of this, he gave an account of a female patient with a very painful, open and ulcerated tumor who "was living an utterly miserable life." He told the patient that a permanent cure could not be expected, but advised her to have the breast removed on account of the pain. In a different case, he and a colleague came to the conclusion that the best thing "for the suffering sick woman" was to remove her breast, not for the sake of a permanent cure but "to free the sick woman from her present suffering."[44] In such cases, he advised his students, the physician could undertake an operation "even without the prospect of a radical cure [...] only to give the patient a respite and an abatement to his present suffering."[45]

New horizons opened up in general surgery and, as a result, also in palliative medicine, in the late nineteenth and early twentieth centuries. The introduction of general anesthesia using laughing gas, chloroform and ether, the reduction of the danger of infection through antiseptics and asepsis, and improved surgical

[41] Ibid., pp. 369–70.

[42] Brodie, Vorlesungen (1847), p. 73.

[43] Ibid., p. 66.

[44] Ibid., p. 75.

[45] Ibid.

techniques changed the situation profoundly. The danger of postoperative infection was drastically reduced. Anesthesia allowed surgeons to operate carefully and without haste. "What a different picture now!" wrote Capellmann, describing the change. "The patient in a calm chloroform sleep, without pain, without will, without resistance. In the greatest calm, with safety and care, the operation can be carried out."[46] In addition to this came improved instruments such as the electric knife.[47]

When cancer was treated surgically, most interventions were palliative because patients generally entered medical treatment when their cancer had reached a stage at which any attempt at a radical therapy seemed hopeless. Through a palliative operation, one could in these cases at least hold the growth of the tumor in check and in the words of Edward Lund, free the patient from misery "occasioned by the constant presence of a large ulcerating and offensive surface" or "take off the pressure upon nerves, and thus diminish the amount of agonizing pain."[48]

Depending on the kind of tumor and its location, different palliative operative procedures were developed. When a tumor caused an occlusion of the esophagus, of the pyloric orifice at the exit of the stomach or of the intestines, surgery was frequently the only viable option. Without an operative intervention, terrible suffering awaited the patients. In the case of obstructed intestines, they were likely to develop painful colics. Eventually the intestine might putrefy and burst, or they might vomit the fecal matter from the mouth. Still today, physicians call this last symptom *miserere* ("have mercy"), an unusually emotional term with an obvious religious connotation.[49] In such cases, the timely creation of an artificial intestinal opening or an *anus praeternaturalis* could prevent the worst.[50] It spared the patient this "repulsive" consequence.[51] In the 1880s, even procedures for intestinal resection with a retained natural anus were developed. Here, the obstructed section was removed and the cut surfaces were sewn back together.[52] Similar procedures were developed for a constriction of the esophagus. Such palliative operations, which cleared the digestive tract, could, according to Linkenheld, throw "a final ray of light on the long time of suffering of the emaciated, skeleton-like patient." With a "face full of

[46] Cf. Capellmann, Pastoral-Medicin (1895), p. 46.

[47] Snow, Palliative treatment (1890), p. 18.

[48] Lund, Palliative medicine (1880), pp. 21–2.

[49] The term derives from the biblical expression "Miserere mei, Deus", "have mercy on me, God"; when their neighbour died in this manner, vomiting feces, Georg Handsch's teacher, Ulrich Lehner, around 1550, still told him in fact that this was called "Miserere mei deus" (ÖNB, Cod. 11240, fol. 37r).

[50] Maurice Recouly, De la valeur de l'anus iliaque comme opération palliative dans le cancer de la partie terminale du gros intestin (S[igma] iliaque, rectum), med. diss., Paris: Henri Jouve 1902; Linkenheld, Palliative Operationen (1894), pp. 416–9.

[51] "To live with an artificial anus and a cancer in the area of the rectum and anus", Finet quoted M. Beaudoin, "that means just not being dead" (Prosper Finet, De la valeur curative et palliative de l'exérèse dans le cancer du rectum, med. diss., Paris: G. Steinheil 1896, p. 75).

[52] Ibid.

thanks", a patient who lay dying was said to have said "Thank God, things can go down again."[53]

In the case of advanced cancer of the tongue, a palliative removal of cancerous tongue tissue could have very beneficial effects that countered the often utterly unbearable nerve pain in the mouth, face, and ears as well as the foul, putrid smell of the secretions that were released from the decomposing tongue tissue.[54] Around 1900, the ligation of blood vessels was a highly discussed subject. The blood vessels that led to and nourished the tumor were blocked off in order to reduce the size of the tumor without removing it entirely.[55]

Intense pain, especially when major nerve trunks were affected, could also be combatted with neurosurgery. The success of chordotomy, the surgical interruption of pain-conducting tracts in the spinal cord, often verged "on the miraculous," to use the praising words of M. Kirschner in 1938. The risks were something the patient and his relatives could "accept given the probability that the sick person will hereby be freed from the terrible pains that would otherwise carry on uninterrupted until his death."[56]

In patients with brain tumors one could attempt to diminish the increasing intracranial pressure that frequently resulted in intense headaches, convulsions and other major neurological symptoms. This could be done by opening the skull or by performing a lumbar puncture to let out cerebrospinal fluid. The risks were very high, however, —many a patient died during the intervention—and the success was usually at best modest.[57] In 1935, Hans-Joachim Ahrens summarized his statistical analysis with the words, "there is likely no other field in all of surgery that shows such discouraging results."[58]

More promising, on the other hand, were attempts to combine palliative surgery with radiotherapy, be it X-rays or radium implants, the latter becoming increasingly significant for cancer treatment in the early twentieth century.[59]

---

[53] Linkenheld, Palliative Operationen (1894), p. 419.

[54] Edward Lund, On the removal of the entire tongue by the Walter Whitehead method, with full details of the operation and after-treatment, London–Manchester: Churchill and Cornish 1880; Snow, Palliative treatment (1890), pp. 18–9.

[55] Max Berl, Zur palliativen Behandlung des inoperablen Uteruscarcinoms, med. diss., Munich: Gerstenberg [1910], pp. 8–9; Gabriel-Adolphe-Léon Planque, De la ligature palliative, atrophique, de l'artère linguale dans les tumeurs malignes de la langue, med. diss., Bordeaux: Barthélemy et Clèdes 1912.

[56] M. Kirschner, Zur Bekämpfung der Krebskrankheit, in: Der Chirurg 12 (1940), pp. 177–92, hier pp. 191–2.

[57] Jean-Auguste Schneyder, De la ponction lombaire comme thérapeutique palliative dans les tumeurs de l'encéphale, med. diss., Bordeaux: Imprimerie du Midi, E. Trénit 1908; Francis Trocmé, De la thérapeutique palliative dans les tumeurs de l'encéphale, méthodes décompressives (ponction lombaire et trépanation palliative), med. diss., Paris: Henri Jouve 1909.

[58] Hans-Joachim Ahrens, Die palliative Trepanation bei Gehirndruck, med. diss., Marburg: Hamel 1935, p. 23.

[59] Max Berl, Zur palliativen Behandlung des inoperablen Uteruscarcinoms, med. diss., Munich: Gerstenberg [1910], pp. 14–6; John V. Pickstone, Contested cumulations. Configurations of cancer treatments through the twentieth century, in: David Cantor (ed.), Cancer in the twentieth century, Baltimore: Johns Hopkins University Press 2008, pp. 164–96.

A wide range of remedies were also available for an external, palliative treatment of tumors. They were able in many cases to hold in check the odious smell and the sanious secretions. These remedies included menthol solutions: pepsin, which is still used today, and iodoform, which was used until very recently.[60]

6.2 Nursing

The question of appropriate nursing care and general emotional support for the dying also gained far greater significance in medical writing from the end of the eighteenth century onward. To the extent that they addressed the issue at all, early modern authors had more or less limited themselves to urging relatives and nurses not to give up, not even if "according to their judgment there was little hope," and to adhere to and enforce the doctors' orders until the end. In this sense, the Eichstädt doctor Jakob Oetheus explained in 1574 that it often happened "that the sick person is so tender and soft or else recalcitrant that he will not suffer anything or will not bear the slightest pain. In this case, it is not necessary for the nurses to pay court to the patient constantly." Rather, they should, if necessary, be "hard with words." Also, bedside attendants were not, as many did, to give the moribund patient "whatever he desires or happens to think of."[61]

Medical writings in the late eighteenth and early nineteenth century mark a profound change in this respect. The particular physical and emotional needs of the dying increasingly began to come into focus, and with this, the requirements of good nursing. A major influence behind this change was undoubtedly the lively debate on *euthanasia medica*, in the comprehensive sense of securing terminal patients a "good death." At the same time, there was an increased recognition in the medical profession that nursing care was an important element of medical treatment in its own right, which led to the founding of nursing schools and a growing number of textbooks on nursing.[62]

In 1792, Ignatius Zach published the first treatise that was devoted exclusively to the assistance of moribund patients, with detailed instructions on how to offer relief depending on the patient's disease. For example, if they were suffering from shortness of breath, they were to be put in a position that made breathing as easy as possible. Dying patients were also not to be tormented, for example, by being forced

[60] Snow, Palliative treatment (1890), pp. 24–5.

[61] Oetheus, Gründtlicher Bericht (1574), fols 126r-v and fol. 131r.

[62] On nursing care for dying patients in the nineteenth century see Nolte, Pflege (2010b), eadem, Umgang (2006a), pp. 165–74 and eadem, Todkrank (2016); for general introductions into the history of nursing see Sylvelyn Hähner-Rombach (ed.), Quellen zur Geschichte der Krankenpflege, mit Einführungen und Kommentaren, Frankfurt: Mabuse 2008; Birgit Panke-Kochinke, Die Geschichte der Krankenpflege (1679–2000). Ein Quellenbuch, Frankfurt: Mabuse 2003; dated but still useful is Adelaide Nutting and Lavinia L. Dock, A history of nursing (orig. 1907), Tokyo–Bristol: Synapse/Thoemmes 2000.

to eat or drink. On the other hand, their death was not to be hastened by removing their pillows or by simply forgoing out of misguided piety wine or other strengthening medicines that were not unpleasant to ingest. If swallowing was difficult, liquids could be administered drop by drop. Further, one was to ensure that the dying patient did not suffer under the burden of numerous spectators, who also spoiled the air in the sickroom.[63]

The authors of works on *euthanasia medica* also regularly urged their colleagues to do everything in terms of nursing care "which is needed by the dying patient for relief."[64] They praised the merits of the good nurse,[65] his or her experienced, sensible services that were sometimes preferable to the loving hand of a wife or daughter.[66] They recommended adjustable beds for an optimal position, and demanded that these were to be, if necessary, available on loan.[67] Everything soiled, "which has perhaps exited involuntarily" had to be removed from their bed,[68] naturally within reason so as not to unnecessarily burden the dying person by rearranging the bed.[69] One was to make sure that there was fresh air, and "ward off everything that might trouble them."[70] One was always to try to moisten the mouth and the dry throat, to wipe off the sweat, warm the cooling limbs, to shoo away flies.[71]

The patients' emotional needs and preferences were also taken into consideration. "The feelings and emotions of the patient, under critical circumstances," Thomas Percival declared, "require to be known and be attended to, no less than the symptoms of their diseases."[72] "Even the prejudices of the sick are not to be contemned [sic!], or opposed with harshness. For though silenced by authority, they will operate secrety and forcibly on the mind, creating fear, anxiety, and watchfulness".[73]

More concretely, some authors put great emphasis on the beneficial effects of good and not excessive company, of soft music and pictures, sculptures and flowers.[74] According to Wolfart, what was especially beneficial was "to lovingly hold the dying person's hand or hands, to breathe upon his forehead, to wash his forehead,

63 Zach, De cura (1792); on Zach's treatise see the medical dissertation by Philipp Feldle, Palliativpflege im 18. Jahrhundert. Ignatius Zachs "De cura, quam moribundis debent, qui aegrotis sunt a ministerio" (1792), Duisburg-Cologne: WiKu-Verlag 2013.

64 Lebrecht, Arzt (1821), p. 104.

65 Vogel, Euthanasia (1834), p. 600.

66 Richter, Euthanasia (1841), p. 365.

67 Jahn, De euthanasia (1839), p. 19.

68 Paradys, Rede (1796), p. 570.

69 Jahn, De euthanasia (1839), p. 18.

70 Paradys, Rede (1796), p. 570.

71 Puchelt, Umriss (1826), p. 522; Jahn, De euthanasia (1839), p. 21; E[rnst F.] Gurlt, Krankenpflege, in: Albert Eulenburg (ed.), Real-Encyclopädie der gesammten Heilkunde, Vienna–Leipzig: Urban & Schwarzenberg 1887, pp. 239–318, here pp. 317–8.

72 Percival, Medical ethics (1803), p. 9.

73 Ibid., p. 11.

74 Jahn, De euthanasia (1839), p. 24; Baltes, De euthanasia (1842), p. 22.

temples, pit of the stomach, hands and feet with wine or other pleasant-smelling waters, all of them remedies to increase the vital power." In this way, the physician does not appear "as a tormenter, but rather as a helper who, in the spirit of the savior directs the dying person onward in a friendly manner."[75]

A further topic that was occasionally taken up was the care for the bereaved—a very important element of palliative care today. H.E. Richter advised doctors to console them and calm them by assuring them that they had done everything they needed to. The doctor was to encourage diversion and distraction and to advise them to move if necessary into a different room. He was not to approach them "too early and too eagerly" for permission to perform an autopsy on the corpse. If "resting after the exhaustion, a change of air or psychological remedies" could not eradicate the symptoms of a looming disease, he was to be on hand with medical help and advice.[76]

General handbooks and textbooks on nursing began to dedicate sections or whole chapters to the right way of dealing with the dying.[77] Krügelstein, in 1807, recommended that doctors and caregivers carefully ensure that dying people lie with their heads elevated and advised them to give them diluted wine, sweetened fruit juice or buckhorn jelly from time to time so as to keep the mouth moist and to ease breathing.[78] In the 1830s by Max Florian Schmidt, who taught nursing in Vienna, gave similar advice,[79] and works on pastoral medicine promulgated recommendations of this kind among the clergy.[80]

Such recommendations were not just abstract demands put forward in the literature. They also found their way into instructions for nursing personnel in hospitals. The *Instructions for Nursing Personnel* of the Nuremburg hospital, for example, demanded in 1855 that "sick people who are in the throes of death be given relief if possible by raising them to a higher position, wiping the sweat, administering beverages etc."[81]

English writing on "medical euthanasia" at the end of the nineteenth century continued to devote considerable attention to adequate nursing. For William Munk in 1887 the aim of nursing in dying patients was above all to help secure a calm, natural, undisturbed death. He opposed the common practice of darkening the death room and demanded, thinking of those suffering from lung complaints, that fresh, cool air be let into the room. One should not, he wrote, burden the dying against their will with blankets, nor should one disturb them unnecessarily. It was better in his view to let them lie in peace, unless their reclining position was obviously

[75] Wolfart, Betragen am Sterbebette (1819), p. 62.

[76] Richter, Euthanasia (1841), p. 367.

[77] Scholand, Menschenfreund (1837), pp. 1–13 ("Von der Behandlung der Sterbenden").

[78] Krügelstein, Handbuch (1807), pp. 424–5.

[79] Salzburg Museum, Salzburg, Hs 2194, handwritten lessons for nurses; I have not been able to consult Schmidt's—possibly largely identical—printed work Unterricht für Krankenwärter, Vienna 1831.

[80] Capellmann, Pastoral-Medicin (1895), pp. 277–8.

[81] Stadtarchiv Nürnberg, C11/I, 124.

uncomfortable. He was vehement in his protest against the "common practice" of forcing all manner of liquids on dying people even when they were not able to swallow anymore.[82]

In 1894, Oswald Browne made the care of the dying the subject of a lecture for nurses, which was later published. It was the most comprehensive work on the subject to that date, and we still can find many of his recommendations in handbooks on palliative care today. According to Browne, nursing handbooks had wrongly neglected the care of the dying. For him, being in the position of helping dying people leave their life on Earth as easily and peacefully as possible was among the greatest privileges of the nurse. It was important to keep an eye on the fatally ill patient and pay attention to many small details. Restless hands could indicate a full bladder; a catheter could provide relief. If the mouth was dry, the patient could be spoon-fed ice water, homemade lemonade, tea with a little lemon, or crushed ice, all of which was experienced as very soothing most of the time. For stimulation, they could be given a little wine, or, following Henry Halford's recommendation, small amounts of brandy softened with cinnamon water and egg yolk. As Munk had already recommended, food and drink were only to be given as long as the patients could still close their lips and swallow without delay. In most cases, a time would come before the person's death in which nature would make it clear that no more nourishment was to be administered. And when it came to bathing or changing the clothes or linens, taking the temperature or even performing physical examinations, the dying patient was not to be burdened anymore, but rather only those tasks were to be performed that truly served to make the patient comfortable.[83]

In comparison with the (very limited) pre-modern medical writings on the appropriate nursing of the dying, a remarkable change becomes apparent. Whereas physicians had once upbraided the "ignorant" bedside attendants who granted dying patients' wishes without any respect for the doctor's orders, they now gave preference to the wishes and desires of the dying: "As the most supreme general rule in the positioning of the dying," wrote Martin Mendelsohn in 1897, "one is to follow precisely the wishes and the will of the patient and to yield to him completely in this regard, even if what he demands is not in agreement with medical theory." This general rule applied to food and drink as well: "everything that the moribund patient asks for [must be] granted to him, even if it seems inappropriate or not salubrious; only that which is directly harmful must be denied."[84]

---

[82] Munk, Euthanasia (1887), pp. 88–93, cit. p. 93.

[83] Browne, Care of the dying (1894).

[84] Mendelsohn, Ueber die Euthanasie (1897), pp. 37–8; similarly already Richter, Euthanasia (1841), p. 365.

7 The Doctor as an Emotional and Spiritual Caregiver

The literature on medical terminal care in the nineteenth century did not merely declare it an important task of the doctor to make sure that nurses or others in the sickroom adequately addressed the special needs of the dying. Doctors themselves, too, were expected to stand by the dying patients' side, to support and console them in a comprehensive sense, above and beyond concrete therapeutic measures. Early modern writers had already underlined how helpful and beneficial the physician's mere presence at the bed of the dying patient could be, even when his medicines were no longer capable of bringing any improvement.[1] Now, however, the "psychological or moral treatment,"[2] the "psychological procedure,"[3] the *cura psychica,*[4] was declared an indispensable element of end-of-life care. In the *Encyclopédie méthodique* of 1824, in the entry on "Médecine palliative," the most powerful "palliative" was said to be that, which affects the soul, which belongs to the "art of psychological treatment."[5] In this sense, writers on palliative care and "medical euthanasia" tended to assign the doctor an additional role as a provider of emotional and spiritual support and consolation. One anonymous author in 1806 wrote that when it came to providing relief in the final hours, the doctor should not "be merely a mechanic who fixes his patients as one would a defective machine." Rather, a doctor was needed who "with warmth connects to the suffering heart of the dying person, who knows how, depending on the circumstances, to give fresh courage to it or to calm it."[6] The doctor was to meet the terminally ill patient with "true sympathy,"

[1] Zacchia, Quaestiones (1651), pp. 392–3.

[2] Anonymus, Vom Verhalten (1806), col. 544; see also Puchelt, Umriss (1826), p. 522.

[3] Richter, Euthanasia (1841), p. 366.

[4] Heinzelmann, De euthanasia medica (1845), p. 22.

[5] Encyclopédie méthodique. Médecine, vol. NOY-PHT, Paris: Panckoucke 1824, pp. 283–4; on the then very influential notion of *Médecine morale* see Elizabeth A.Williams, The physical and the moral. Anthropology, physiology, and philosophical medicine in France, 1750–1850, Cambridge: Cambridge Univ. Press 1994.

[6] Anonymus, Vom Verhalten (1806), col. 538 and col. 541.

M. Stolberg, *A History of Palliative Care, 1500–1970*, Philosophy and Medicine 123,
DOI 10.1007/978-3-319-54178-5_7

"noble and unshakeable conduct" and a "soft and charming manner of speech," as Lebrecht put it in 1821 in a section on the *Behavior of the Doctor Toward the Dying*.[7]

Even the administering of medication was attributed with a beneficial influence on the soul above and beyond its effect on the body. Around 1800, Christian August Struve asserted that although "not much [could] be done in particular" about most of the symptoms that accompanied diseases, "the doctor's efforts to liberate the patient from a burdensome circumstance flatter him so much, and he feels a great relief when he uses a remedy against a certain complaint, even if it is only in his imagination."[8]

The "psychological" care for the dying at the same time made it easier for doctors to deal with the painful experience of therapeutic failure. If an effective treatment were no longer possible, what helped them in August Stöhr's words were "tact and the full psychological knowledge of the experienced practitioner [...] to play this pitiful role with assurance until the end and to hold his own in front of the patient and any bystanders in such a way that he commands respect."[9]

Insofar as they made the emotional and spiritual care of patients one of their tasks, doctors were laying claim, sometimes very explicitly,[10] to an area of activity that had previously been the acknowledged domain of clergymen. Driving the clergy out of this traditional, prominent role resonated with the wishes of at least some members of the medical profession at the time. At the end of the eighteenth century, an increasingly fervent critique of the pastoral care of the dying could be heard in medical circles. It focused principally on what some doctors saw as an exaggerated, indeed fanatical zeal of certain clergymen who confronted dying patients with dramatic images of the torments of hell that awaited them after their sinful lives. This was in blatant contradiction to the *cura psychica* that physicians considered appropriate. In their opinion, the clergymen disturbed the dying patients' peace of mind and thus also negatively affected their physical condition and, in the worst case, hastened the approach of death.[11]

John Gregory, at the end of the eighteenth century, was still moderate in weighing the pros and cons: "The conversation of a clergy-man of cheerful piety and good sense, in whom a sick man confides, may sometimes be of much more consequence in composing the anguish of his mind, and the agitation of his spirits, than any medicine; but a gloomy and indiscreet enthusiast may do great hurt, may terrify the patient, and contribute to shorten a life that might otherwise be saved."[12] Johann Peter Frank was more vehement in his *System einer vollständigen medicinischen Polizey (System of a Complete Medical Policy)*. In a section with the tellingly drastic heading *Von Mißhandlung sterbender Menschen (On the Maltreatment of Dying People)* he conceded that good pastoral care could have a thoroughly good

[7] Lebrecht, Arzt (1821), pp. 102–7, ("Verhalten des Arztes zum Sterbenden").

[8] Struve, Kunst (1799), part 2, p. 248.

[9] Stöhr, Handbuch (1882), p. 246.

[10] Ibid.; Reil, Entwurf (1816), p. 577.

[11] Collner, Specimen (1799), p. 9; Hellwag, De euthanasia (1841), p. 16.

[12] Gregory, Lectures (1772), p. 36.

influence. However, often, he continued, the clergymen were too insistent and did not allow the patient to die in peace. According to what would become an oft-quoted description, Frank had heard clergymen:

> drawing a full breath and screaming with their mouths right up to the patient's ear, so that a half-deaf healthy person on the street could have understood them easily: I have seen such words be screamed like this for days, and I have also seen two clergymen taking turns for such a well-meaning purpose. What does a poor patient have to endure, not even considering the fear?[13]

Even in the heathen lands, Macdonald concluded, dying people suffered in some respects less than in Christian countries with their "monstrous absurdity of a future eternal punishment."[14]

According to the widespread concern among physicians, the mere presence of a clergyman could have a negative impact on a patient's health because he made the seriousness of the patient's situation abundantly clear. The fact that strong affects had far-reaching effects on the body was still generally recognized in the early nineteenth century and seemed to be confirmed time and again by experience. Seen this way, the fear of death and the grief that was provoked in the thus-far hopeful patient, when a clergyman was called, threatened to shorten the patient's life. Moreover, in their efforts to move the dying person to repent or return to God, clergymen according to the doctors' lamentations often did not mince words. They confronted dying patients with their fast-approaching death and thus robbed them of their life-preserving hope. Schaffrath, for example, wrote with disgust about a "fanatic" priest who, 10 days before she died, "announced ruthlessly to a young consumptive woman, who was leaving behind four small children, that her death was inevitable."[15]

Some authors considered physicians better sources of solace even in spiritual matters. According to Gossweiler, the "doctor as a human being and a Christian [could often] let more moral-religious consolation flow into the soul of the dying patient, especially as regards its continuance after death, than the clergyman."[16] Schaffrath saw things in a similar manner. In the case of the clergyman, one assumed that it was his duty to speak of matters of faith. If doctors, who were suspected by many of lacking faith, spoke of these matters, it not seldom had all the greater effect.[17]

Of course, for the medical critics, the focus was not only on the actual behavior of the clergyman at the deathbed. In their attempt to protect the dying from "superstition and clericalism,"[18] these critics also unmistakably had the larger societal and

---

[13] Frank, System (1788), pp. 646–671, here p. 660; see e.g., Collner, Specimen (1799), pp. 10–11; Heinzelmann, De euthanasia medica (1845), p. 12.

[14] Keith Norman Macdonald, On death, and how to divest it of its terrors, Edinburgh: Maclachlan and Stewart 1875, p. 8.

[15] Schaffrath, Euthanasie (1869), p. 22; Schaffrath had this story from his father.

[16] Gossweiler, Erinnerungen (1838); similarly Richter, Euthanasia (1841), p. 366.

[17] Schaffrath, Euthanasie (1869), p. 23.

[18] Richter, Euthanasia (1841), p. 365.

political influence of religion and the church in view. In the nineteenth and early twentieth centuries, a growing number of doctors held philosophical views that were more or less secularized or stood at a remove from religion. And for many physicians, the different popular rituals and practices at the deathbed that were perpetuated by clergy, especially in the Catholic context, seemed particularly offensive, retrogressive and superstitious: the death bells, for example, that made the parish aware of someone's death, or the ringing of the so-called Loreto's bells, which were to keep the devil away from the dying person.[19]

[19] Frank, System (1788), esp. pp. 655–62; Richter, Euthanasia (1841), p. 365.

The Perspective of Patients

8

How the severely ill and dying perceived their situation and the nursing and medical care they received, both at home and in institutions, is so far been known only in very broad terms and mostly only for the upper classes. Sources that could throw a more nuanced light are unfortunately scarce. The pre-modern tradition whereby relatives gave accounts of the last days of a deceased person lost significance at the time. Personal testimonies that document the personal experience of illness and approaching death are few and far between. From the late nineteenth century, we can gain important insights from fictional writing, especially when authors were able to draw on their own experiences as doctors, patients or relatives. However, for the great rural populations and the countless urban workers, tradesmen and servants we have to rely almost exclusively on the often biased accounts of more educated contemporaries. Ultimately, for the most part, we can only draw conclusions indirectly, trying to conclude from what we know about the circumstances of death what the experience of dying may have been like.

Until well into the twentieth century, the great majority of people died at home, with their families. The circumstances in which people spent their last weeks and days varied greatly, depending on the social situation of the individual. Our modern, at times romantic image of dying in earlier centuries reflects almost exclusively the world of the nobility and the middle classes. But most people did not enjoy that degree of affluence. Many people, in this age of industrialization, urbanization and pauperism, spent their last days without any comfort, in rooms or even on beds or bags of straw that they had to share with others. They might not have the money to buy painkillers or other medication and in the worst case they died on the street.

Apart from the general living conditions, the character and the course of the disease undoubtedly had a great influence on the experience of dying and death. In spite of all efforts and improvements cancer, consumption and dropsy, that is the most commonly diagnosed chronic and often fatal illnesses, continued to be accompanied in many cases by excruciating pain and other tormenting symptoms as well as by a dramatic general physical decline. The notion of severe, terminal illnesses as a medium of spiritual refinement, that we find expressed in nineteenth-century

M. Stolberg, *A History of Palliative Care, 1500–1970*, Philosophy and Medicine 123,
DOI 10.1007/978-3-319-54178-5_8

fictional writing,[1] especially in the depiction of consumption, is deeply out of touch with everyday realities, whereby sick patients lay writhing and exhausted day in, day out or struggled, in fear, for air, hardly able to find sleep, and in the end died a wretched death. There was hardly room for thoughts of higher things. With good reason, Florence Nightingale, the pioneer of professional nursing, criticized as out of touch with reality the association of the deathbed with an "almost seraphic [...] lucidity of intelligence."[2]

In the late nineteenth and early twentieth centuries, literary depictions increasingly took a step back from an aestheticizing, romantic perspective of consumption and other illnesses, as part of a larger trend toward realism and expressionism. In fact, now they sometimes emphasized the ugly and offensive aspects. While in Theodor Fontane, the dying process remains, to use Katharina Faber-Castell's words, "strangely abstract" because "the physical component is lacking,"[3] Theodor Storm makes things much clearer. "I saw nothing but the old woman struggling to no avail with her pain," he has the narrator say in *A Confession,* "who with hands splayed out buffeted the air as if she wanted to call for help, her jaws banging together but producing no sound except for nightmarish noises which I would not have hitherto thought possible among the living."[4] In Thomas Mann's *The Magic Mountain* Mallinckrodt's wife "in number fifty" is described as "a perfect Lazarus and Job in female form." Her skin is "covered in large tracts by an itching eczema, with open sores here and there, even in the mouth."[5] After she had left her husband and children, her lover too separated from her, perhaps, as she thought, because "he too had been revolted by her illness."[6] The "once-charming Scotswoman" was so afflicted by "gangrene of the lungs", "a green and black pestilence," that she spent the entire day breathing a vaporized solution of carbolic acid "lest she go out of her head from sheer physical disgust."[7] Overpowered by intolerable pain, nausea and exhaustion, many a dying person at the time would have had hardly any room for perceptions and thoughts other than the urgent wish to have the suffering finally end.

While fatal suffering reduced many sick people to their physical existence, the suffering of the terminally ill and dying—and this is true both then and now—is more than physical, as long as the pain or the severest of other symptoms do not overshadow everything else. Physical pain, as Ernestine von Krosigk put it

[1] Cf. Sontag, Illness (1978).

[2] Florence Nightingale, Notes on nursing, London sine anno (orig.: 1859), p. 56.

[3] Katharina von Faber-Castell, Arzt, Krankheit und Tod im erzählerischen Werk Theodor Fontanes, med. diss., Zürich: Juris-Druck 1983, p. 83.

[4] Storm, Bekenntnis [1887] (1988), pp. 596–7.

[5] Mann, Magic mountain (1929), p. 395; on Mann's "antiromantic disillusionment" in the *Magic mountain* see Brigitta Schader, Schwindsucht. Zur Darstellung einer tödlichen Krankheit in der deutschen Literatur vom poetischen Realismus bis zur Moderne, Frankfurt: Lang 1987, pp. 127–50.

[6] Mann, Magic mountain (1929), p. 396.

[7] Ibid., p. 546.

succinctly in 1834, is "perhaps not always the greatest, and certainly not always the only suffering the sick person will experience." One might at least temporarily succeed in taking something of the sharpness out of pain. But "a quiet sadness, a noticeable dismal displeasure and also likely irritable flares of anger, depending on the character of the sick person, are the great evils that accompany almost without fail the state of illness, and they often abate more slowly than the pain itself." They are what "darken indescribably the patient's days of suffering."[8] Vogel wrote from his own experience of the "sick person's often morose, surly, stubborn, recoiling mood."[9]

The Scottish poet William Soutar (1898–1943), drawing on his own experience, gave an exemplary description of such changes in his state of mind in his *Diaries of a Dying Man*:

> The feeling of helplessness and frustration during a spell of breathlessness hurts one's pride and one grows angry. In our temporary weakness we tend to become childish; and not a few times my face has automatically puckered up as if I were about to cry: in the humiliation of extreme weakness one might actually cry like a child.[10]

In the end, he was so short of breath and weak that he could not even pull back his pillow by himself when it slipped. This, he noted "made me quite irritable for a bit. I really must try to control these irritable exhibitions."[11] On the weekly change of pillows he commented:

> It seemed incredible that a man of my age should act like a bairn and be brought by frustration to the verge of tears. I must be weaker than I know, surely; and as weak in will as in body—for there is no indication yet of this increasing stoic calm that I imagined I would gradually achieve.[12]

Something else that had problematic effects on the experience and mood of dying patients was the continuing practice of concealing a negative, fatal prognosis. When the doctor and everyone else did all they could to veil the seriousness of the situation, they left the patient still hoping, and shortened the period of grief and despair. Yet this practice of concealment was also deeply unsettling. Patients knew that their physicians and relatives were likely to lie to them. Once dying patients had seen through this "comedy," which, as Arthur Schnitzler put it, "has always been played with varying degrees of success,"[13] they were all the more left to their own devices, and their loneliness and isolation risked becoming even more painful. This culture

[8] Krosigk, Umgang (1834), p. 106.

[9] Vogel, Euthanasia (1834), p. 600; drawing on his extensive personal experience with pulmonary diseases, Stuertz made a similar statement (Nietner, Zur Tuberkulose-Bekämpfung (1913), pp. 33–53, here pp. 38–9).

[10] Soutar, Diaries (1954), p. 198, September 9, 1943.

[11] Ibid., p. 199, September 12, 1943.

[12] Ibid., p. 202, September 26, 1943.

[13] Schnitzler, Sterben [1892] (1961), p. 175.

of lying robbed them of the possibility of sharing their fear and grief and they might even feel under pressure to hide from families and friends that they had seen through their game.

In the nineteenth and early twentieth centuries, death and dying for many people also came to signify a confrontation with fundamental, existential questions of meaning that was more forceful, more direct and more personal than it had been before. Making a case for a right to euthanasia, Roland Gerkan wrote in 1913 that, in the name of science, the belief in the beyond that "makes the agonizing months and years of dying bearable for the miserable," had been destroyed and that no replacement had been offered.[14] For many people religion with its rituals continued to provide a source of consolation and confidence. But growing segments of the population were becoming alienated from the established churches and the traditional beliefs that accompanied them. In German lung clinics, Gerkan wrote, workers were said to have ridiculed devout Catholics who made the sign of the cross before eating. Here, for some, not the Bible but the socialist journal *Vorwärts* was the central point of reference,[15] and the priest might find it difficult make his message heard.[16]

In confessional nursing, this could lead to intense conflict. Drawing on the accounts of middle-class female volunteer visitors to the sickbed as well as on letters sent to the motherhouse in Kaiserswerth by deaconesses who nursed patients in their homes, Karen Nolte has shown just how much these pious and dutiful women sometimes harassed their patients in their avid desire to save their souls. In extreme cases, in order to keep the mind of the dying patients clear and open to conversion, they even refused to administer narcotics. To their great regret, however, the deaconesses experienced how some severely ill patients refused to hear their pious words or even lapsed into blasphemy.[17]

People who found no satisfactory answers in religion were likely to be much more radical in posing questions about mortality and the meaning of human life. In the early nineteenth century, Henry Halford expressed a certain understanding for the fact that some men in heathen antiquity consciously starved themselves to death when they were severely ill, thus sacrificing a life "that was only painful, without the consolation of that sure and certain hope for a better life in the beyond" which was promised by the Christian religion.[18] Fictional writing in the late nineteenth and early twentieth centuries addressed this intensive search for meaning and the loneliness that came with it in various ways. A despairing Mr. Reffold in Beatrice Harraden's *Ships that Pass in the Night* asks the heroine Bernhardine: "Do you

[14] Roland Gerkan, Euthanasie, in: Das monistische Jahrhundert 2 (1913), pp. 169–74, cit. pp. 170–1.

[15] Speech by Dr Liebe (Waldhof, Eigershausen) in: Nietner, Zur Tuberkulose-Bekämpfung (1912), pp. 37–41, here p. 38.

[16] Johannes Handrick, Seelsorge und Politik in Heilstätten für tuberkulosekranke Männer, in: Die Tuberkulose 11 (1931), pp. 221–3.

[17] Nolte, Wege (2006b), pp. 46–7; eadem, Pflege (2010b), pp. 98–9.

[18] Halford, On the deaths (1842), pp. 163–6.

believe we get another chance [...]? Or is it all ended in that lonely little churchyard here?" Yet Bernhardine has no answer: "How do I know? [...] How does anyone know; but it is all a great mystery—nothing but a mystery."[19] The experience of what seemed a meaningless, undeservedly torturous illness could for its part raise the old theodicy question and even promote doubts about the existence of God. "Suffering viewed without the context of anything else," wrote Haeberlin in 1919, is perceived by the suffering person "as cruelty, as meaningless [...] which tortures and torments him."[20] In this situation, the physician, according to Haeberlin, had to assume an important task. By acting on the patient's soul, he had to move the patient toward "affirmation and values" and help him to accept his suffering as the most inner necessity. Then the patient "who only possessed his suffering before and who saw no escape from the violence that constrained and fettered him" could learn "perhaps by readjusting his outlook and the life of his soul, even when experiencing an illness from which his life will not victoriously exit, to gain values, values that in these circumstances nevertheless, or indeed all the more, carry within them the potential to expand and deepen his being."[21]

[19] Harraden, Ships (1894), p. 83; on Harraden's work see Pohland, Sanatorium (1984); I owe this passage to Katrin Max.

[20] Haeberlin, Vom Beruf (1919), pp. 89–90.

[21] Ibid., pp. 83–4.

9 Ethical Controversies

The declining force of religious norms in Western societies had lasting effects also on the way in which ethical questions concerning the treatment of the dying were viewed and handled. Human life became increasingly removed from the exclusive power of God. Especially in the question of shortening life the deep cleft between lay beliefs and the professional deontology of the doctors persisted. This cleft now divided not only learned doctors from the plain folks with their "popular" practices but highly educated lay people, too, put themselves at a distance to the traditional medical idea that the physician, under all circumstances, had to do everything he could to maintain and, if possible, prolong the patient's life.

At first, the right to set an end to a life that seemed unbearable was discussed above all in the context of suicide.[1] For hundreds of years, suicide had been considered a particularly severe sin, one that did not even leave the sinner the possibility to repent.[2] In the eighteenth century, however, some intellectuals began to call the reprehensibility of suicide into question.[3] For David Hume (1711–1776), the well-known Scottish philosopher, there was no reason to prolong a miserable existence out of a vain fear of offending the maker. To the universe, the life of a man was of no greater importance than that of an oyster. If age, sickness or misfortune made life a burden that was worse than death, then suicide was in our interest, indeed, it was a duty to ourselves.[4]

[1] See also Derek Humphry and Ann Wickett, Euthanasia from the Renaissance through the early twentieth century, in: Loreta M. Medina (ed.), Euthanasia, Detroit: Thomson Gale 2005, pp. 38–46.

[2] Cf. Vera Lind, Selbstmord in der Frühen Neuzeit. Diskurs, Lebenswelt und kultureller Wandel am Beispiel der Herzogtümer Schleswig und Holstein, Göttingen: Vandenhoeck und Ruprecht 1999.

[3] Good survey in Ursula Baumann, Vom Recht auf den eigenen Tod. Die Geschichte des Suizids vom 18. bis zum 20. Jahrhundert, Weimar: Böhlaus Nachfolger 2001.

[4] David Hume, Dialogues concerning natural religion and the posthumous essays *Of the immortality of the soul* and *Of suicide*. Ed. by Richard H. Popkin, Indianapolis-Cambridge: Hackett 1980, p. 104.

M. Stolberg, *A History of Palliative Care, 1500–1970*, Philosophy and Medicine 123,
DOI 10.1007/978-3-319-54178-5_9

Such ideas resonated increasingly. It was said, wrote Ulrich in 1780, that death was the greatest evil, but "the greatest evil, which we do not feel, can be more desirable to our thinking selves than a condition of consciousness in which the evil overwhelms what little good there is."[5] Certainly, wrote Knüppeln in 1790, there were duties to others, being the father of a family or holding an office, "but someone who has been abandoned by everyone," whose existence is no good to anyone or whose suffering is fruitless should at least have the right to leave the world. After all, severe pain robbed the weakened person of the use of his will and his reason in the end. He stopped "being a human being before he died and, by taking his life, does nothing more than leave a body that has become a burden to him, and in which his soul no longer lives."[6] K. J. Bischof made similar arguments in 1797. Enduring physical or psychological suffering ultimately destroyed freedom, "self-determination", and the ability to act in accordance with "the laws of reason." With this, the purpose of existence and the "value of life" were negated and "the remaining physical existence, which does not deserve to be called life," became "the greatest evil of all."[7]

As Kevin Siena has shown for England, the mere wish to end one's life was for some eighteenth century authors just the symptom or effect of mental illness. In court records and medical treatises, however, there are many cases of patients whose suicide was explained and justified by the argument that they had wanted to put an end to their agony.[8] Contemporary lay writers were sympathetic with such views. One anonymous diarist commented on the self-inflicted death of two patients in the Bussorah factory, a colonial trading post: "I believe every one of us at times would have done the same, had we been possessed of the means of accomplishing it." Like himself, the two patients had fallen ill with a very painful, epidemic fever that left them screaming like animals. One had shot several bullets into his chest; the other had opened his veins and bled to death.[9]

[5] Johann Heinrich Friedrich Ulrich, Moralische Encyclopädie, vol. 3, Berlin: Joachim Pauli 1780, pp. 629–30; however, for a more sceptical stance see Georg Wilhelm Block, Vom Selbstmord, dessen Moralität, Ursachen und Gegenmitteln, Aurich: Winter 1792, who justified suicide in principle but warned that it was impossible to know, whether one would really be unhappy until the end of one's life.

[6] Julius Friedrich Knüppeln, Ueber den Selbstmord. Ein Buch für die Menschheit, Gera: Bekmannsche Buchhandlung 1790, p. 96 and pp. 106–7; see also ibid., pp. 126–7.

[7] K. J. Bischof, Versuch über den freiwilligen Tod, Nürnberg: Raspesche Buchhandlung 1797, esp. pp. 78–80, p. 138 and p. 219.

[8] Siena, Suicide (2009).

[9] Anonymus, Case of a gentleman labouring under the epidemic remittent fever of Bussorah, in the year 1780. Communicated by John Hunter, in: Transactions of a Society for the Improvement of Medical and Chirurgical Knowledge, vol. 1, London: J. Johnson 1793, pp. 53–90, cit. p. 86.

9.1 Active Euthanasia

Having established that life for those with advanced, agonizing illnesses was senseless and having found a justification for suicide in these cases, the related question gained increasing prominence as to whether one was allowed to consciously put an end to the lives of others when they were suffering from agonizing physical pain. Until very recently, historians assumed that, among physicians, active euthanasia became an option that could publically be discussed and endorsed only around 1900.[10] As I have shown elsewhere in greater detail, however, it was already around 1800 that the walls began to crumble.[11] As early as 1792, Zach related that an unnamed doctor whom he described as quite well known at the time posed the question whether, in hopeless cases, it would not be better to free the patient from his raging pains and agonies and to accelerate inevitable death.[12] In England, some physicians had the reputation of doing this tacitly with deadly doses of opium.[13]

It was not long before some doctors professed publically their espousal of a deliberate shortening of life. In 1800, Carl Theodor Kortum, a medical practitioner in Stolberg near Aachen, described from his own experience the different course which consumption could take. For some patients, the complaints improved. However, others fell victim to their disease, suffering terrible agonies—and Kortum felt that the doctor could not stand idly by and watch:

> How terrible is the sight of the dying person for those standing by, the person who, after the expectoration of sputum has come to a halt, the ability to swallow has almost entirely stopped, and even the power of consciousness has already in large part escaped, who often lies for another two times 24 hours with a constant, boiling rattle in his chest, and is there anything desirable left for such a person aside from a gentle resolution that comes as soon as possible?

Kortum's answer was clear and unambiguous:

> A moderate dose of poppy juice, e. g. 20 drops of laudanum liq. infallibly shortens such agony by extinguishing the weak vital flame entirely, and it is, in my opinion, morally permitted in such cases.

---

[10] Some authors have interpreted a well-known passage in Thomas Morus' *Utopia* as a plea for active euthanasia or assisted suicide. *Utopia* clearly was not meant to be understood as political program, however. Like other "utopias" it was a thought experiment (Thomas Morus, A fruteful and pleasaunt worke of the beste state of a publyque weale, and of the neweyle called Utopia. Transl. by Raphe Robynson, London 1551 (repr. Amsterdam–New York: Da Capo Press 1969).

[11] Michael Stolberg, Two pioneers of active euthanasia around 1800, in: The Hastings Centre report 38 (2008), n. 6, pp. 19–22; idem, Aktive Sterbehilfe um 1800: "Seine unbeschreiblichen Leiden gemildert und sein Ende befördert". Eine ärztliche Debatte und ihre Hintergründe, in: Deutsches Ärzteblatt A 106 (2009), pp. 1836–8; see also idem, Aktive Sterbehilfe und Eugenik vor 1850. Frühformen, Ursachen, Entwicklungen, Folgen, in: Ignacio Czeguhn, Eric Hilgendorf and Jürgen Weitzel (eds), Eugenik und Euthanasie 1850–1945, Baden–Baden: Nomos 2009, pp. 9–26.

[12] Zach, De cura (1792), pp. 26–7.

[13] Berridge and Edwards, Opium (1987), p. 82; Jalland, Death (1996), pp. 85–6.

Kortum left it open as to whether he himself had acted in this way with individual patients but his remark that this dose "infallibly" shortened the patient's agony certainly suggests this.[14]

Kortum was not alone. In 1801, the well-known Berlin surgeon Christian Ludwig Mursinna published the medical history of a military officer from Stettin whom he had treated several years before at the Berlin Charité for an aggressive cancerous ulcer on his lower lip. A different surgeon had previously removed the parts that were affected by the cancer, but the cancerous ulcer had continued to erupt, becoming "significantly larger, more malignant and cankerous." The patient, now discouraged and infirm, ultimately rejected any further treatment and requested only "resolution, meaning an acceleration of death." Mursinna responded to this wish only to a limited extent. The man died months later, after the cancer had taken possession of half the tongue and penetrated deep into the throat. But Mursinna, looking back, made a remarkable admission: "He would have died even later had I not given him opiates so often and thus alleviated his indescribable suffering and promoted his end." Mursinna left it open as to whether he had consciously accelerated death, or whether he had only accepting the risk of this whilst seeking to fight the patient's pain—some medical ethicists today would speak of "indirect euthanasia" in this case. What is beyond doubt, however, is that, in his own assessment, he had shortened his patient's life and apparently he saw no reason to justify his course of action or indeed apologize for it.[15]

Kortum and Mursinna's published these statements not in treatises on medical ethics or the professional duties of a physician but in little articles that were devoted to concrete, practical questions. Probably only few physicians read these provocative passages. By all appearances, Kortum und Mursinna were crucial, however, in prompting an oft-quoted, fiery crie de coeur against active euthanasia that a leading representative of the German medical profession, Christoph Wilhelm Hufeland, made public in 1806. Hufeland was almost certainly familiar with Kortum's and Mursinna's articles. He was the publishing editor of the journal bearing his name, the *Hufelandsches Journal,* in which Kortum's article was published, and Hufeland worked, as did Mursinna, at the Berlin Charité. With arguments that still shape the discussion today, Hufeland insisted on the fundamental incompatibility between active euthanasia and the doctor's profession, and warned of a slippery slope: Every physician, he wrote, had sworn, "to do nothing that might shorten the life of a man." Certainly, a well-meaning doctor could fall into doubt sometimes when a patient was being tormented by incurable afflictions and was asking for death. He might wonder whether it were not allowed or even a duty to "free the miserable person from his burden somewhat sooner." Yet such action, according to Hufeland, "would be highly unjust and punishable. It annuls the very nature of the physician." The doctor was allowed

---

[14] Kortum, Kleine Aufsätze (1800).

[15] Mursinna, Etwas über den Gebrauch des Cosmischen Mittels (1801).

> to do nothing other than maintain life; whether it is happiness or unhappiness, whether it has value or not, this is none of his business, and if he arrogates to include this consideration in his business, the consequences will be incalculable, and the physician becomes the most dangerous person in the state; because if the line is crossed just once, if the physician feels entitled to decide about the necessity of a life, then all it takes is a step-by-step progression to apply [this criterion, M.S.] of worthlessness, and consequently the lack of necessity of a human life, to other cases as well.[16]

Among the medical profession, Hufeland's line of argument remained the dominant position on active euthanasia for decades to come. Only very few, isolated cases of active euthanasia by physicians are documented for the entire nineteenth century. The earliest known case, from France, is connected to the name of the famous Louis Pasteur (1822–1895) and was described by Léon Daudet (1867–1942) in his memoirs. In 1886–87, when Daudet was 20 years old, he witnessed the case of six Russian farmers in the Parisian Hôtel Dieu, who had all been bitten by a rabid wolf. Pasteur's serum treatment, which had just revolutionized the treatment of rabies, did not produce any results. The farmers' condition became hopeless. According to Daudet they, "grotesquely contorted, with bulging eyes, frothing mouths," clung to the railings of their beds or rolled on the floor, a corner of their blanket between their teeth. When the cramps temporarily subsided, they begged the doctors to put an end to their agonies. The doctors took their request seriously. After consulting with the head pharmacist, Pasteur decided to grant their wish. The five who were still alive—one had died in the meantime—were given a deadly pill. Then, Daudet continued, a silence fell over the house and they cried.[17]

In the late nineteenth and early twentieth centuries, the cultural context changed fundamentally. There emerged—principally among lay people at first—a vigorous debate about the right of being granted active euthanasia. In retrospect, a key text appears to have been a lecture, later published, given in 1870 by the author Samuel D. Williams, Jr. to the Speculative Club in Birmingham. Using the title *Euthanasia,* Williams declared it a medical duty to administer in cases of hopeless or painful diseases chloroform or comparable medication if the patient wished "so as to destroy consciousness at once, and put the sufferer to a quick and painless death."[18] Energetically, he turned against the objection that this contradicted the "sacredness" of human life. After all, even "amid the most civilized countries of Europe, 'the sacredness of man's life' is thrown to the winds, the moment national or political passion grows hot, or even when mere material interests are seriously threatened."[19]

[16] Hufeland, Verhältnisse (1806); see also idem, Von dem Rechte des Arztes über Leben und Tod, in: Journal der practischen Heilkunde (1823), n. 1, pp. 3–28.

[17] Daudet, Devant la douleur (1915), pp. 62–3.

[18] Williams, Euthanasia (1870), p. 212.

[19] Ibid., p. 215.

The familiar term "euthanasia" had taken on a new meaning: the deliberate, active ending of suffering and life.[20] The consequences of this have been described many times.[21] Taken up by others, Williams's theses soon found a resonant echo far beyond Birmingham. While the editors of the newspaper *Spectator* criticized Williams severely, the philosopher Lionel Tollemache took a stand for him.[22] A lively discussion developed, which soon spread to other countries. The newspapers reported spectacular "mercy killings."[23] Writers made them the central subject of their novels and plays.[24] The first drafts of laws sent waves through parliaments in Germany and the United States.[25]

[20] A short time before Williams went public with his ideas, William Lecky had already written of the ancient "conception of suicide as an euthanasia, an abridgment of the pangs of disease, and a guarantee against the dotage of age" (William Edward Hartpole Lecky, History of European morals, vol. 1, London: Longmans, Green & Co. 1869, p. 233).

[21] The history of euthanasia (in the sense of voluntary euthanisia and mercy killing) has been traced by numerous authors, especially for the time since the late 19th century; see e.g., Ranaan Gillon. Suicide and voluntary euthanasia: Historical perspective, in: A. B. Downing (ed.), Euthanasia and the right to die, London: Peter Owen 1969, pp. 171–92; Stanley Joel Reiser, The dilemma of euthanasia in modern medical history. The English and American experience, in: John A. Behnke and Sissela Bok (eds), The dilemmas of euthanasia. New York: Anchor Press and Doubleday 1975, pp. 27–49; Fye, Active euthanasia (1978); Elkeles, Aussagen (1979), pp. 126–35; N. D. A. Kemp, N. D. A., Merciful release. The history of the British euthanasia movement, Manchester: Manchester University Press 2002; Dowbiggin, Life unworthy (2005); Benzenhöfer, Euthanasia (2010); see also Helmut Ehrhardt, Euthanasie und Vernichtung "lebensunwerten" Lebens, Stuttgart: Enke 1965; I. van der Sluis, The movement for euthanasia 1875–1975, in: Janus 66 (1979), pp. 131–72; Gerald J. Gruman, An historical introduction to ideas about voluntary euthanasia. In: Omega 4 (1973), pp. 87–138; Ezekiel J. Emanuel, The history of euthanasia debates in the United States and Britain, in: Annals of internal medicine 121 (1994), pp. 793–802; Edward J. Larson and Darrel W. Amundsen, A different death. Euthanasia and the Christian tradition, Downers Grove, Ill.: InterVarsity Press 1998; Harold Y. Vanderpool, Life-sustaining treatment and euthanasia: Historical aspects, in: Stephen G. Post (ed.), Encyclopedia of bioethics, 3rd edn, New York: Macmillan Reference 2004, pp. 1421–32; Shai J. Lavi, The modern art of dying. A history of euthanasia in the United States, Princeton-Oxford: Princeton University Press 2005; Lewis, Medicine (2007), pp. 198–228.

[22] Lionel Tollemache, The cure for incurables, in: The fortnightly review N. S. 13 (1873), reprinted in idem, Stones of stumbling, London: W. Rice 1893, pp. 1–30, postscript of 1893, pp. 30–1; cf. Benzenhöfer, Der gute Tod? (2009), pp. 134–8.

[23] Tollemach, Cure, pp. 10–11; Henri Bouquet, L'euthanasie, in: Revue générale des sciences pures et appliquées 44 (1933), pp. 532–4; Zumstein, Le débat (1986), p. 91; my thanks to the author—now a film-maker—for letting me see this work, which was unfortunately never published.

[24] See e.g., Heyse, Auf Leben und Tod (1886); Storm, Bekenntnis [1887] (1988); Nassauer, Sterben (1911); Ricarda Huch, Der Fall Deruga, Berlin-Vienna: Ullstein & Co. 1917; cf. Mayer, Euthanasie (1982); Herbert Viefhues, Das Motiv der "Euthanasie" in der fiktionalen Literatur—zugleich ein Beitrag zu einer metaphorischen Verstehensweise der Ethik, Bochum: Zentrum für Med. Ethik 1992; Käser, Arzt (1998), pp. 150–78; Yahya Elsaghe, Sterbehilfe, Glaubensverlust und Religionsersatz in Theodor Storms *Bekenntnis*, in: Zeitschrift für Religions- und Geistesgeschichte 63 (2011), pp. 23–44.

[25] An early survey can be found in Sicard, Essai (1913), pp. 8–9.

In Germany, the young Adolf Jost demanded in 1895 that physicians be allowed to kill the incurable if the patient himself requested it.[26] Ernst Haeckel, who had gathered experience as a medical student in the Julius-Spital in Würzburg, spoke in 1904 in favor of allowing the killing of the "hundreds of thousands" of incurables, "namely the mentally ill, the leprous, the cancerous and so forth" who "in the modern culture states [are being] artificially kept alive without any use for themselves or for the whole." For Haeckel, one had the right, if not the duty, to "put an end to the severe suffering of our fellow men, if severe illness without hope of recovery makes their lives intolerable and when they themselves ask us for 'deliverance from evil'"—just as people sometimes, if necessary, gave a merciful death to dogs and horses.[27] Those afflicted would be spared suffering and pain and society great financial expenditures "if one would finally decide to free the fully incurable from their unspeakable torments through a dose of morphine!"[28] The German Monist League, founded in 1906 by proponents of Haeckel's ideas, became a driving force in Germany in the discussion around legalizing voluntary euthanasia. In 1913, Roland Gerkan, who suffered from a lung complaint, wrote a draft of a law in the magazine *Monistisches Jahrhundert* that would grant the right to "*Sterbehilfe (Euthanasie)*" if a specialist in forensic medicine and two further specialists at the request of the sick patient confirmed "the overwhelming probability of a fatal outcome."[29]

When Gerkan spoke of "Sterbehilfe," that is literally of "help with dying," he used a term that was in the process of becoming a common synonym for "euthanasia" in the German language.[30] In earlier times, the term "Euthanasie" in German would have been paraphrased with expressions such as "easing death" or "making death easier."[31] But as Heyn explained in 1921, "Sterbehilfe" now did not refer simply to forgoing "medications that prolong life and thereby agony;" rather, it meant the deliberate "initiation of death in the case of a sick person who is irretrievably lost but not yet actually dying." And if the first case was to be described as "passive" euthanasia, one had better use quotation marks.[32]

[26] A. Jost, Das Recht auf den Tod. Sociale Studie, Göttingen: Dieterich 1895; for a brief overview of the German developments see Benzenhöfer, Euthanasia (2010).

[27] Ernst Haeckel, Die Lebenswunder. Gemeinverständliche Studien über biologische Philosophie; Ergänzungsband zu dem Buche über die Welträthsel, Stuttgart: Kröner 1904, p. 132 and pp. 134–5.

[28] Ibid., pp. 134–5.

[29] Roland Gerkan, Euthanasie, in: Das monistische Jahrhundert 2 (1913), pp. 169–74, cit. pp. 170–1.

[30] Gerkan may even have coined the term "Sterbehilfe". His text is the earliest source I have been able to find so far that uses it. By 1915, at the latest, it had entered legal terminology: Dr Kaßler, Das Recht auf Sterbehilfe (Euthanasie), in: Deutsche Juristenzeitung 20 (1915), cols 203–4; Dr v. Olshausen, Zum Recht auf Sterbehilfe, in: Medizinische Klinik 11 (1915), p. 739; W. Hanauer, Euthanasie, in: Therapeutische Monatshefte 31 (1917), pp. 107–12.

[31] Choulant, Anleitung (1836), p. 183.

[32] Heyn, Ueber Sterbehilfe (Euthanasie) (1921).

At first, it was principally lay people who demanded a legalization of voluntary euthanasia. In a sense, they stood in the tradition of the popular belief that it was legitimate to shorten the process of suffering and dying, by means of a sudden removal of the patient's pillows. In fact, according to ethnographic surveys, undertaken at the time, these practices continued to be known and accepted in the wider population.[33] As late as 1897, Mendelsohn declared that the removal of the pillows of the dying was a "widespread" custom.[34] Some observers associated the practice even more so than in earlier times with the rural lower classes,[35] but in Great Britain, where the public discussion about killing by request emerged in the late nineteenth century, and even in British cities, such practices were apparently still very well known, as Munk reported in 1887, drawing on 40 years of experience in medical practice in East London.[36] There is some evidence of them even in personal testimonies from the educated classes. When Frank Rogers lay dying of "cerebral softening" in 1886, Sabina Rogers asked whether she should take the pillow out from under his head, which her nephew Arthur correctly interpreted as meaning that she wanted to accelerate her husband's demise.[37] According to Hastings's *Encyclopaedia*, removing the pillow was still "a very wide-spread custom" in Europe around 1930 and was practiced in the belief, "that it abridges the sufferings of the dying and is therefore an act of kindness."[38]

For these reasons, the demands for killing by request that were put forth in lay circles at the end of the nineteenth century were less revolutionary than they may seem at first glance. Now, however, these demands were founded on completely different philosophical prerequisites. In the place of the "folk" practices, which in retrospect occasionally bordered on the symbolic-ritualistic, came the call for a medicalized killing by professional physicians by means of appropriate medications and narcotics.

Only a small minority of doctors, around 1900, supported the legalization of active euthanasia. In France, Jules Regnault opposed in 1905 the *sensiblerie* of modern civilization, in which one tried to prolong the suffering of the severely ill as long as possible. If the incurably ill patient so desired, one should be allowed to end his life.[39] In 1913, the Parisian *Gazette médicale* kindled a heated debate in its letters

[33] Cf. G[ottfried] Lammert, Volksmedizin und medizinischer Aberglaube in Bayern und den angrenzenden Gebieten, Würzburg: F. A. Julien 1869, p. 101; E. H. Meyer, Badisches Volksleben im neunzehnten Jahrhundert (reprint of the 1900-edition), Stuttgart: Kommissionsverlag K. Theiss 1984, pp. 580–3.

[34] Mendelsohn, Ueber die Euthanasie (1897), p. 38; around the same time, the practice was described as "not rare" in certain areas in Capellmann, Pastoral-Medicin (1895), p. 278.

[35] Krügelstein, Handbuch (1807), p. 420; Choulant, Anleitung (1836), p. 189; Jahn, De euthanasia (1839), p. 19.

[36] Munk, Euthanasia (1887), p. 95.

[37] Jalland, Death (1996), p. 95, based on the manuscript notes of Arthur Rogers.

[38] J. Hastings (ed.), Encyclopaedia of religion and ethics, vol. 4, Edinburgh: Clark 1935, p. 415.

[39] Jules Regnault, Assassinat médical ou suprême charité, in: La Revue (1905), pp. 472–87, according to Zumstein, Le débat (1986), pp. 36–7.

to the editor, in which individual physicians spoke up in favor of legalizing voluntary euthanasia.[40] In 1919, the French military doctor Charles Binet-Sanglé even called it "barbaric, cruel and inhuman" that one denied the incurably ill the right to suicide. Using the telling title *L'art de mourir,* he demanded state-run "euthanasia institutes" in which specially employed "euthanizers" would kill the incurably ill with laughing gas. A requirement was that three "euthanizers" had to be in unanimous agreement about the unfavorable prognosis.[41] In Germany, Heyn wanted to see as permissible the "painless shortening of life" in cases of cancer and tuberculosis, the "two worst scourges of humanity," but also with other terminal illnesses such as chronic heart or nerve failure, advanced *tabes dorsalis* (literally: dorsal or spinal consumption) or severe diabetes, if the sick person requested it.[42] In England, Harry Roberts sympathized with this proposal, provided the patient himself wished for his end and was not being killed because this was cheaper or more pleasant for everyone else. For in that case unwanted infants or run-down grandparents might be killed.[43]

On the other side, physicians who opposed the legalization of voluntary euthanasia insisted on the intrinsic uncertainty of diagnosis and prognosis, even in the case of the most severe illnesses. It was always possible in their view that one or the other sick patient could have been saved whose life was put to a premature end by active euthanasia.[44] And they considered active euthanasia to be incompatible with the medical profession.[45] The physician's motto was "war on death!" ("guerre à la mort!"), declared Boulai in 1914: This was how he justified his existence.[46] Along similar lines, the French physician Henri Bouquet stated that in every moment of a doctor's professional life death was the enemy that he fought. "Do not ask of him that he accelerate his inevitable triumph, regardless of the circumstances."[47]

Some critics put forward the alternative possibility of a palliative alleviation of suffering. Henri Bouquet for example explained, "Today we have methods and medications […] that allow us to suppress pain in the most agonizing diseases or at least to alleviate it, and every day we discover new ones."[48] According to Hans Lieske, if a doctor was "overcome by pity over the agony of a sick patient" and was thus tempted "to shorten the path of the approaching savior Death," then he was still left with "the possibility of alleviating the dying person's final hours by numbing

---

40 Gazette médicale de Paris 1914, pp. 16–7, 47–8, 71–2, 96, 128–9, 152–3, 184–5 and 233.

41 Binet-Sanglé, L'art de mourir (1919), pp. 32–3 and pp. 145–52.

42 Heyn, Ueber Sterbehilfe (Euthanasie) (1921), pp. 260–1.

43 Harry Roberts, Voluntary death, in: idem, Euthanasia and other aspects of life and death, London: Constable 1936, pp. 3–18.

44 See e.g., Dr v. Olshausen, Zum Recht auf Sterbehilfe, in: Medizinische Klinik 11 (1915), p. 739.

45 Sicard, Essai (1913).

46 Letter to the editor of the Gazette médicale de Paris, January 21, 1914.

47 Henri Bouquet, L'euthanasie, in: Revue générale des sciences pures et appliquées 44 (1933), pp. 532–4, cit. p. 534.

48 Ibid.; a similar early statement can already be found in Sicard, Essai (1913), p. 50.

the pain."[49] To Haeckel, Maeterlinck and other authors this position indicated a general change of heart on the part of medical professionals in the early twentieth century. Even if some doctors hesitated to administer narcotics due to a fear of the dangers associated with them, Maeterlinck found, it nevertheless became increasingly common with hopeless cases to—as no one had dared just shortly before—"if not shorten the throes of death, then put the dying person to sleep."[50]

As Hufeland had in the early nineteenth century, some critics also saw a danger of deliberate abuse.[51] Their warnings would prove to be all too justified, in Germany in particular. Here, some authors, drawing on eugenic and social Darwinist convictions, were quick to extend the demand for a legalization of voluntary euthanasia. They wanted to see the killing of the mentally ill and handicapped legalized, without the expressed wish of those in question. This, they claimed, was for the patients' own good as well as for the good of society as a whole. *Die Freigabe der Vernichtung lebensunwerten Lebens (Legalizing the Annihilation of Life Not Worth Living)* was the programmatic title of a famous and influential book by Karl Binding and Alfred Hoche, who gave decisive impetus to such ideas in the 1920s. Against the demands of an "overwrought concept of humanity and an overestimation of the value of existence as such," they advocated in particular for the killing of "the incurably idiotic." For Binding and Hoche, these people were a "terribly heavy burden" for their relatives and for society, and they did not have a will that one would have to ignore or break.[52] In Nazi Germany, such demands were applied, as is well-known, with horrific consequences and without a legal basis, first between 1939 and 1941 in systematic, thoroughly bureaucratized mass murders, above all in the so-called *Aktion T4*,[53] and later—more difficult to discern in the sources—without central coordination, locally, in institutions and homes, sometimes with the distinction blurred between deliberate killing, conscious undernourishment and allowing that patients starved to death.[54]

Due their primary interest in the genesis of the National Socialist "euthanasia" program, histories of the debates on active euthanasia before 1933 have, understandably, often focused on authors such as Jost, Haeckel, Binding and Hoche. Their statements are of course central to an understanding of the developments after 1933 and the skill with which Nazi propaganda linked the idea of mercy killing for

---

[49] Hans Lieske, Dem Tode verfallen. Eine juristische Geschichte, in: Fortschritte der Medizin 35 (1917/18), pp. 126–7.

[50] Maeterlinck, Vom Tode (1913), p. 8.

[51] Hans Lieske, Dem Tode verfallen. Eine juristische Geschichte, in: Fortschritte der Medizin 35 (1917/18), pp. 126–7.

[52] Binding and Hoche, Freigabe (1920), p. 62 and p. 31.

[53] Recent overview in Maike Rotzoll et al. (eds), Die nationalsozialistische "Euthanasie"-Aktion "T4" und ihre Opfer: Geschichte und ethische Konsequenzen für die Gegenwart, Paderborn: Schöningh 2010.

[54] Hans-Walter Schmuhl, Rassenhygiene, Nationalsozialismus, Euthanasie. Von der Verhütung zur Vernichtung "lebensunwerten Lebens", 1890–1945, Göttingen: Vandenhoeck und Ruprecht 1987, pp. 220–4; Süß, Der "Volkskörper" (2003), pp. 314–69.

terminally-ill patients suffering from agonizing pain—an idea that was acceptable to many people at the time—with a justification for mass-murdering the disabled and the mentally ill, for example in Wolfgang Liebeneiner's successful film *Ich klage an* (*I Accuse,* 1941) may serve as a warning to this day. Studying the debates about voluntary euthanasia before 1933 only in the light of the atrocities afterwards risks paying insufficient attention, however, to those whose concern was strictly voluntary euthanasia, based on the expressed wish of mentally fully competent patients who saw no meaning in enduring weeks or indeed months of possibly horrendous suffering before their death. Conversely, the organized murder in the course of the *Aktion T4* must not lead us to hasty generalizations with regard to how "common" terminally ill and dying patients were handled in that period. National Socialist medical politics distinguished between those who were valuable to the state and to society for racial or economic reasons, and those who were "inferior."[55] When they suffered from a severe, chronic, or potentially terminal illness, the mentally ill or disabled and those considered "racially inferior," could not expect major efforts to keep them alive or to alleviate their complaints. Beginning in the 1930s, Jewish patients were hardly admitted to general hospitals anymore. Even sick forced laborers, in spite of their economic significance, only exceptionally received thorough treatment as resources became increasingly scarce.[56]

This does not necessarily apply to the rest of the population in Nazi Germany, however. There is little evidence, in fact, that the terminally ill and dying, in general, were deliberately left to their fate or that their lives were even shortened on purpose. The search for effective preventative measures and treatments to fight the two most important causes of chronic, terminal infirmities that is cancer and tuberculosis was moved forward with much determination in Nazi Germany in particular.[57] In magazines such as *Die Tuberkulose (Tuberculosis)* or the *Monatsschrift für Krebsbekämpfung (Monthly Journal for the Fighting of Cancer)* numerous articles presented the most recent research on the prophylaxis, diagnosis and treatment of these illnesses. In retrospect, there were some very questionable experiments with "biological" treatments, but there were also some experimental and empirical studies that still seem "modern" today, for example demonstrating the carcinogenicity of tobacco smoke.[58] In any case, even physicians such as Binding, who demanded a legalization of the "destruction of life not worth living," at the same time wanted to establish clear limits on "euthanasia" for those from the remaining population who

[55] See also Fridolf Kudlien, Fürsorge und Rigorismus. Überlegungen zur ärztlichen Normaltätigkeit im Dritten Reich, in: Norbert Frei (ed.), Medizin und Gesundheitspolitik in der NS-Zeit, Munich: Oldenbourg 1991, pp. 99–111.

[56] Süß, Der "Volkskörper" (2003), p. 293; Wolters, Tuberkulose (2011), pp. 90–2. In the Pfaffenwald camp alone almost 400 "Ostarbeiter" died between 1942 und 1945; most of them had been diagnosed with tuberculosis (Susanne Hohlmann, Pfaffenwald. Sterbe- und Geburtenlager 1942–1945, 2nd edn, Kassel: Bibliothek Gesamthochschule 1988, pp. 81–5).

[57] Wolters, Tuberkulose (2011).

[58] A. H. Roffo, Krebserzeugende Tabakwirkung, in: Monatsschrift für Krebsbekämpfung 8 (1940), pp. 99–102; cf. Robert Proctor, The Nazi war on cancer, Princeton: Princeton University Press 1999; Wolters, Tuberkulose (2011).

were hopelessly ill or wounded. Accordingly to Binding, a deadly injection of morphine was not to be expressly permitted unless death was certain and imminent, in which case only the most "parochial pedant" could speak of "a noticeable shortening of the lifetime of the deceased."[59]

Winfried Süß, who in his extensive analysis of Nazi health politics also studied how the chronically ill, care-dependent and dying were dealt with, found that for the time before 1939 there are no clear indications of a systematic neglect or even killing of "normal" patients with severe chronic illnesses. He concludes that a discrimination of old and chronically ill patients was "not common" and was also not seriously considered in the medical literature.[60] Süß and Kenan H. Irmak[61] have, however, found some evidence that the situation worsened significantly for elderly patients in need of a high level of care during the last 2 years of the war amidst an increased scarcity of resources. As a way of protecting them against air raids, but also to free up the beds so they could be used as urgently needed emergency beds, thousands of them were taken, often against their will, to secondary hospitals—so-called war infirmaries—and other makeshift facilities outside the cities. These patients now also filled the beds in asylums, whose previous inmates had been systematically killed. In these places, the medical and nursing care was apparently minimal and in some the mortality rate was extremely high. In isolated cases, old patients, after having been moved to an asylum, were murdered, and there are indications that relatives preferred to care for their very care-dependent family members at home for fear that they would be killed in an asylum.[62] Further, beginning in November 1944, not only the chronically ill were to be taken to such care facilities, but all patients of general hospitals who did not recover within 4 weeks.[63]

In the war years, particularly severe cases—those who were terminally ill and dying—were increasingly excluded from regular healthcare. In July 1943, the Reich minister of health and director of the Reich Chamber of Physicians, Leonardo Conti, banned hopeless patients from admittance to hospitals for their last days of life.[64] As early as at the outset of 1942, Munich gynecologist Otto Eisenreich received the explicit approval from the director of the health department in the Bavarian Ministry of the Interior for his refusal to admit moribund female cancer patients to his clinic: "We cannot afford to admit people with sanious carcinomas to our clinic, just because they are poor devils, and thereby take the beds of other, more urgent cases."[65] Toward the end of the war, the exclusion of the chronically ill from the healthcare system reached an apex, as Süß has found, in the "establishment of

[59] Binding and Hoche, Freigabe (1920), pp. 18–19.

[60] Süß, Der "Volkskörper" (2003), pp. 292–310, cit. p. 297.

[61] Irmak, Der Sieche (2002), pp. 230–2.

[62] Ibid., p. 378.

[63] Süß, Der "Volkskörper" (2003), pp. 298–310.

[64] Bundesarchiv Berlin, R18/3791, letter from Conti to the *Reichsverteidigungskommissar*, July 5, 1943, cit. in Süß, Der "Volkskörper" (2003), p. 300.

[65] Stadtarchiv München, Gesundheitsamt/118, minutes of a conference about the medical care of civilians, February 23, 1942, cit. in Süß, Der "Volkskörper" (2003), p. 300.

special death houses for terminal patients, with the most limited medical care." As an example, Süß names the St. Josef convent in Neuß, which had 150 beds for the chronically ill but temporarily also 60 beds for moribund cancer patients.[66] Just how widespread such facilities were and to what degree they perhaps did after all offer palliative treatment and care for the dying requires further investigation, however.

A major group that did fall victim to a massive and deliberate underprovision of healthcare were those tuberculosis patients who were branded as "asocial." Beginning in 1930 in Thuringia and, by 1939, across the Reich, they could be forcibly admitted to sanitariums, which were generally closely connected to mental institutions. This was the fate of only a fraction of tuberculosis patients, but ultimately anyone could fall into the category of "asocial" for resisting treatment and/or being isolated, because he or she did not experience subjective complaints or could not afford treatment in a hospital or sanitarium. Some of the sanitariums to which these patients were forcibly admitted did not conceal the fact that no medical intervention was carried out to slow the progress of illness, that patients were fed a starvation diet, and/or that they became forced laborers. The mortality rate of these inmates was accordingly high. Like many psychiatric patients, many of the sanitarium inmates also fell victim to National Socialist "euthanasia."[67]

9.2 Unintentional Shortening of Life and the Limiting of Therapy

There were, as we have seen, isolated opposing voices, but generally doctors practicing in the nineteenth and early twentieth centuries continued to reject the deliberate shortening of the lives of terminally ill and dying patients. A commonly repeated warning went further still: It was wrong for a doctor to contribute to shortening someone's life even indirectly, involuntarily, in his attempt to alleviate suffering. As Anthony Carlisle stated in 1818, the physician had no right to make even the slightest chance of an unexpected recovery futile by administering opium or shortening the life of a sick person even by a fleeting moment.[68] When administering narcotics, claimed Goetz similarly in 1841, the most important thing was to make sure that they did not do more harm than good, and that the thread of life was not cut earlier than was right.[69] Schrader pointed out in 1842, in the context of the palliative treatment of uterine cancer, that careful attention had to be paid to make sure that the medical treatment did not worsen the malady and that "the fatal outcome [was] not hastened."[70] Reimann went so far as to categorically condemn "euthanasic

[66] Süß, Der "Volkskörper" (2003), p. 300.

[67] Wolters, Tuberkulose (2011), pp. 62–93.

[68] Anthony Carlisle, An essay on the disorders of old age and on the means of prolonging human life, 2nd edn, London: Longman 1818, p. 108.

[69] Goetz, De euthanasia (1841), pp. 18–19.

[70] Wilhelm Schrader, De carcinomate uteri, med. diss., Berlin: Nietack 1842, p. 30.

medication" that was used for the "purported mitigation of death"—first and foremost opium—as having the "most pernicious and harmful effect on the severely ill." Such medication, he claimed, advanced death and caused the transition from life to death to be only more painful.[71] Eulenburg's widely read *Real-Encyclopädie der gesammten Heilkunde* (*Complete Encyclopedia of Medicine*) of 1886 likewise stated that as long as there was a glimmer of hope, it was the doctor's duty to do everything that was medically possible "without any regard for euthanasia," meaning a death that was as gentle and pain-free as possible. Even in cases that were beyond hope, the physician was not allowed to do anything in the slightest "that might contribute to shortening life."[72]

Some laypeople thought otherwise. In his discussion of "so-called euthanasia, the mitigation of dying in the case of the hopelessly ill, who spend the remainder of their lives in great physical agony," the jurist Oppenheim explicitly made a point of granting the physician the right to administer narcotics even if this "possibly or even likely hastened death." "Alleviating suffering," he claimed, "was the major task of the physician here compared to which a possible shortening of life becomes irrelevant."[73]

Yet even Joseph Bullar, someone who emphatically spoke out in favor of the palliative administration of opium, wrote that he hesitated to give it to a patient who had death written all over his face and was about to suffocate. Bullar was concerned that "the opiate should stop respiration altogether and at once." Therefore, he first gave him only brandy and only later, when the patient asked for it, careful, small doses of an opium preparation that brought the patient instant relief without killing him. This practice of administering several carefully dosed, small amounts was also the recommendation he had for his colleagues.[74]

In 1896, Scipione Riva-Rocci, wrote in a very personal tone about a dying pneumonia patient, giving a vivid account of his own crisis of conscience in this situation. Especially in cases of a protracted death agony, he had often wondered whether it might be permissible to alleviate the patients' suffering during the last moments of their lives by sedating them with a little morphine. On the other hand, the dosage required for this might compromise the function of the heart and nervous system and have fatal consequences. Perhaps one had to accept that risk when the patient was still fully conscious and experienced the agony of dying in all its extent. Once a patient was already losing consciousness, however, or when the throes of death were perhaps harder to bear for the family than for the dying person himself, the doctor was not allowed to do anything that might hasten death.[75]

[71] Reimann, Schädlichkeit ([1843]), pp. 28–37, cit. p. 28.

[72] Dr Samuel, Euthanasie, in: Albert Eulenburg (ed.), Real-Encyclopädie der gesammten Heilkunde, Leipzig 1896, pp. 640–1.

[73] L. Oppenheim, Das ärztliche Recht zu körperlichen Eingriffen an Kranken und Gesunden, Basel: Schwabe 1892, p. 30.

[74] Bullar, Opium (1856), p. 268.

[75] Riva-Rocci, Cura (1896), p. 470.

It is difficult to say whether, in their daily practice, physicians did in fact show that kind of restraint. According to contemporary observers, some doctors at the sickbed certainly did risk shortening life by giving opiates and other palliative remedies.[76] It might scarcely be the case, wrote Olfers in his *Pastoralmedicin,* that doctors gave a remedy with the intention "of cutting short a sick person's suffering through death." But they did administer narcotic remedies in such doses "as would doubtlessly expedite death."[77] Considering the prevalent medical reservations against any form of shortening life, the question remains whether doctors believed this was the inevitable result of giving opium. After all, doctors who used opium and morphine more generously with terminally ill patients could calm their conscience by reminding themselves of the relatively common experience that these medicines in many cases actually helped prolong life.[78] Adolf Gottstein for example held the view that, possibly, "a vigorous, truly soothing dosage" may often even delay death—and thus the doctor's conscience could rest at ease.[79]

Closely connected to the issue of an unintentional shortening of life was the question of whether, in hopeless cases, a doctor was permitted to forgo life-sustaining remedies. As in the eighteenth century, the question arose principally from the common warning of the dangers of *dysthanasia* or *kakothanasia* caused by medical intervention. The exhortation to forgo healing attempts that threatened only to increase the suffering of a dying person was among the core messages of the *euthanasia medica* literature of the nineteenth century. According to Gmelin, it was even "the main point of so-called euthanasia to abstain from torturing the dying, for whom there is no hope, with supposed supporting remedies until their last breath."[80] As early as 1798, John Ferriar had demanded that the doctor who was unable to help his patient should at least protect him from unnecessary suffering, instead of tormenting the dying person "with unavailing attempts to stimulate the dissolving system, from the idle vanity of prolonging the flutter of the pulse for a few more vibrations."[81]

Ferriar's reference to "idle vanity" of course expresses a value judgment: he clearly did not consider it the task of the doctor to prolong a person's life at all cost. In this vein, Hennemann cautioned his colleagues not to prolong the suffering of hopeless patients without their "well-considered consent."

> Not life is the deity for which our art builds altars; it is health—and while the artist of healing cannot be authorized to lead the lamentable person, whose torments can be ended only by death, into death's arms, the artist is nevertheless obliged to first seek the well-considered

[76] Williams, Euthanasia (1870), p. 216.

[77] E. W. M. Olfers, Pastoralmedicin. Die Naturwissenschaft auf dem Gebiete der katholischen Moral und Pastoral. Ein Handbuch für den katholischen Clerus, 2nd edn, Freiburg: Herder 1893, p. 175.

[78] E.g. Schaffrath, Euthanasie (1869), p. 14.

[79] Gottstein, Heilwesen (ca 1926), p. 286.

[80] Gmelin, Allgemeine Therapie (1830), p. 75.

[81] Ferriar, Treatment (1798), p. 193.

consent of the lamentable person when it comes to trading [life's end] with a miserable existence.[82]

It appears though that this was a minority view, one that continued to lose influence in the course of the nineteenth century. There were other authors who warned of the dangers of dysthanasia and cacothanasia as caused by medical intervention, but at the same time they were critical of forgoing therapeutic measures as long as these might still prolong the patient's life. Considering the limited diagnostic and prognostic capabilities of the time, however, it was rarely possible to determine with absolute certainty that that they did not, in certain cases, withhold a treatment that still might have kept the patient alive for a while. For this reason, Reimann, for example, was strictly against "treating [a seemingly hopeless case] merely euthanasically, as this might be one of the few patients that we are wrong about, whom we would be able to save still by exerting an ongoing and vigorous influence."[83] And there were others who urged doctors "to preserve life as long as possible, to be miserly about minutes."[84]

This remained an issue until the patient's last breath. Today the discussion about the use of life-prolonging measures is regarded by many as a modern phenomenon. But while the possibilities of today's intensive care were were beyond imagination back then, people believed they had remedies at their disposal that effectively stimulated the life forces and thus prolong life even when someone lay dying.[85] These were for the most part pungent "stimulants," such as camphor, musk or castoreum, ammonium and naphtha. In the experience of doctors, these remedies had brought back to life many a patient for a certain time. Even in completely hopeless cases, when it was only a matter of hours before death arrived, some doctors, as Richter worded it critically, tried their luck with such remedies.[86] According to Riva-Rocci's account, this practice was very common, so much so that the smell of camphor more or less belonged to the deathbed and was familiar to patients and their families as something which signaled that death was at the doorstep.[87] Franz Kafka, too, in 1924, only a few hours before he died, was denied the lethal morphine shot he had asked for and instead was injected with camphor.[88] The practice of administering camphor to the dying is also reflected in literary depictions of the time. In Klabund's

[82] Hennemann, Kakothanasie (1830), p. 179; this is a very early example of the use of an expression—"wohlüberlegte Zustimmung" ("well-considered consent")—which comes close to the modern expression "informed consent".

[83] Reimann, Schädlichkeit ([1843]), p. 14.

[84] Anonymus, Arzt (1838), p. 231.

[85] Heinzelmann, De euthanasia medica (1845), p. 19; references to such medicines can already be found in the early modern period; see e.g. Detharding, De mortis cura (1723), p. 87 (Detharding, like Wedel, recommended above all amber).

[86] Richter, Euthanasia (1841), p. 366.

[87] Riva-Rocci, Cura (1896), p. 470.

[88] Jörg Zittau, Matt und elend lag er da. Berühmte Kranke und ihre schlechten Ärzte, 2nd edn, Berlin: Ullstein 2009, p. 136.

Die Krankheit (*The Disease,* 1917) the "little Japanese man" working at the sanitarium as an assistant states at the bed of dying Sybil: "I will give her a camphor injection." And he adds: "Incidentally, this is only about prolonging life for a few more hours." "You mean keeping her dying," replies his sidekick Thorax.[89] When Joachim Ziemßen lies dying in Thomas Mann's *Der Zauberberg* (*The Magic Mountain,* 1924), Privy Councilor Behrens, the medical director of the sanitarium, comments: "The heart is giving out rapidly, lucky for him and for us; we can do our duty with camphor injections and the like, without much chance of drawing things out."[90]

9.3 Conflict Between Doctors and Laypeople

By all appearances, many laypeople in the nineteenth and early twentieth centuries were much more open than most doctors to letting people die when death seemed inevitable and indeed to shortening the life of a dying person intentionally. Even someone with the rank of Duke of Rutland wrote in 1840 that it was questionable whether prolonging the suffering of Princess Augusta was desirable given that the fatal outcome of her disease was beyond doubt.[91] Conflicts were inevitable. In his 1913 work *La mort* the Belgian philosopher Maurice Maeterlinck addressed the issue openly:

> All doctors consider it their principal duty to draw out as much as possible even the most desperate death struggle with its terrible convulsions. [...] They are so sure of themselves; and the duty they feel bound by leaves so little room for doubt that compassion and reason, blinded by tears, reign themselves in and shrink from a principle that everybody accepts and worships as the highest principle of human conscience.

Thus, some doctors stingily counted the "drops of charity and of peace"—this obviously refers to narcotics—which they "should administer lavishly. [...] They are afraid of breaking the final resistance, that is, the most futile and most painful convulsions of a life that is not yet willing to give in to the approaching rest."[92] As Maeterlinck saw it, doctors in this way put the family in the position of powerless supplicants: "Who has not felt the urge twenty times at the deathbed, indeed, who has not dared to throw himself down at their feet and ask them for mercy?" The doctors held that, even if in the majority of cases, life could be "prolonged for only several days or a few months at the most," "the hundred thousand torments were not

---

89 Klabund, Krankheit (1917), pp. 69–70; cf. Déirdre Mahkorn, Die Darstellung von Krankheit im Werk Klabunds, Cologne: typescript med. diss. 2003; Max, Literarische Texte (2008); Caroline Korf, Davoser Sanatorien im Spiegel der Literatur: Tuberkulose bei Franke, Klabund und Marti, Norderstedt: GRIN Verlag 2008.

90 Mann, Magic mountain (1929), p. 675.

91 Letter from John Henry, Duke of Rutland to Henry Halford, September 19, 1840, cit. in William Munk, The life of Sir Henry Halford, London 1895, pp. 240–1.

92 Maeterlinck, Vom Tode (1913), pp. 6–8.

in vain." Others called this nothing more than "a long death." In this case, medical knowledge ultimately only served to make patients "die more painfully than ignorant animals. One day, science will go up against its own fallacy and no longer hesitate to shorten our agony."[93]

Accounts written by patients and relatives illustrate the tensions and conflicts that arose from the doctors' restraint.[94] Time and again, the sick, in their already weakened state, found themselves exposed, almost powerless, to the pressuring of doctors, even if it was sometimes trivial, as in the case of the author Sophie Cottin, who complained that her doctors considered it their duty to prolong her agony by giving her strengthening bouillons.[95]

The French composer Hector Berlioz in his memoirs described with great urgency his painful experience of powerlessness when faced with a doctor's insistence on prolonging life at all cost:

> I lost my older sister Nanci. She died of breast cancer after six months of terrible suffering that wrenched heartbreaking cries from her night and day. [...] And not a single doctor had the humanity ["humanité"], to put an end to this martyrdom by giving my sister a bottle of chloroform to breathe. This is something that is done to save a patient the pain of a surgical operation that lasts a quarter of a minute, and yet one refrains from using this remedy to relieve someone of a torment of six months. When there is proof, certainty, that no remedy, nothing, not time either can heal a terrible illness, when death is obviously the greatest good, is liberation, joy, blessedness!...

Indeed, "with pain like this, you have to be a barbarian or a fool or both to not choose the safe and mild remedy that we have today and put an end to it. The savages are wiser and more humane."[96]

These contrasts between the physicians' insistence on keeping patients alive as long as possible and the wish of the family to let the terminally ill die in peace are powerfully evoked in the fiction of the day as well. In Paul Heyse's novella *Auf Tod und Leben* (*A Matter of Life and Death,* 1884) young Lucile says,

> I'll admit that I often shook my head when I saw how doctors thought it their duty to hold back a lost life that was running pitifully through their hands, doing so with all their effort and art, for weeks, days and hours, how they prolonged suffering only to eke out a little more of the poor existence that had lost all value; how they were miserly with the last breaths, as if wanting to extend the stay of execution of a condemned person at any cost. Is this not one of the cruelest, most thoughtless prejudices of human society?[97]

With bitter irony, Thomas Mann portrayed this attitude in his novel *Buddenbrooks* (1901). The dying Frau Consul implores her doctors to give her a remedy to help her

---

[93] Ibid., p. 6.

[94] See also Jalland, Death (1996), p. 92.

[95] Bibliothèque Nationale, Paris, NAF 15985, 1807.

[96] Hector Berlioz, Mémoires [...] comprenant ses voyages en Italie, en Allemagne, en Russie et en Angleterre 1803–1865, Paris: Ed. du Sandre 2010, pp. 469–70.

[97] Heyse, Auf Leben und Tod (1886), pp. 284f; cf. Käser, Arzt (1998), pp. 150–78.

sleep: "'I want—I cannot—let me sleep! Have mercy, gentlemen—let me sleep!'" "But the physicians knew their duty: they were obliged, under all circumstances, to preserve life just as long as possible; and a narcotic would have effected an unresisting and immediate giving-up of the ghost. Doctors were not made to bring death into the world, but to preserve life at any cost. There was a religious and moral basis for this law, which they had known once, though they did not have it in mind at the moment. So they strengthened the heart action by various devices, and even improved the breathing by causing the patient to retch." The sick woman died a short while later.[98]

Showing a similar critical attitude, the physician and writer Max Nassauer (1869–1931) in his *Sterben...ich bitte darum!* (*Dying ... yes, please!*, 1911) has his protagonist, who suffers from cancer, comment on the doctors' "hangman's art" at his father's deathbed:

> The doctors tried to help him day and night. They managed to keep the man alive for ten more days. With injections and other things. And they knew from the start that he could not be saved, that he would not regain consciousness. They made no pretence of it. Let me tell you, this was an unforgettable horror for us, his wife and us children. Day by day, night by night, hour by hour, the man who wanted to die, and the doctors who prevented it. [...] This was the most horrible thing I ever experienced, these ten days, these ten nights, the way my father died.[99]

9.4 A Right to Know? Dealing with Fatal Prognosis

The question to what degree terminally ill patients should be told about their nearing end remained controversial among physicians of the nineteenth and early twentieth centuries. Thanks to their increasingly dominant position at the deathbed, physicians carried more responsibility than ever in this respect. While British doctors, as Pat Jalland was able to show with family records, tended to speak more openly to their patients,[100] most medical authors on the European continent continued to be reluctant.[101] Works on *euthanasia medica* regularly cautioned their medical readers to practice utmost restraint, even when the patient explicitly demanded to hear the true prognosis, no matter how calm and stoic the patient seemed.[102] The doctor even had to check carefully his gestures, his facial expression and his speech

---

[98] Thomas Mann, Buddenbrooks. The decline of a family. London: Secker 1924 (first German edn. 1901), book 2, p. 172; cf. Grote, Tod (1996), pp. 91–7; Paul, Tod (2005), pp. 53–7.

[99] Nassauer, Sterben (1911), p. 62; on Nassauer's novella see Grübler, Euthanasie (2011), pp. 101–4, and Claudia Meißner, Dr. Max Nassauer. Arzt und Schriftsteller, Aachen: typescript med. diss., TH Aachen 2000, esp. pp. 82–3.

[100] Jalland, Death (1996), pp. 108–16.

[101] For example Thierfelder, Darf der Arzt...? (1843); overviews in Brand, Ärztliche Ethik (1977), pp. 147–50; Karen Nolte, "Telling the painful truth". Nurses and physicians in the nineteenth century, in: Nursing history review 16 (2008), pp. 115–34; see also Nolte, Ärztliche Praxis (2010a), 43–6; Carol, Les médecins (2004), pp. 18–28; Szabo, Incurable (2009), pp. 114–7.

[102] Hoffmann, Inhalt (1969), p. 66.

as well, because all this was closely observed by wary patients—especially women.[103] Even with patients who seemed to possess strength of mind, the doctor risked making a big mistake, explained Leo Lebrecht:

> They plead with him, try everything to squeeze it out of him, as it were. They talk of the necessity of tidying up their business and say that they are prepared for anything, that they await their fate contentedly and calmly. Here the doctor has to be on guard and not let himself be misled by such enthusiasm. Many sick people who boast of awaiting death coolly still retain a little hope of getting well again and would plunge into terrible despair if told their true situation. This not only would make all saving efforts on the side of nature no longer possible but would hasten death itself.[104]

In fact, many a patient who could have lived on had died upon hearing the sad news, claimed Lebrecht.[105] And summing up this notion succinctly, Pugnet asked in 1837, "Does this not mean murdering the patient?" "This is opening his grave and putting him in while he is still alive!"[106]

In addition to the worry that disclosing a bad prognosis would break the vital force and contribute to making the sickness worse, another, new worry was now heard: There had been cases, it was said, of desperate patients killing themselves after learning of their inescapable fate.[107]

On the down-side, this practice of concealment weighed on the doctor-patient relationship. It created an atmosphere of profound distrust. An oft-quoted saying went, "Mentiris ut medicus," "You lie like a physician." As early as 1700, Döbeln had already remarked that people complained that "you seldom learn the truth about the course of the illness from a physician."[108] Inevitably the patients would try to read the doctor's facial expression or deduce the true prognosis from the doctor's actions, as when he prescribed only simple, mild remedies which might indicate that he did not want to burden the terminally ill person unnecessarily but could, of course, also reflect his judging the disease to be of little importance.[109]

From the late eighteenth century, some writers began to insist on the unwelcome effects of concealment. As the Görlitz doctor and apothecary Christian August Struve (1767–1807) explained, "Certainty about one's condition" was always

---

[103] Hellwag, De euthanasia (1841), pp. 15–16; Stubendorff, De euthanasia medica (1836), p. 24.

[104] Lebrecht, Arzt (1821), pp. 101–2.

[105] Ibid.

[106] J. François Xavier Pugnet, Beobachtungen und Erfahrungen aus dem Gebiete der praktischen Heilkunst, 2 vols, Aarau: Sauerländer 1837, quoted, without page numbers, in Thierfelder, Darf der Arzt […]? (1843), p. 153.

[107] C. B. Tilanus, Over de behandeling van carcinoma (= reprint from: Nederlandsch weekblad voor geneeskundigen (1851/52)), p. 12; Putz, De euthanasia (1843), p. 11. A rich fictional account of the manifold negative effects, which knowing that death is inevitable can have on the patients and those around them, was given by the physician-writer Arthur Schnitzler (Schnitzler, Sterben [1892] (1961); cf. Grote, Tod (1996), pp. 56–76; Paul, Tod (2005), pp. 73–94).

[108] Döbeln, De erroribus (1700), p. 64.

[109] Ibid.

better, "than a changeable back and forth of the mind and emotions."[110] At any rate, the moribund often knew quite well that they were in a bad position, thought Ernestine von Krosigk in 1834. So it was "only empty consolatory prattle, unsympathetic even, to try and reassure a sick person by presenting his malady as something less than it actually is and that he himself senses," she wrote.[111] Gossweiler held that if the words of the doctor "most decidedly contradicted" the sense and the conviction of the sick person, then "distrust and unwillingness" followed.[112] In his novella *The Death of Ivan Ilych* (*Smert' Ivana Ilyicha,* 1886), Leo Tolstoy impressively evoked the resulting insecurity felt by the sick in the late nineteenth century:

> What tormented Ivan Ilych most was the deception, the lie, which for some reason they all accepted, that he was not dying but was simply ill, and that he only need keep quiet and undergo a treatment and then something very good would result. He however knew that [...] nothing would come of it, only still more agonizing suffering and death. This deception tortured him—their not wishing to admit what they all knew and what he knew, but wanting to lie to him concerning his terrible condition, and wishing and forcing him to participate in that lie. Those lies—lies enacted over him on the eve of his death and destined to degrade this awful, solemn act to the level of their visitings, their curtains, their sturgeon for dinner—were a terrible agony for Ivan Ilych.[113]

At that time, in the late nineteenth century, criticism of this dominant culture of concealment was also beginning to gain momentum among doctors. More and more authors voiced their doubt that sharing the prognosis would have disastrous consequences on the course of a disease. Duncan, in a talk for the London Abernethian Society in 1886, stated his conviction.

> It is said that a knowledge of the truth has an injurious effect on the progress of many diseases. I do not believe it. [...] I am among those who believe that the truth communicated to an inquiring doubting patient has a decidedly beneficial therapeutic effect, at least in the majority of cases.[114]

The patients "need to be told the truth" the Danish doctor Emil Hornemann demanded. "It is the doctor first and foremost who has to remind them of death."[115]

This tendency toward more openness also reflected a profound change in the medical understanding of the relation between the body and the soul. In the nineteenth century, the affects or "movements of the soul" came to be interpreted primarily as actions of the soul or psyche and were no longer identified as concrete disruptions of the material, physical movement of the life spirits and the blood. This

---

[110] Struve, Kunst (1799), Teil 2, p. 246.

[111] Krosigk, Umgang (1834), p. 108.

[112] Gossweiler, Erinnerungen (1838), p. 36.

[113] Leo Tolstoy, The death of Ivan Ilych, transl. by Louise and Aylmer Maude, Grand Rapids: Christian Classics Ethereal Library [sine anno], p. 27.

[114] Matthews Duncan, Concerning medical education 1886, pp. 16–17, cit. in Browne, Care of the dying (1894), p. 23.

[115] Hornemann, Vom Zustande (1881), pp. 14–16, cit. p. 14.

meant that the centuries-old conviction that strong negative affects almost inevitably caused the physical condition of the severely sick to worsen lost ground.

Added to this came a new ideal, a new norm that was being established: the patient's right to full access to information. As early as the late eighteenth century, James Boswell quoted the ill Samuel Johnson, speaking about doctors who lied to patients. "You have no business with consequences; you are to tell the truth."[116] "Surely an adult has a right to know the state of his own body and its prospects," was also the conclusion of M. Duncan. "He consults you to know what is the matter, what he should do, what he may expect. You have no right to mystify or deceive him, even under the specious pretext of doing what is best for him."[117]

To be sure, most medical writers still continued to advocate concealment or at least great restraint, around 1900,[118] which they saw as an important element of "psychological treatment."[119] Only very few patients actually wanted to know the full truth, claimed Silas Weir Mitchell. While he never found that news of a bad prognosis shortened patients' life, it made them more miserable in most cases. Doctors should be open only if the patient persisted in asking him directly.[120] If the patient had to attend to the salvation of his soul or had to put important worldly matters in order, the doctor was to tell him the truth "in a gentle manner," thought Alfred Moll, still qualifying this statement by adding that the doctor had to be very careful, unless the terminal patient asked him unambiguously for his prognosis.[121] Haeberlin wrote that the doctor must not "before the patient's eyes tear away the veil of hope that nature had sparingly put over the future," because "he might kill when killing hope." This was all the more true as the doctor could never be sure of his prognosis.[122] Accordingly, Ostermann cautioned in his instructions on the "care of the dying" that one was to avoid in the presence of the sick "making even the faintest remark about their condition or about the nearing end."[123] And Haeberlin for his part held that even the family did not have to be told everything. The doctor was to "present them with both the favorable and the serious prospects" and inform them "that he could only talk about probabilities."[124]

The dissemination of medical knowledge among laypeople became a further argument against communicating a bad prognosis openly. Krecke admitted that every person had "a right to learn essential information" about the nature of his

[116] James Boswell, Boswell's Life of Johnson, vol. 4, ed. by George Birkbeck Hill, revised by L. F. Powell, Oxford 1934, p. 306, conversation on June 13, 1784.

[117] Matthews Duncan, Concerning medical education 1886, pp. 16–17, cit. in Browne, Care of the dying (1894), p. 23.

[118] Elkeles has arrived at the same conclusion; see Elkeles, Schweigsame Welt (1989), pp. 72–4.

[119] Max Berl, Zur palliativen Behandlung des inoperablen Uteruscarcinoms, med. diss., Munich Gerstenberg [1910].

[120] Silas Weir Mitchell, Doctor and patient, Philadelphia: Lippincott 1888, pp. 46–52.

[121] Moll, Ärztliche Ethik (1902), pp. 121–124 and pp. 188–9.

[122] Haeberlin, Vom Beruf (1919), pp. 91–2.

[123] Ostermann, Krankenpflegelehrbuch (1928), pp. 327–8.

[124] Haeberlin, Vom Beruf (1919), p. 92.

condition, but "knowledge of medical matters" had meanwhile "penetrated lay circles so deeply and the encyclopedia is often consulted so thoroughly after a medical consultation that the patient can get into quite a desperate emotional state if given too much information." Particularly with cancer, it was thus better to be content with vague circumscriptions and refer, for example, to a "lump in the uterus, in the stomach, in the chest" that just might become malignant later on.[125]

To what degree unfavorable prognoses were communicated in everyday life can only be roughly discerned from largely anecdotal accounts or general remarks found in contemporary sources. There are many indications that, as late as the nineteenth and early twentieth centuries, doctors and relatives mostly tried to hide the foreseeable end from the moribund. In 1817, Osiander wrote about a young patient who had heard someone say—perhaps the doctor, a friend or an attendant—that he would hardly outlive the night. Obviously, the sick man had heard what was not meant for his ears. Until only a few hours before his death, they had tried to keep the truth from him.[126] When the treatment given to Louis Benoît Coppens, who suffered from a lung disease, was no longer effective, the attending doctor put the patient's sister in the picture, saying that if there were any family matters the sick man had to settle, he should do so promptly. The sick man himself was left in the dark, and the sister, too, apparently kept the bad news to herself, while her brother, on his own account, arrived at "the cruel certainty" that he would not recover from his illness.[127] Henry Halford as well hesitated until the last moment to tell his dying patients the plain truth. In the case of the terminally ill Duke of York, he was even supported in this by the King, George IV, who voiced his grave concern that the ill duke might become depressed and discouraged at the slightest indication that he was in danger. Even 2 weeks before the duke died, Halford was only willing to allow a friend of the duke to tell him that he had detected in the face of the doctor signs of increased concern.[128] At times, relatives and doctors entered into something like a conspiracy to pull the wool over the eyes of a terminally ill family member. For example, in 1832, the husband of a patient of Samuel Hahnemann, "deeply grieved" about the unfavorable prognosis for his sick wife, asked the founder of homeopathy to write a second letter that he could show his wife. The letter was to say that the illness of his wife, while "not minor, was not life-threatening either."[129]

When it came to the rural population and workers, by contrast, contemporary writers described the ways a fatal prognosis and approaching death were handled—depending on the perspective—as either more natural or more brutal. Krecke

[125] Krecke, Vom Arzt (1932), p. 100.

[126] Friedrich Benjamin Osiander, Über die Entwicklungskrankheiten in den Blüthenjahren des weiblichen Geschlechts, part 1, Tübingen: Bey dem Verfasser 1817, pp. 119–20.

[127] Archives Générales du Royaume, Brussels, family archive Van Male de Ghorain n. 382 /3 "Récit de la maladie et des derniers jours de Louis Benoît Coppens, relatés par sa soeur, 1836".

[128] Letter from Halford to C. H. Taylor, August 18, 1826, in William Munk, The life of Sir Henry Halford, London: Longmans, Green & Co. 1895, pp. 160–2.

[129] Institut für Geschichte der Medizin der Robert Bosch-Stiftung, Stuttgart, Hahnemannarchiv, B 32466, letter from E. J. Wehli, Vienna, April 12,1832.

advised doctors with patients in the countryside to conceal the true nature of an illness even from the family, so they would not throw the bad prognosis at the sick. This was because people there did not particularly appreciate "the subtle consideration of the cultured human being and the politeness of the heart."[130] Erich Stern summarized his personal experience in a Swiss sanitarium for the wealthy and in a people's sanitarium in France, saying that families belonging to the less privileged classes were "generally much calmer and natural in the face of death" than members of "socially superior circles." In the private sanitariums, one sought to conceal death, and the patients hardly talked about it either. In people's sanitariums with their lower-class patients by contrast, the dead were carried out of their rooms openly and the sick talked about "who is feeling badly and who will die" and about "how long this or that patient may still have to live."[131]

[130] Krecke, Vom Arzt (1932), p. 108.

[131] Erich Stern, Die Psyche des Lungenkranken klinisch-psychologische und sozial-psychologische Untersuchungen über den Einfluß der Lungentuberkulose und des Sanatoriumslebens auf die Psyche des Kranken, 2nd revised edn (orig. Halle 1925), Berlin–Charlottenburg: Carl Marhold 1954, p. 66.

Institutional Care 10

One of the most profound changes in how dying was approached and how medical end-of-life care was administered—changes that came about between 1800 and 1970 and continue to have a shaping influence today—was the growing significance of inpatient institutions and the development of modern palliative care units and hospices for the dying. Some modern authors declared the medieval and early modern "hospitals" and "hospices" to have been the precursors of these modern institutions.[1] For centuries however, "hospitals" were almost exclusively for the care of a small, predominantly poor minority of people who had noone who was able or willing to take care of them. These houses were a refuge for people who were unable to work, for the lame, the blind and the deaf, for the insane and epileptics as well as for people with severe, chronic physical ailments. In larger institutions a doctor or surgeon might make regular visits but most "hospitals" were not primarily medical institutions and they certainly were not set up to provide medical care to dying patients. Residents often lived in them for many years, until they died. In relation to the number of beds, the annual number of deaths was therefore usually very small.

The pre-modern "hospices" or "hospitia" as well had little more than the name in common with the eponymous modern institutions. The word "hospice", just like the word "hospital", derives from the Latin *hospes,* meaning "host" (or also "guest").[2] The hospices of centuries past were primarily hostels or inns for pilgrims and travellers, which is why they were often built along travelling routes and pilgrim trails, at mountain passes and bridges. These were not institutions in which the dying were afforded an alleviation of their agonies. "The idea that hospices, as places concerned specifically with the care of the dying have a history stretching back into

[1] E.g., William E. Phipps, The origin of hospices/hospitals, in: Death studies 12 (1988), pp. 91–9.

[2] Cf. Charles Talbot's comments on the history of the term in Goldin, A protohospice (1981), pp. 387–9; in modern Dutch the term "Gasthuis" is still commonly used for "hospital".

M. Stolberg, *A History of Palliative Care, 1500–1970*, Philosophy and Medicine 123,
DOI 10.1007/978-3-319-54178-5_10

early times is misleading, and serves little purpose in advancing our understanding of such care in the past," David Clark has correctly noted.[3]

Sometimes, more specifically, the pre-modern French *hospices*—with the stately Hôtel Dieu de Beaune serving as a very popular example—are declared precursors of the modern hospices for the dying, yet they have little in common with them. In Beaune and elsewhere, the designation "hospice" was used largely synonymously with "hôpital."[4] The term still today means "old-age home" and "nursing home" in the general sense, and so the French phrase "être bon pour l'hospice," refers to being old, not to suffering from a terminal disease. Unlike in England, it was therefore not possible in the 1970s in Canada with its francophone contingent to refer to institutions for the dying as "hospices" as it would have been misunderstood by the French-speaking population.

Very few pre-modern hospitals provided medical care for the curable sick on a major scale.[5] Featuring prominently among these are the large hospitals of northern Italian cities, such as the Santa Maria Nuova in Florence or San Francesco in Padua.[6] North of the Alps, there were also a few institutions that acted to a considerable degree as providers of health care proper. The Heilig-Geist-Spital in Nuremberg, for example, at the behest of its founder, reserved 128 beds for the curably sick.[7] Close to one third of its patients in the seventeenth century were released within 3 weeks of their admission.[8] The Frankfurt Heilig-Geist-Spital, too, admitted roughly one third of its patients—as far as we can tell from the records—on the grounds of an illness.[9] The Julius-Spital in Würzburg was designed from its very beginning to offer amongst others medical care for the sick.[10] However, these were exceptions.

---

[3] Clark, Cradled to the grave? (1999), p. 66; see also Talbot in Goldin, St. Luke's House (1981), p. 389; J.-M. Nuñez Olarte, Care of the dying in eighteenth-century Spain—the non-hospice tradition, in: European journal of palliative care 6 (1999), pp. 23–7.

[4] See e.g., Curchod de Necker, Hospice de Charité (1780); Olivier Faure, Genèse de l'hôpital moderne. Les hospices civiles de Lyon de 1802 à 1845, Lyon: Presses Universitaires de Lyon 1982.

[5] Special cases were plague lazarettos, which served primarily to protect the rest of the population from contagion, and the hospitals for the treatment of patients with syphilis or the "French disease".

[6] John Henderson, The Renaissance hospital: healing the body and healing the soul, New Haven: Yale University Press 2006; Matheus, Funktions- und Strukturwandel (2005); Carlos Watzka, Vom Hospital zum Krankenhaus. Zum Umgang mit psychisch und somatisch Kranken im frühneuzeitlichen Europa, Cologne: Böhlau 2005; Alain Montandon (ed.), Lieux d'hospitalité. Hospices, hôpital, hostellerie, Clermont–Ferrand: Presses universitaires 2001; Gisela Drossbach (ed.), Hospitäler in Mittelalter und Früher Neuzeit. Frankreich, Deutschland und Italien. Eine vergleichende Geschichte, Munich: Oldenbourg 2007.

[7] Knefelkamp, Pflege (2005), p. 187.

[8] Ibid., pp. 187–8.

[9] Robert Jütte, Das Frankfurter Hl. Geist-Spital im 16. und frühen 17. Jahrhundert. Aufgabe und Funktion einer bürgerlichen Fürsorgeanstalt, in: Hessisches Jahrbuch für Landesgeschichte 33 (1983), pp. 145–67.

[10] Andreas Mettenleiter, Das Juliusspital in Würzburg, vol. III: Medizingeschichte, Würzburg: Stiftung Juliusspital 2001, p. 5.

This would change fundamentally beginning in the late eighteenth century with far-reaching consequences for terminal and dying patients. The hospital gained more and more significance as a medical institution. Many of the older hospitals now focused increasingly on the admission of the curable sick. Furthermore, numerous new hospitals were founded. Tellingly, in German, they were now often referred to explicitly as *Krankenhäuser*, meaning "houses for the sick." These new hospitals were intended from the outset to serve the curable sick. A major driving force behind this development was social and economic change. Urbanization and industrialization, on the one hand, and the dissolution of old guild structures, on the other, brought numerous unmarried workers, journeymen and domestic servants to the cities. When they fell ill, they often had no one to care for them. Yet their swift recovery was in the best interest of their masters as well as of the municipal authorities. The masters wanted to have their manpower back, while the authorities sought to prevent sick workers from adding to the hordes of beggars and vagabonds, which at the time came to be increasingly seen as a problem for public security and order. In some German cities of the late eighteenth century, so-called *Gesellen- und Dienstboten-Institute*, i.e. domestic servants and journeymen funds, were set up, constituting an early form of modern health insurance. Domestic servants and journeymen paid compulsory contributions into these funds. In return, they were entitled to free inpatient care in hospitals which, in some places, were in fact financed in large part with the contributions.[11]

This development was accompanied by a self-confident therapeutic optimism on the part of hospital physicians. The growing physiological and pathological knowledge and new theories such as Brownianism or, in Germany, a medical theory that was influenced by Schelling's natural philosophy, pointed toward a future in which doctors would be able to cure almost any illness. Even an official compendium for hospitals in Paris stated in 1832 that, "the number of diseases that were once quickly identified as incurable is getting smaller by the day."[12] From today's perspective, the theories of the day seem highly speculative and the resulting therapeutic approaches hardly fit to improve treatment. But the doctors, at the time, believed in these possibilities and had their minds set on making the hospital a place for the curative treatment of patients.

This distinct curative function of the hospital had paradoxical consequences for the relevance of the hospital as a place of dying, consequences to which historians have not paid much attention so far: The more the hospital focused on treating only patients whose diseases were considered curable, the more it also became a place of dying. The mortality rate as such was sometimes decidedly low, especially at the new hospitals that were established for curable patients from the start. Most journeymen and domestic servants were young and often presented with simple acute

[11] For a survey see Alfons Labisch and Reinhard Spree, Krankenhaus-Report 19. Jahrhundert. Krankenhausträger, Krankenhausfinanzierung, Krankenhauspatienten, Frankfurt: Campus 2001.

[12] F.-S. Ratier, Formulaire pratique des hôpitaux civils de Paris, ou recueil des préscriptions médicamenteuses employées par les médecins et chirurgiens de ces établissemens, Paris: J.-P. Baillière 1832, p. 14.

illnesses, from which they recovered quickly. For the years 1821–1829, the Würzburg Julius-Spital, for example, had an average mortality rate of 5.9%.[13] Especially the new, large, urban hospitals now cared for many times the patients per year, however, than would have been admitted to the traditional type of hospital—and some of these patients were bound to die. With a total of more than 10,000 patients per year there would have been, even with a very low mortality rate, between one and two deaths every week. And at some hospitals of the new, curative type, the mortality rate was considerably higher than in Würzburg. At the Paris Hôpital Saint Antoine, which had been opened in a former abbey in 1796, 3933 of the 21,860 patients who were admitted between 1803 and 1813 died there. This amounts to an average of one patient per day. Death in these institutions had literally become an everyday occurrence.[14]

The importance of the hospital as a place of dying grew dramatically in the second half of the nineteenth century. Far into the nineteenth century, many people avoided going to the hospital if they could afford to. In many places, hospitalization originally even required a certificate of poverty and was seen as dishonorable.[15] As Lampe explained in Petersburg in 1789, an "utter dislike of all public institutions" was even felt by impoverished but formerly better-off patients.[16] When sick people from a somewhat wealthier background went to a hospital because the institution had a good reputation, as did the Paris *Hospice de Charité,* this was considered worth mentioning.[17] This changed in the course of the nineteenth and early twentieth centuries. The number of patients in hospitals continued to multiply. Industrialization and urbanization caused a steep increase in the numbers of men and women, who had no one to look after them when they got sick. At the same time, hospitals became increasingly attractive as institutions that offered the best-possible medical expertise and treatment. More and more of the financially better off also went to the hospital believing they would find the best doctors there and receive the best medical treatment. Inevitably, in a certain number of serious cases, no medical effort could prevent a fatal outcome, however. Mortality rates were frequently low but with the massive rise in the number of admissions, the importance of the hospital as a place of dying also continued to grow dramatically. Increasingly, people people from all walks and life—an not only the poor and destitute—no longer died at home, among family, but in the hospital.

---

[13] Johanna Bleker, Eva Brinkschulte and Pascal Grosse (eds), Kranke und Krankheiten im Juliusspital zu Würzburg 1819–1829. Zur frühen Geschichte des allgemeinen Krankenhauses in Deutschland, Husum: Matthiesen 1995, appendix. My thanks to Johanna Bleker for giving me to access the raw data.

[14] Pastoret, Rapport (1816), pp. 227–8.

[15] Cf. Jean Imbert, Mourir à l'hôpital, in: Jean-Pierre Bardet and Madeleine Foisil (eds), La vie, la mort, la foi, le temps. Mélanges offerts à Pierre Chaunu, Paris 1993: Presses Universitaires de France, pp. 345–37, esp. p. 353, with contemporary references.

[16] Lampe, Nachricht (1789).

[17] Curchod de Necker, Hospice de Charité (1780), p. 5.

10.1 No Room for Hopeless Cases

The hospital's transition from a facility that offered a refuge for a wide range of poor and needy people to a medical institution meant not only that life ended in the hospital for far more people than in previous times. It also had far-reaching and largely negative effects on how incurable and dying patients were cared for. While most traditional hospitals had not primarily admitted patients for medical treatment, they had opened their doors, to some degree at least, also to those who suffered from chronic and ultimately fatal diseases. The more hospitals came to be reserved for the curable sick, the less many of them had room for hopeless cases. These cases might be admitted initially, but as we learn from contemporary accounts, when the doctors could no longer help, it was common practice to discharge these patients as incurable, no longer served by the mandate of the hospital.[18] Some terminally ill patients had nowhere to go and lived in the street, such as a certain Jane, who was discharged from St. George's Hospital as "incurable" and soon after died one cold January night in the street.[19] Even patients who had gone in for a serious surgical intervention had to be prepared to be shown to the door if the treatment turned out to be ineffective—and be it only because the doctor did not want to be faced on a daily basis with the consequences of his failed treatment, as some critical voices claimed.[20]

The main reason for the rejection or discharge of incurable and hopeless cases was that the beds were needed for the many acute patients. Yet, by the end of the nineteenth century, also another, new reason emerged, namely the hospital's concern with its reputation. The mortality rate increasingly became the standard for measuring the quality of care at a hospital. "There are hospitals that refuse to admit those patients because they don't want to have bad results," observed Sanders in 1875. It was known that the mortality depended crucially on the kind of clientele that was admitted, and that the number of sick people "who entered a hospital in a state beyond hope and died within 24 hours" varied greatly.[21] At the same time, no one was willing to risk acquiring the reputation of a "death cave," as was the case with the Hôtel Dieu in Paris, which, around 1800, was known throughout Europe for its high mortality rate. Therefore, at the *Hospital for Consumption and Diseases of the Chest* in London, for example, efforts were made to prevent the terminally ill from being admitted. There was no benefit to the patients, it was claimed, and their death meant a rise in expenditures and caused the mortality at the hospital to rise "in an unfair manner."[22]

---

[18] Lund, Palliative medicine (1880), p. 9.

[19] Westminster Abbey Library and Muniment Room, Westminster Coroner's Inquests, 1760–1799, January 16, 1765, cit. in Siena, Suicide (2009), p. 61.

[20] See Nolte, Wege (2006b), p. 42, on the ways in which F. B. Osiander dealt with one of his female patients.

[21] Sander, Krankenhäuser (1875), p. 7; similarly already Curchod de Necker, Hospice de Charité (1780), pp. 18–19.

[22] Husson, Hôpitaux (1862), p. 259.

As we have seen, medical writers in the late eighteenth and early nineteenth century, more than ever, declared the care for the dying an important duty of doctors. Yet the hospital, the very institution that was becoming the site of best available medical care, was inaccessible to most people with an advanced, terminal disease. This problem did not go unnoticed. The situation seemed irreconcilable with the kind of well-ordered, enlightened poor relief and healthcare that was championed by many municipal governments and territorial princes in the late eighteenth and early nineteenth centuries. A range of solutions to this problems emerged.

In some places, the hospitals' admissions restrictions on incurable and dying patients were more or less simply ignored. Numerous hospitals were destined for the curable sick but ended up with a certain percentage of incurable and dying patients. This could happen all the more easily since the prognosis at the time was often uncertain, even for seriously ill patients. Patients were admitted to a hospital with the hope that they would be cured and only with time this hope proved elusive. The decision was especially difficult in the case of strokes. Quite often, strokes resulted in death within only few days or else were at the beginning of years of lingering illness but sometimes patients quickly improved under medical treatment.

Some hospitals went one step further. In addition to their curable patients, they deliberately accepted patients suffering from consumption or cancer in advanced stages, patients for whom there was no realistic prospect of a successful cure from the start. In the city hospital of Passau, for example, around 2000 patients were treated between 1837 and 1843. Most of them were acute patients, but there were also 75 consumptive patients, 36 of whom died at the hospital. Apparently most of them had come to the hospital in a very advanced stage of their illness. In the words of the hospital doctor, "obsolete" cases also predominated among dropsical patients, "incurable individuals" who, "in their last stage sought refuge and accommodation in the hospital."[23] At the Hôpital Saint Antoine in Paris, 100 out of 442 deaths in the year 1807, or close to 25%, were attributed to advanced consumption and other chronic diseases of the lung, 21 more patients died of hardened tumors and cancer and 18 of organic heart diseases.[24] At the Allgemeines Krankenhaus in Vienna, as many as 758 of 1214 deaths were caused by tuberculosis.[25] In some locations, pressure from the general public played a role, too. The hospital in Lyon, for example, despite its curative focus, admitted many chronically ill patients as well, and when in the end they were turned out onto the street, this sometimes met with fierce protests, and in some cases the hospital was forced to readmit them.[26]

---

[23] F. X. Bernhuber, Jahresberichte über die während eines Zeitraumes von sechs Jahren im Stadt-Krankenhause zu Passau aufgenommenen Kranken und behandelten Krankheitsformen, Landshut: Commissions-Verlag der Krüll'schen Universitäts-Buchhandlung 1843, pp. 54–60.

[24] Pastoret, Rapport (1816), pp. 227–8.

[25] Oppert, Hospitäler (1872), pp. 293–4.

[26] Cf. Olivier Faure, Genèse de l'hôpital moderne. Les hospices civiles de Lyon de 1802 à 1845, Lyon: Presses Universitaires de Lyon 1982, pp. 60–2.

There were also institutions that explicitly offered some of their beds for hopeless cases and the dying. In Würzburg, for example, the local government permitted on a provisional basis, in 1791, against the resistance of the hospital management, that moribund patients be admitted to the Julius-Spital. The government conceded that the incurable and moribund were,

> not quite suited to the Julius-Spital, especially as those who go on living there for several years can take away the room from other, curably ill people. Nevertheless, we have no qualms about tentatively allowing those to be admitted who, according to the doctor's probable estimation, have no more than six weeks to live.[27]

In the mid-nineteenth century, the Hospitalklinik in Göttingen, too, explicitly admitted patients who came to die. In this case, the reasons were not only humanitarian reasons at play, however. They patients were to be anatomized later.[28]

Occasionally, the medical care of incurably sick and dying patients could even become the principle task of a hospital whose mandate was officially curative. An impressive example is the Hundertsuppe, the new hospital for the poor, established in Nuremberg in 1780.[29] Its founders dedicated it to the impoverished curable sick who could not be cared for adequately at home. The house was to close a gap in the city's healthcare, giving this group of ill people a better prospect of getting well by offering good medical care. However, in practice, the hospital became the earliest known inpatient facility that, like a modern hospice, served primarily as a sanctuary for the dying. Of the first 24 patients admitted, 21 died in the hospital, most of them within a few days or weeks.[30] Subsequently, the proportion of patients who were considered "cured" and discharged rose somewhat, yet mortality remained very high. Of the 526 patients who were treated in the first 30 years, between July 1770 and June 1800,[31] 366 or almost 70% died. Thrity six patients were transferred to other institutions, their outcome remaining unknown, or they left early. And yet, the institution was called a *Krankenhaus,* a "house for the sick," for good reason. Half of all admitted patients were under 44 years of age and most of them had been diagnosed with a clearly outlined, usually severe illness. It was the patients and their families who, it appears, perceived the new hospital as mainly a sanctuary for the dying and chose it for this reason. A "large part, even the majority of admitted people," explained the hospital doctor, came "so they will not have to die without

[27] Archiv des Julius Spitals Würzburg, Akt 4005, fol. 6v, cit. in Andreas Mettenleiter, Das Juliusspital in Würzburg, vol. III: Medizingeschichte, Würzburg: Stiftung Juliusspital 2001, pp. 56–7.

[28] Conrad Heinrich Fuchs, Bericht über die medicinische Klinik zu Göttingen im Jahre 1853/54, Göttingen 1855, p. 203, cit. in Nolte, Wege (2006b), p. 40.

[29] For a more detailed account of the Nürnberg "Hundertsuppe" see Stolberg, Europas ältestes Sterbehospiz? (2009).

[30] Another patient was dismissed after 2 months but she was readmitted in 1772 and also died in the hospital (Stadtarchiv Nürnberg C 23/I 2).

[31] Ibid.; the admission books list altogether 556 patients; 30 of them had already been previously in the hospital, in some cases up to three times.

any support, lying on the bare ground and suffering a thousand torments, but will at least have a bed in which to come to life's end."[32] The representative of the city's local alms office accordingly rejected the criticism that mortality was too high and that it proved the hospital's low quality of care. This "proof," he wrote, "would only have weight if many sick people were admitted there to be cured." But the majority of patients did not at all come "to be cured, but to die under charitable care." He explained that many of the poor were "admitted merely for purposes of the final end, so the suffering during the last days of their life can be made more bearable and [so that] they do not have to part with this world lacking all necessities and in a desperate way."[33]

10.2 Hospitals for the Incurable Sick

When the admittance restrictions for chronic and incurable patients were circumvented, people who had a terminal prognosis could find a final sanctuary even in hospitals with a curative mandate. However, these institutions risked blocking beds that were urgently needed for acute patients. Over time, this situation created the political pressure and initiatives to establish special institutions for desperate and dying patients who required medical treatment due to their symptoms.

The roots of such institutions reach far back into the early modern period.[34] Starting around 1500, a number of Italian cities saw the development of institutions known as *ospedali degli incurabili*.[35] The name is somewhat misleading. The mandate of these institutions was decidedly medical. They served above all to care for patients suffering from the French disease which was spreading all over Europe at the time. The symptoms were frequently described as highly dramatic. Sometimes the entire body became dotted with chancres and those afflicted appeared to be rotting alive. But the disease was not considered incurable. The main treatment was with mercury ointments and fumes or else with guaiac wood, both of which were believed to give good results. From the Ospedale degli incurabili in Florence, a list is extant from later times, a statistical document that bears the paradoxical title "incurabili guariti", that is, "cured incurable patients."[36]

Yet, even after the treatment with mercury preparations, the illness often progressed and many patients ultimately succumbed to it. Patients with the French

[32] Stadtarchiv Nürnberg, D15 S14 Nr. 13, letter of justification from Dr. Baier, fall 1801 (copy without a date).

[33] Ibid., report from the *Stadtalmosenamt*, October 2, 1801.

[34] See my brief overview in Michael Stolberg, Fürsorgliche Ausgrenzung. Die Geschichte der Unheilbarenhäuser (1500–1900), in: Historia hospitalium 27 (2011), pp. 71–8.

[35] The best account of the early history of these institutions is still Langasco, "Ospedali degli incurabili" (1938); esp. for Venice and its territory see also Bernard Aikema and D. Meijers, Nel regno dei poveri. Arte e storia dei grandi ospedali veneziani in età moderna, 1474–1797, Venice: Arsenale 1989, pp. 131–148.

[36] Archivio di Stato, Florence, Ospedale della Santissima Trinità detto degli Incurabili 90, Incurabili guariti 1749–1781.

disease were sometimes very disfigured and their transpirations alone were thought to be contagious. Particularly in early modern Italiy, where the large urban hospitals were dedicated primarily to acute patients relatively early on, it was difficult for them to find a hospital bed. In light of this situation, the *ospedali degli incurabili* answered a serious demand.[37] The foundation of the Ospedale degli Incurabili in Rome, for example, was justified explicitly by pointing to the many incurable sick who had been forced into vagrancy for years.[38]

With time, some of the Italian *ospedali degli incurabili* opened their doors not only to people suffering from the French disease but also admitted people with other incurable diseases.[39] In this respect, the boundaries were fluid between these institutions and traditional hospitals for the old, the lame, the blind and others in need of long-term care. This was the case even more so with comparable institutions outside of Italy. The Josephs-Spital, founded in 1624 as a royal court hospital in Munich, was instituted as a place for men and women suffering from incurable, internal and external illnesses or defects who could "not be treated or only with difficulty" in the other hospitals in town.[40] Other than this, the hospital each year also admitted a certain number of people suffering from the French disease as well as other patients with festering ulcers, who would receive medical treatment over the course of several weeks.[41]

The *hospices des incurables,* which were founded during the early modern period in several French cities, served to an even greater degree as institutions that provided care for a wide variety of people in need.[42] As Pastoret wrote in 1816, they were meant "for old age, for children, for incurable diseases."[43] The best-known example is the Hospice des incurables in Paris.[44] Founded in the seventeenth

[37] Thus, according to Langasco, "Ospedali degli incurabili" (1938), the Pammatone hospital in Genua, a city where also one of the first *ospedali degli incurabili* had been established, only accepted patients with diseases that were considered curable.

[38] According to founding charter (Langasco, "Ospedali degli incurabili" (1938), p. 32).

[39] Brian Pullan, The Counter-Reformation, medical care and poor relief, in: Ole Peter Grell, Andrew Cunningham and Jon Arrizabalaga (eds), Health care and poor relief in Counter-Reformation Europe, London – New York: Routledge 1999, pp. 18–39, esp. pp. 21–7.

[40] Founding charter, cit. in Anselm Martin, Geschichtliche Darstellung der Kranken- und Versorgungsanstalten zu München mit medizinisch-administrativen Bemerkungen aus dem Gebiete der Nosokomialpflege, Munich: Franz 1834, pp. 253–4. I am largely summarizing the major results of the detailed research on this institution by Hannes Langrieger, which he unfortunately never published.

[41] Bayerisches Hauptstaatsarchiv, Munich, GL Fasc. 2721, Nr. 645, report of 1705.

[42] Little research has been undertaken so far on the French *hospices des incurables* outside of Paris; however, on Lyon see Olivier Faure: L'hôpital et les incurables au XIXe siècle: l'exemple de Lyon, in: Handicaps et inadaptations (1990), pp. 71–8.

[43] Pastoret, Rapport (1816), p. 250.

[44] Cf. Alain Dauphin and Marc Voisin (eds), De l'hospital des incurables à l'hôpital Laennec 1634–2000, Paris: Hervas 2000; P. Bourée, Heurs et malheurs de l'hospice des incurables, in: Histoire des sciences médicales 8 (1974), pp. 535–9; François Joulet de Châtillon, De l'origine de l'hospice des incurables, Paris: Imprimerie nationale 1885; in 1793 the institution was divided into the Incurables hommes and the Incurables femmes.

century, its statutes stipulated that it had to offer a last refuge to the chronically sick or to invalids who would otherwise showcase their ailments in the streets for everyone to see. Those who were to be admitted were people with paralyses and contractures, with badly healed fractures or chronically dislocated joints, with large growths, with distinct hernias, with prolapses of the uterus or the rectum but also patients with cancer and dropsy. They often stayed for many years.[45] By the 1690, the hospital had a designated doctor who, as noted in 1720, visited once every 8 days; the patients had to pay for his services themselves.[46] The hospice also had its own infirmary for the treatment of acute patients.[47] However, the institution was not primarily meant to offer medical treatment or even care for the dying.

As can be gathered from the lists of different diseases and ailments that were considered incurable at the time, some "incurable" patients—like those suffering from the French disease before them, in the sixteenth-century—required constant and at times intensive medical attention, for example treatment of their ulcers or their agonizing pain. In the eighteenth and nineteenth centuries, the perception grew that caring for this group of people was a problem that needed to be solved. New and increasingly medicalized institutions were created specifically for these patients, and significantly, they were first established predominantly in places where the existing "hospitals" or "houses for the sick" had come to focus more or less exclusively on the treatment of curable illnesses early on. The prototype of this development was the Royal Hospital for Incurables in Dublin, which began its work in May 1744 with 24 beds.[48] It was founded on the initiative of the Charitable Musical Society a few years after the Steevens' Hospital, the Mercer Street Hospital and the Charitable Infirmary had been opened in the same city, all of which were for the benefit of the curable sick. The new institution by contrast, which moved to its final location in the borough of Donnybrook in 1792, opened its doors specifically to patients suffering from various incurable diseases. Excluded from admission to the general hospitals, they were received here to be "palliated."[49] Their illnesses might be incurable, but they were still "susceptible of more or less relief from the physician's skill, and of much soothing from Christian sympathy."[50] Local doctors and surgeons provided medical care, and soon the demand was so high that only a fraction of all applicants met with success in the weekly intake sessions.[51]

---

[45] Carl Maximilian Andrée, Neuester Zustand der vorzüglichsten Spitäler und Armenanstalten in einigen Hauptorten des In- und Auslandes. Part 1: Die Spitäler und Armenanstalten von Paris, Leipzig: Barth 1810, p. 228 and p. 235.

[46] H. Feulard, L'hôpital Laennec, ancien hospice des incurables (1634–1884). Notice historique, Paris: Imprimerie Grandremy & Henon 1884, p. 42; Husson, Hôpitaux (1862), pp. 301–2.

[47] Pastoret, Rapport (1816), p. 250.

[48] Cf. Brady, History (1875); Helen Burke, The Royal Hospital Donnybrook. A heritage of caring 1743–1993, Dublin: University College 1993.

[49] Gentleman [sic] and citizen's almanack 1748, p. 67.

[50] Brady, History (1875), p. 30.

[51] Gentleman [sic] and citizen's almanack 1748, p. 67; Ibid. 1758, p. 71.

In the years to come, the institution expanded and, following its relocation to a new building, had beds for a total of 84 patients in six wards. Five hundred and fifty nine patients had been cared for by 1780.[52] The financial resources did not allow for more. In the nineteenth century, when the available number of places became increasingly inadequate to the growing demand in the city, priority was given to patients with especially malignant cancers or advanced consumption, and, in general, precedence was given to everyone whose suffering was particularly intense and whose medical treatment and care at the hospital could be expected to bring considerable relief.[53]

In other places, too, the plight of the incurable sick with their need for treatment began to be recognized. In the Imperial city of Augsburg, starting in 1718, the town council repeatedly underlined the necessity of an *Incurabelnhaus*. Finally, in 1738, such an institution was officially authorized and endowed with the requisite financial means. Formed from two previous institutions, the leper house St. Servatius and the plague hospital St. Sebastian,[54] the new institution was to admit, according to a memorandum by the city physician Octavianus Floß, the blind, the lame as well as epileptic patients. In addition, those suffering from an incurable stone disease and those who were "afflicted with internal or external cancer or other incurable regular and fistulous sores that were intolerable due to their smell" were to be cared for until their death by nurses and to be given medical treatment by the town physicians.[55]

Bamberg, too, established not only the much admired Allgemeines Krankenhaus, but also, in 1806, a separate hospital for incurables. Its main initiator was Adalbert Friedrich Markus, the doctor in charge of the Allgemeines Krankenhaus, one of the most famous doctors and hospital reformers of his day.[56] He was convinced that a hospital for incurables would also provide a welcome opportunity for doctors in training to gain experience with serious, chronic illnesses.[57] In Regensburg, it was decided in 1821 to erect the Armen Kranken Versorgungshaus, a house for the care of the poor sick to serve "incurables of both sexes and religions" with 40 beds.[58]

---

[52] Gentleman's and citizen's almanack 1780, p. 86.

[53] Brady, History (1875), p. 29; Helen Burke, The Royal Hospital Donnybrook. A heritage of caring 1743–1993, Dublin: University College 1993, p. 46.

[54] This institution is extensively documented in Stadtarchiv Augsburg, St. Servatius 22, 23 und 24. My account is based to a considerable degree on the results of archival research by Hannes Langrieger.

[55] Stadtarchiv Augsburg, St. Servatius 22. It is unclear to what degree these admission rules were heeded in actual practice. From October 1811 until February 1813 we find—among 20 inmates who were mentioned in different sources—only two women with cancer of the breast viz. of the womb.

[56] Cf. Adalbert Friedrich Markus, Über die Einrichtung klinischer Anstalten, in: Magazin für specielle Therapie und Klinik 1 (1803), pp. 425–46; Wolfgang Grünbeck, Der Bamberger Arzt Dr. Adalbert Friedrich Markus, Erlangen–Nürnberg: typescript med. diss. 1971.

[57] For a detailed account see Langrieger, Medizinische Versorgung (2010).

[58] Staatsarchiv Amberg, Regierung des Regenkreises, Kammer des Inneren 883, establishment of a hospital for the poor in Regensburg, 1821–22, extract from the minutes of the session May 21, 1821; on the origins and the further development of this institution see Langrieger, Platz (2008).

Great Britain and North America saw a wave of new facilities for incurable patients from the middle of the nineteenth century. Separate wards established and special institutions were founded, mostly supported by private initiatives and often with religious intentions. They admitted patients who had no prospect of being cured but who, until their death, as it was put, required medical treatment to make their suffering at least more bearable. In 1854, Andrew Reed, a nonconformist clergyman, opened the first institution of this kind in England, the Royal Hospital and Home for Incurables, in Putney near Wimbledon.[59] According to its statutes, it was to provide "a final home for such as would otherwise be the rejected and outcast of mankind."[60] Similar institutions followed, such as The British Home and Hospital for Incurables in 1861. The professed goal was to alleviate with good care and medical treatment the suffering of incurably sick people, to the extent that they were not helped by poor relief efforts.[61] The USA during the late nineteenth century likewise saw the founding of hospitals for incurable patients, specifically in New York, Washington, Baltimore and Philadelphia. Small beginnings sometimes led to large institutions that accommodated more than 100 patients.[62]

As this brief overview shows, the majority of nineteenth and twentieth-century homes for incurables were not primarily a refuge for terminal patients. Some patients suffered from palsies, rheumatism or arthritis and other chronic but usually non-life-threatening diseases. In this respect, there were no clear-cut distinctions between almshouses, nursing homes and homes for the infirm, all the more so as the importance of medical care in all of these institutions increased significantly.[63] However, annual reports, patient lists and admissions statistics make it clear that many of them accepted—or even privileged—patients who suffered from advanced cancer or consumption. In this sense, these institutions for incurable patients also take a central place in the prehistory of today's hospice for the dying.

[59] The Royal Hospital for the permanent care and comfort of those who by disease, accident, or deformity, are hopelessly disqualified for the duties of life, London: Printed by Reed and Pardon 1855.

[60] Ibid., pp. 18–25, statutes; see also the later accounts by visitors in J. C. Parkinson, Gordon Calthrop and Anonymus, Three visits to the Royal Hospital for Incurables, West Hill, Putney Heath, London: Board of Management 1870.

[61] Mrs. Clarke, Helpless. A history of the British Home for Incurables, at Clapham, now removed to Streatham, for 32 years, London: Deverell Bros. 1894; for a detailed account see Cook, The incurables movement (2006); the house was moved, in 1863, from Clapham Rise to Streatham.

[62] A. H. Campbell, A brief record of God's wonderful care of Faith Home for Incurables: April 1st, 1873 – April 1st, 1900, Brooklyn, N.Y.: Bowles [ca 1900]; St Barnabas Hospital for Chronic Diseases, Constitution and bylaws of the Home for Incurables, New York: E. D. Crooker 1887; Alta E. Thompson, Fiftieth anniversary of the Home for Incurables of the City of Baltimore 1883–1933, Baltimore: Community Fund Member [1933 (?)].

[63] Irmak, Der Sieche (2002), pp. 220–30.

10.3 Institutions for Cancer Patients

Considering the often quite heterogeneous clientele of the homes for incurables, future research will have to reveal to what extent individual institutions in practice lived up to the expectation that they would provide intensive medical, surgical and nursing care, and to what extent they can be regarded as institutions for end-of-life care of a medical nature. There is, however, no doubt about the medical function of a growing number of institutions that were dedicated specifically to the main chronic and frequently fatal diseases: the hospitals for cancer patients and consumptive or lung patients.

The medical care of cancer patients came with particular challenges. When tumors began to ulcerate and disintegrate, disfiguring the face or body, or even beginning to give off festering, putrid secretions, cancer patients became a heavy burden even to hospitals and homes for incurables. Since the late eighteenth century, the drive for a spatial separation of cancer patients on aesthetic and hygienic grounds joined hands with a growing therapeutic optimism. While previously cancer, except in its early stages, had been seen as the epitome of incurable diseases, there was now a growing hope that it might be cured even in its later stages.

Some institutions established special departments for cancer patients or housed them in separate buildings.[64] To date the Hôpital Saint-Louis, established in 1742 on Rue de Saint-Denis in Reims, may be considered the oldest known hospital serving cancer patients exclusively. It had its beginnings in an endowment by the canon Jean Godinot, who gave two beds for penniless cancer patients. Further endowments and donations followed. In 1786, the institution boasted 12 beds funded with endowments for the use of patients suffering from disintegrating cancer, eight for women and four for men. The medical care was overseen by the doctor of the Hôtel Dieu, while a head nurse and two maids cared for the patients on site.[65]

The department for cancer patients established in 1792 at the Middlesex Hospital in London, focused even more on medical treatment.[66] Founded as the Middlesex Infirmary in 1745, as an institution for the poor sick and lame, it came to lack funding and as a result several wards stood empty around 1790. This was the situation in which a benefactor, Samuel Whitbread, offered a considerable sum to furnish one of the vacant wards for 10–12 cancer patients and to pay for the running costs.[67] The institution was to serve primarily as a final refuge for "the more distressing and speedily destructive cases." In addition, patients showing a milder or slower

[64] Husson, Hôpitaux (1862), p. 290; Oppert, Hospitäler (1872), p. 90.

[65] Cf. Pol Gosset, L'hôpital des cancérés. Fondation du chanoine Godinot (1740), in: Union médicale du Nord-Est (1926), pp. 17–26. Until 1841 the house was subject to the administration of the Hôtel Dieu and afterwards to that of the former Hôpital Saint-Marcoul.

[66] For a detailed account with extensive quotes from original documents see Wilson, Middlesex Hospital (1845), pp. 128–60.

[67] Whitbread maintained his anonymity until his death. Initially he promised a single payment of 3400 pounds but ultimately he established a fund the profits of which could be used to pay for the costs of running the institution.

progression who were still able cope with everyday life were to be treated in an outpatients department for as long as their admittance to the wards could be avoided. Caring for the patients was not the only aim. The focus on cancer patients was to facilitate research on the best ways to treat cancer and to offer an opportunity to train medical students in this field. The plan was to keep a detailed record of each patient's history and specific circumstances, along with "the effects of medicines and of operations, when necessary."[68]

The cancer ward opened on 19 June 1792. According to the statutes, cancer patients with disintegrating ulcerating tumors, those requiring surgery and those whose cancer had begun to grow again following surgery were permitted on the ward for an unlimited time, until they either improved or passed away. In 1811, thanks to another endowment, it was possible to set up several more beds for cancer patients in one of the other wards as well. Around 1870, the hospital had beds for 36 cancer patients.[69]

New therapeutic procedures continued to be tested, above all at the suggestion of those in charge, who were not medically trained. They wanted to test procedures which some physicians elsewhere claimed yielded good results.[70] The treatment with a vegetable diet, suggested by a Dr. Lambe, was among the more harmless attempts. Others were very painful. In 1816, for example, eight patients with hardened, scirrhous carcinoma and eight with open cancerous ulcers were used to test the benefit of a localized pressure treatment. The treatment showed no positive effect, in fact the doctor's opinion was that in many cases it seemed even to speed up the dying process. Physicians in general were skeptical about these kinds of experiments. In the 24 years between 1792 and 1816, they complained, no specific remedy for cancer was discovered, despite all efforts. In the 1840s doctors considered the Middlesex Hospital to have found its principal purpose in significantly alleviating suffering rather than in curative treatment.[71] Exuberant therapeutic optimism had given way to palliative realism.

Starting in the middle of the nineteenth century, an increasing number of independent hospitals were founded in the United Kingdom specifically for cancer patients. Caroline Murphy has traced their history in detail.[72] Her research shows that these institutions were founded as part of a more general trend toward specialized institutions. Like the cancer ward at the Middlesex Hospital, they were usually inspired by the hope of being able to develop better cancer therapies by concentrating cancer patients in one place. But they were also a refuge for patients in the advanced stages of the disease.

---

[68] Wilson, Middlesex Hospital (1845), pp. 129–33, letter by John Howard to the "medical gentlemen" of the hospital, cit. p. 130 and p. 131.

[69] Oppert, Hospitäler (1872), p. 212.

[70] According to the complaints of the commission, cit. in Wilson, Middlesex Hospital (1845), pp. 150–9.

[71] Report of a commission headed by Charles Gower, June 1816, cit. in. Wilson, Middlesex Hospital (1845), pp. 142–5, here p. 145.

[72] Murphy, Friedenheim (1989).

In 1851, William Marsden founded the London Cancer Hospital, later named the Royal Marsden Hospital, after his wife had died of ovarian cancer.[73] This hospital is said to have served around 50,000 patients in the years leading up to 1900, many of them as outpatients. Inoperable, hopeless cases remained there until their death and the death rate was accordingly high.[74] Similar institutions were founded in other cities, such as the Liverpool Cancer Hospital (1862), the Glasgow Cancer Hospital (1890) and the Manchester Cancer Pavillon and Home (1892).[75] The latter also served a small number of paying patients until they died. To be admitted, one had to be among the "very severe, often fast-progressing cases."[76] Founded in 1893 in Bradford, the St. Catharine's Home for Cancer and Incurables was designed for hopeless cases exclusively from the start; it first had 10 and then 25 beds.[77]

In the early twentieth century, new type of cancer hospital was established, which combined the features of a modern research institution with those of a medical treatment center for cancer patients. The institution in Moscow, initiated by the surgeon Leon Leweschin, was to offer a place where "the unlucky patients [were to] find humane relief and appropriate medical care," as A. Dworetzki wrote, while, at the same time, "the most varied trials for the most radical therapies of carcinoma were to be carried out"—making it "a true institute for cancer research and cancer treatment."[78] In Germany at around the same time, the Institut für Experimentelle Krebsforschung (Institute for Experimental Cancer Research) was founded in Heidelberg, which was associated with a home for cancer patients, the so-called Samariterhaus.[79] Numerous and varied therapeutic procedures were tested there, ranging from passive and active immunization to treatment with toxins to chemotherapy.[80] Close to 2500 patients were treated in inpatient care during the first 5 years. Approximately 1500 patients occupied the three 10-bed halls for class-III patients, and another almost 1000 class-I and II patients were admitted, because, in the words of the medical director, they appreciated "the benefit of careful nursing and good treatment." This was true even of "wholly desperate patients, who had become impossible to care for at home."[81]

In summary, it can be said that the cancer hospitals of the nineteenth and early twentieth centuries typically, albeit with varying emphasis, combined curative and

[73] Ibid.; Anonymus, The Royal Marsden Hospital, in: The cancer bulletin 14 (1962), p. 53.

[74] Scheffler, Cancerhospitäler (1900); Murphy, Friedenheim (1989), pp. 223–4.

[75] Scheffler, Cancerhospitäler (1900); Murphy, Friedenheim (1989), pp. 224–5; the later, more "neutral" name was The Christie Hospital and Holt Radium Institute (cf. Anonymus, The Christie Hospital and Holt Radium Institute, Manchester, in: The cancer bulletin 13 (1961), p. 11).

[76] Scheffler, Cancerhospitäler (1900), p. 20.

[77] Ibid.

[78] A. Dworetzki, Die neue Moskauer Klinik für Krebskranke, Münchener medizinische Wochenschrift 50 (1903), pp. 277–9; Goldblum-Abramowicz, Versorgung (1908), p. 17.

[79] Vincenz Czerny, Das Heidelberger Institut für Experimentelle Krebsforschung, I. Teil, Tübingen: Laupp'sche Buchhandlung 1912.

[80] Ibid., p. 61.

[81] Ibid., p. 11 (cit.) and p. 66 (table).

palliative functions. Their purpose was to give sufferers who had no hope of a cure a refuge and a measure of medical care, while at the same time hope was invested in the scientific investigation of cancer and the development of new therapies. The available beds of course were far from sufficient, considering the increasing prevalence of cancer. In many towns and even more so in the country, people in the advanced stages of a cancer illness had nowhere to go for care. If they were not looked after by relatives or friends, they had to struggle along on their own or, like so many of the sick poor in England, spent their last days in a workhouse.

10.4 Institutions for the Consumptive

Even more than cancer hospitals, institutions for patients consumption or pulmonary tuberculosis were committed to curative treatment. It was known that even after months of coughing and bringing up blood, many patients improved and could—at least temporarily—be released, which physicians and officials understandably attributed to the treatment these patients had received.[82]

London in 1872 already had four such institutions and one of them, the Royal Chest Hospital, dated back to 1814.[83] The demand was great as the general hospitals in London opposed the admission of this particular patient group with particular vigor.[84] Some of the new tuberculosis hospitals were large institutions. The Brompton Hospital, operating since 1846, had 210 beds and there were even plans for expansion in the 1870s. The hospital did not primarily practice palliative care, yet mortality was very high because it admitted many patients in advanced stages.[85]

In the late nineteenth and early twentieth centuries, large numbers of tuberculosis sanitariums were founded all across Europe.[86] This movement was especially successful in Germany, not least of all because there even members of the working class were covered by social and health insurance and could stay at one of the many people's sanitariums for several months. Early in the twentieth century, these

---

[82] Thomas Beddoes, Observations on the medical and domestic management of the consumptive; on the powers of digitalis purpurea; and on the cure of schrophula [sic], London: Longman & Rees 1801.

[83] Extensive archival documentation has survived in the London Metropolitan Archives; see also Dietrich-Daum, "Wiener Krankheit" (2007), p. 22.

[84] Oppert, Hospitäler (1872), pp. 91–2.

[85] Ibid., pp. 218–20.

[86] For a good contemporary survey see Handbuch der Architektur. IV.Teil. Entwerfen, Anlage und Einrichtung der Gebäude. fifth half-volume, n. 2, 2nd edn Stuttgart: Bergsträsser 1903, pp. 126–87; see also Flurin Condrau, Lungenheilanstalt und Patientenschicksal. Sozialgeschichte der Tuberkulose in Deutschland und England im späten 19. und frühen 20. Jahrhundert, Göttingen: Vandenhoeck & Ruprecht 2000; Sylvelyn Hähner-Rombach, Sozialgeschichte der Tuberkulose. Vom Kaiserreich bis zum Ende des Zweiten Weltkriegs unter besonderer Berücksichtigung Württembergs, Wiesbaden: Steiner 2000; Dietrich-Daum, "Wiener Krankheit" (2007), pp. 192–207.

institutions were already treating around 30,000 patients annually.[87] As the name "sanitarium" or "sanatorium" (both from Latin *sanitas* or *sanare*, for "health" or "healing") indicates, these institutions aimed primarily at an active treatment of patients who were considered curable. With treatment that commonly lasted 13 weeks, the attempt was made to cure patients or at least improve their condition enough for them to go back to work. Besides the "rest cure," preferably done in the fresh mountain air, and dietetic approaches, there were also invasive procedures, in particular the attempt to immobilize and thereby restore the affected lung by creating an artificial pneumothorax, i.e. by letting external air enter the thorax through an opening which caused the lung to collapse on that side.[88] Consequently, the tuberculosis sanitariums can only be understood as institutions of palliative medicine to a very limited degree. As fictional accounts like Thomas Mann's *The Magic Mountain* suggest, patients at private sanitariums often remained there until the bitter end,[89] but many sanitariums for the less affluent did not even admit severe cases or else released them as incurable. According to a compilation of data from 40 German tuberculosis sanitariums, only 304 of 20,399 patients died there in 1922, a mortality rate that was even lower than that of the general population.[90] There were only some places where a much higher percentage of patients with tuberculosis spent their last days in a sanitarium and died there. One such exception was Hamburg, where, in 1896, 40.7% of all registered deaths from tuberculosis occurred in sanitariums, and in 1912 the number had risen to 56.4%, or 720 of 1277.[91]

In many places, patients with advanced consumption could only hope to be admitted to a general hospital when they became increasingly weak and short of breath and, toward the end, were largely confined to their sickbed. At the Barmen hospital, for example, 287 of the 542 consumptive patients admitted between 1868 and 1872 died—more than every second patient.[92] The medical literature and organizations such as the *Deutsches Central-Komité zur Errichtung von Heilstätten für Lungenkranke* (German Central Committee for the Establishment of Sanitariums for Lung Patients) demanded that sanitariums be opened up to severe cases and that specialized tuberculosis hospitals be built. Alternatively, special departments or pavilions could be set up as part of the general hospitals, as places where severely suffering lung patients would recover or at least experience "an alleviation of their

[87] Prof. Dr. Jacob, Die Tuberkulosefrage auf dem Internationalen Hygienekongress in Brüssel, insbesondere mit Rücksicht auf die gegen die deutschen Heilstätten gerichteten Angriffe, in: Bericht über die I. Versammlung der Tuberkulose-Ärzte, Berlin, 1. bis 3. November 1903, ed. by Prof. Dr. Pannwitz, Berlin: Dt. Central-Komite zur Errichtung von Heilstätten für Lungenkranke 1904, p. 8.

[88] Dietrich-Daum, "Wiener Krankheit" (2007), pp. 210–11.

[89] Speech by Chefarzt Ritter in: Nietner, Zur Tuberkulose-Bekämpfung (1913), pp. 21–33, here p. 25; Klabund, Krankheit (1917), pp. 69–70; Mann, Magic mountain (1929).

[90] Hellmuth Ulrici, Jahresbericht deutscher Lungenheilanstalten 1922, in: Beiträge zur Klinik der Tuberkulose und der spezifischen Tuberkulose-Forschung 57 (1924), pp. 332–41.

[91] Speech by Chefarzt Ritter in: Nietner, Zur Tuberkulose-Bekämpfung (1913), pp. 21–33, here p. 23.

[92] Sander, Krankenhäuser (1875), pp. 29–30.

complaints, and impeccably good care."[93] In all this, the concern was not only with the wellbeing of the patients themselves but also with the protection of the public. Many doctors had for a long time believed that consumption was a contagious disease, and their belief became certainty with the discovery of the tuberculosis bacterium in 1882. To protect the public and in particular the children of consumptive patients from contracting the disease, the call was for patients with advanced symptoms to be isolated.[94] In Germany at least, these demands were increasingly met. In 1913, according to Nietner, Germany had 222 care homes and special hospital wards to serve advanced cases, and their number grew steadily. Yet, in many places, there were still not nearly enough beds and "the majority of sufferers in advanced stages continued to be at home, where they [had to be] isolated as much as possible."[95]

10.5 The First Hospices for the Dying

The general hospitals and the homes for incurables as well as the institutions and hospital wards specialized in cancer and diseases of the lungs did not primarily serve the dying, in fact some of them were rather ill equipped to deal with dying patients. Institutions that would correspond to today's understanding of "hospice for the dying" or "hospice for the terminally ill" developed slowly and only in some places.

In the research literature on the subject, contradictory and in some cases blatantly incorrect information about the earliest examples of hospices for the dying can be found. As explained above, the French *hospices* had little more in common with today's hospices for the dying than the name. Some have declared the *hospice* founded in Lyon in 1843 and run by Les Dames du Calvaire under the directorship of Jeanne Garnier as the oldest institution to be specialized in the care of the dying.[96] However, a closer look reveals that the *hospice* in Lyon was a home for women in need of nursing, in particular for those who suffered from chronic ulcers and had to be bandaged regularly. This was certainly not an institution specialized in the care of the terminally ill and dying.[97] Grace Goldin's claim that the Irish Sisters of

[93] Wilhelm von Leube, Spezialkrankenhaus für Tuberkulöse in den vorgeschriebenen [sic! presumbably for "fortgeschrittenen", i.e. „advanced" M. S.] Stadien der Erkrankung. Tuberkulosekrankenhäuser ("Heimstätten", "Invalidenheime") – Krankenhauspflege, in: B. Fränkel (ed.), Der Stand der Tuberkulose-Bekämpfung in Deutschland, Berlin: Selbstverlag des Deutschen Central-Komités 1905, pp. 252–61.

[94] Ibid., p. 255; Speech by Chefarzt Ritter in: Nietner, Zur Tuberkulose-Bekämpfung (1913), pp. 21–33; Joh. Dvořák, Über die Frage der Errichtung von Isolierabteilungen oder Krankenhaussanatorien in allgemeinen öffentlichen Krankenhäusern in Österreich, in: Zeitschrift für Tuberkulose und Heilstättenwesen 2 (1901), pp. 487–97.

[95] Field, Palliative medicine (1994).

[96] E.g., Saunders, Evolution (1988), p. 169; David Clark, Palliative care history: A ritual process, in: European journal of palliative care 7 (2000), n. 2, pp. 50–5; Lewis, Medicine (2007), p. 20.

[97] See, by contrast, S. Reymond, L'œuvre des Dames du Calvaire 1842–1914, Lyon: Mémoire de maîtrise d'histoire 2001; Jérôme Desfourneaux, Jeanne Garnier: Du soin aux incurables aux soins palliatifs, Lyon: med. diss. 2002.

Charity established a hospice for the dying in Australia as early as the 1830s has turned out to be unfounded as well.[98] This institution, the Sacred Heart Hospice in Darlinghurst, Sydney, in fact opened its doors only in 1890.[99] If there is one institution before 1870 that could be described as a prototype of the modern hospice for the dying, it is the abovementioned Hundertsuppe in Nuremberg, a hospital whose primary if not exclusive task was already in the late eighteenth century to care for the terminally ill and dying though it was not founded for that purpose.

Decisive steps toward the development of a separate type of institution for the terminally ill and dying, in the sense of a modern hospice for the dying, were taken above all in the English-speaking regions during the late nineteenth century. In the middle of the nineteenth century in England, there was a public debate about the insufficient medical and nursing care for the terminally ill and dying in public health institutions. In 1860, the chairwoman of the Workhouse Visiting Society addressed the regional poor commissioners in a circular letter and also gave talk to the public at large, which was subsequently published. Emphatically, she pointed out that there was a serious gap in the health care provided to the impoverished masses. Less severe cases, she said, were well cared for but those suffering from incurable cancer, dropsy, consumption and such, who were in need of particularly good care and treatment, lacked suitable institutions. She went on to state that, in England alone, around 80,000 people fell victim to these diseases every year, 50,000 of whom were poor people. A portion of them ultimately died in the hospitals but many did not find admission, because, barring a few exceptions, many of the hospitals did not accept long-term and incurable cases. Thus, many of those pitiful individuals spent their last days in "abject misery," with poor relatives or, and this applied to the majority, in a workhouse. The author admitted that specialized hospitals for such a large number of hopelessly lost sufferers could not be financed, especially given that they required more intensive care than common patients. But this only meant that it was all the more important for those living in workhouses—which otherwise mainly fulfilled a deterrent, socially disciplining function—to be cared for as best as possible, as sick patients rather than just as poor people. It was imperative, she said, to at least create conditions within the workhouses that came as close as possible to those one would expect in a specialized institution for incurables, for the benefit of those suffering from cancer, consumption, dropsy and other comparable diseases. In the workhouses, she said, they lived in dreadful conditions. Instead of receiving the necessary opiates for their pain and strengthening remedies, people were given only the cheapest, coarsest medication. For food, they had the ever-the-same boiled beef,

[98] Goldin, A protohospice (1981), p. 390.

[99] Cf. Derek Kerr, Mother Mary Aikenhead, the Irish Sisters of Charity and Our Lady's Hospice for the Dying, in: American journal of hospice and palliative care 10 (1993), n. 3, pp. 13–20; Margaret M. Donovan, Apostolate of love. Mary Aikenhead 1787–1858. Foundress of the Irish Sisters of Charity, Melbourne: Polding Press 1979, pp. 230–1; Lewis, Medicine (2007), p. 23.

which three quarters of the sick poor could not even chew. The skin of the bedridden was often covered with horrid bedsores from lying on the hard, bad mattresses.[100]

The oldest institution, however, which is known to have been founded with the explicit aim to care primarily for terminally ill and dying patients was not established in England but in Ireland. The Royal Hospital Donnybrook looked back on a long tradition of offering appropriate care to incurable patients. In 1879, the Irish Sisters of Charity opened Our Lady's Hospice for the Dying in Harold's Cross near Dublin.[101] As a complement to the St. Vincent's Hospital, which the sisters operated in the city, it was designed to serve those who were not only considered hopeless cases but most likely had only little time to live.[102] Our Lady's was also the oldest known institution bearing the English term "hospice" in today's sense of an institution for terminal patients in its name. In 1880, the hospice already had more than 40 beds; in 1889 there were 108. Little is known about the kind and extent of the medical care that was provided. An earlier annual report only speaks generally about increased therapeutic expenses: "The dying cannot be treated as one would common patients; they require the more costly diet and treatment demanded by their weakened condition."[103]

In the late nineteenth century, several institutions were established in the United Kingdom that are rightfully considered important direct precursors of the modern hospice for the dying. These were houses designed first and foremost to serve as a refuge for the dying and were religiously motivated to varying degrees. Concentrated in London, they were the Hostel of God (1892),[104] St. Columba's (1889),[105] St. Luke's Hospital (1893) and St. Joseph's House (1905), operated by the English Sisters of Charity. Also, there was the Friedenheim, which already had eight beds in 1885, and after its move to a larger building in 1892, had 35 beds set aside for the care of patients with terminal consumption.[106]

We have relatively good knowledge of the history and work of St. Luke's, thanks to the work of Grace Goldin and Natalie A. Fleming who examined the surviving

[100] Miss Elliot and Miss Cobbe, Destitute incurables in workhouses. A paper by Miss Elliot and Miss Corbe, read at the social science meeting in Glasgow, September, 1860, London: Nisbet & Co. 1860.

[101] Healy, 125 years (2004); Katherine Butler, We help them home: the story of Our Lady's Hospice, Harold's Cross, Dublin, Dublin: Our Lady's Hospice 1980; in 1870 the Sisters had already established St Patrick's in Cork, which, according to its founder, the physician Patrick Murphy, was designed for patients with incurable cancer but ended up taking care primarily of consumptives (Healy, 125 years (2004), p. 3).

[102] Prospectus of 1879, reprinted in Butler, op. cit., next to p. 22.

[103] Annual report 1880/81, cit. in Healy, 125 years (2004), p. 16.

[104] The house was also known under the name *Free Home for the Dying*; it was founded by the philanthropist William Hoare and the Anglican order *St James's Servants of the Poor* in Clapham Common in London and initially only had 10 beds (The Hostel of God, Annual report 1977/78, p. 4); Clark, Cradled to the grave? (1999), p. 67); since 1980, the house has been known as Trinity hospice.

[105] Clark, Cradled to the grave? (1999).

[106] Lewis, Medicine (2007), p. 21.

annual reports. More than any other institution in London at the time, this was a hospice for the dying in the modern understanding, a "home for the dying," as its appeals for donations called it. It was meant, from the outset, to only admit patients with a limited life expectancy of no more than several months. The driving force behind the foundation of this house was Howard Barrett, who won the West London Mission for his plans and would later act as medical director.[107] The institution admitted mainly tuberculosis and cancer patients: In 1896, 26 patients were diagnosed with tuberculosis and 13 with cancer. The proportion of cancer patients rose while the total number of patients also rose considerably after 1914. In 1918, 91 of 206 admitted individuals had tuberculosis and 110 had cancer. Between 1895 and 1900, the average length of stay until the patient's death, or more rarely until a patient was released temporarily, was between 31 and 58 days.[108] According to the annual report of 1908, only patients with an estimated life expectancy of no more than 4 months were to be admitted. There were even some patients who were released on the grounds that their disease had not yet progressed far enough.[109]

Grace Goldin assumed that St. Luke's was only able to offer good nursing care but no efficient pain management.[110] Considering the leading role of Howard Barrett as a doctor and the potent analgesics and narcotics that were available at the time, there seems to be little support for this assumption. Also, both doctors and patients pointed out the joyful, even jocular atmosphere there, contrasting it with the all too serious, mournful way of dealing with the dying in other institutions.[111] The medical director emphasized that, at St. Luke's, they did not perceive patients as "cases" and instead saw each person as "a human microcosm, with his own features, his own interplay of joys and grief, hopes and fears, his own life history."[112] The visiting hours were relatively generous and it was a conscious choice to forgo strict discipline and avoid the atmosphere of other houses, which had become cold and sterile, as it was put. However, the institution did not have the poorest among the poor in mind. Those who had relied on pauper relief before their illness were rejected.[113] The house was to serve exclusively the "respectable poor," those who had met with adversity because of their disease.

---

[107] Goldin, A protohospice (1981), p. 403. Later it was called *St Luke's Home for Advanced Cases* and since 1953 it has gone by the name of *Hereford Lodge*.

[108] Goldin, A protohospice (1981), p. 407. In 1901, the number soared abruptly to 105, due to several patients who stayed for longer periods of time.

[109] Fleming, Care of the dying (2005), pp. 31–2.

[110] Goldin, A protohospice (1981), p. 407.

[111] Ibid., p. 399.

[112] Howard Barrett in the annual report for *St Luke's* 1909, cit. Ibid.

[113] Goldin, A protohospice (1981), p. 402.

10.6 Dying in an Institution

In part, the growing significance of hospitals and various specialized institutions as providers of inpatient health care for the dying was the result of socio-political measures and, when it came to tuberculosis, also of hygienic regulations that were put in place to prevent epidemics. But most of all, it resulted from the rising demand coming from the population, as people increasingly appreciated these institutions for the professional medical treatment and care they offered, and not just as a welcome refuge. However, patients whose various treatments ultimately met with failure often paid a high price. The prospect of having their life end in the hospital scared them. Even if they lived in absolute squalor, people suffering from a disease decidedly preferred to die at home, as contemporary sources tell us unanimously. Patients who "are wholly incurable and are living their final days," Lampe wrote in 1789 in his plea that outpatient healthcare be made available to the poor, "regardless of all medical help and all care, miss their attentive spouse, their compassionate child or comforting friend, people who undoubtedly refresh them in their suffering more than all medication and all nurses."[114] One hundred years later, Kirchner similarly saw the reason for the low popularity of tubercular sanitariums in the fact that the severely ill tuberculosis patient "considers them a house for the dying, and because he and his family often think it is not right that these advanced and helpless consumptives are removed from their families, becoming, in a sense, outcast the way we experienced with leprosy."[115] According to Stuertz, writing in the early twentieth century, a severely ill person who had the impression, "that he is beyond hope, and that he would merely move to a death house," would "prefer to die at home."[116]

To Stöhr the most important reason for people's fear of dying in a hospital was the anonymous hospital routine:

> The unfortunate person wants something more besides the bed on which to stretch out his emaciated limbs, more than the food and care the law allows him with arithmetic precision: He wants a word of sympathy and comfort, to be understood somewhat as a person, which will help him forget the thought that he figures as a mere number in the large works of this 'city of suffering' operating with a cold regularity, a number that one day will be erased from the board above his head.[117]

Using the example of the large Paris Hôtel Dieu with its 559 beds, a kind of "industrial" dying was also bemoaned by Rainer Maria Rilke in *Die Aufzeichnungen des Malte Laurids Brigge* (*The Notebooks of Malte Laurids Brigge*, 1910). Dying under these circumstances, to Rilke, meant depriving a person of dying "one's own death," a form of dying the narrator's grandfather had still experienced.

[114] Lampe, Nachricht (1789), p. 10.

[115] Speech by Ministerialdirektor Kirchner in: Nietner, Zur Tuberkulose-Bekämpfung (1913), pp. 61–7, here p. 63.

[116] Speech by Oberarzt Stuertz, in: Ibid., pp. 33–53, here p. 34.

[117] Stöhr, Handbuch (1882), p. 290.

> With such high production, a single death isn't carried out with the same care anymore, it's not important. It's all about quantity. Who today is still interested in a carefully done death? Nobody. Even the rich, who after all could afford to die a death with complete attention to detail, are beginning to become careless and apathetic about it; the wish to die one's own death is becoming rare. Before long it will be just as rare as leading one's own life.[118]

Added to this came the omnipresence of death and disease in these houses. For reasons of space alone, patients with different illnesses of varying degrees of severity lay closely together in many hospitals, which meant that they experienced the suffering of their fellow patients at close quarters. In small facilities in particular, complained Lochner, a doctor in mid-nineteenth-century Nuremberg, the dying were a heavy burden on fellow patients. Such houses were "terrible places in this respect," he claimed. In a room with several consumptive patients, the sick person looked in vain for "comfort and reassurance," when "every couple of weeks one or several of his comrades, who had the same complaints and were comforted with more or less the same words, died at his side." In this situation, the sufferer was bound to "despair completely" and "long before his final, most difficult hours."[119]

> If someone like this, in his bleakest physical condition decides to find a nook where he may await his final hour in quiet, undisturbed by the groaning and wailing of the dying or the rawness of his fellow sufferers, who would hold it against him, and who would not gladly lend him a hand![120]

In the large new hospitals of the late nineteenth and early twentieth centuries, the situation was hardly better. "In domestic life, in the presence of people with this illness, we anxiously avoid even the mention of death," Franz Oppert wrote about sufferers of a "chest ailment," yet in a hospital they had to witness "the suffering of their fellow patients and their dying all the time."[121]

The conditions in institutions for tuberculosis and cancer patients were especially burdensome. The "often dismal images" of severely ill and dying tuberculosis patients, said Stuertz, "fresh bleeding, other patients' depressions and frequent evacuation of stool with patients suffering from gastrointestinal tuberculosis causes most fellow patients to get depressed, although a bed screen mitigates the impressions."[122] Added to this came the malodorous sputum, the smell of physical decay that some patients gave off.[123] When, as was the case in some of the older

---

[118] Rainer Maria Rilke, Die Aufzeichnungen des Malte Laurids Brigge, Augsburg: Weltbild 2009 (orig. 1910).

[119] [Georg Friedrich] Lochner and [Ludwig] Bock, Statistisch-medizinischer Bericht über die Kranken- und Versorgungs-Anstalten Nürnbergs, Nürnberg: Bauer and Raspe 1844, p. 31.

[120] Ibid.

[121] Oppert, Hospitäler (1872), p. 92.

[122] Speech by Oberarzt Stuertz in: Nietner, Zur Tuberkulose-Bekämpfung (1913), pp. 33–53, here p. 39.

[123] The bad smell which emanated from tuberculotic patients had already for a some time been considered a sign of consumption; see e.g., Christoph Friedrich Seld, De signis mortis prognosticis. Praes. Andreas Elias Büchner, Halle – Magdeburg: Hilliger 1747, pp. 26–7.

institutions, 20–30 tuberculosis patients shared one large hall, it also made sense to doctors, "that some tuberculosis patients or their families think back to their stay in the large halls of the tuberculosis ward almost with horror, not to mention the irksome disturbance of nighttime peace by the coughing and moaning of fellow patients."[124]

Cancer patients, with their open ulcers, secretions and stench, could present an almost insurmountable challenge even to institutions that were set up specifically for them. For example, one doctor's report on a 79-year-old widow in Regensburg found that "admission to the local infirmary can currently not take place," as she "has carcinoma not only on both breasts, but also the glands in her armpits (glandulae subaxillares) have undergone complete cancerous ulceration."[125]

Some hospitals sought a way out early on by isolating the terminally ill and dying. For St. Wolfgang in the town of Neuburg an der Donau, it is documented that, as early as 1622, the house had both a ward with 12 beds and a separate room for the severely ill.[126] At the large Hospital of Saint John of Jerusalem on the island of Malta, John Howard visited a "hall for the dangerous patients and those who were dying" in the late eighteenth century.[127] An early outline for the new Allgemeines Krankenhaus, a general hospital in Bamberg, even included several separate rooms for the dying.[128] Yet, in many places hospitals had to make do with removing the dying from the sight of the other patients using only folding screens, especially when bed curtains—formerly common in many places—gradually went out of use. In the early twentieth century, Ewald still felt compelled to make the demand for separate death rooms in hospitals. The dying, he held, were distressing to those around them. Letting them "die in the general wards, perhaps with nothing more than a screen in front of their bed, is inhuman and cruel to a high degree."[129]

Many patients also found the thought hard to bear that they might be anatomized after they died.[130] As the number of medical students increased while executions became rare, many universities lacked corpses for their anatomy lessons. Following a decree of 1707, hospital directors in Paris were obliged to make corpses available to professors of medicine for the purpose of anatomical demonstrations and lessons in surgery. This decree was still in force in the early nineteenth century.[131] As it was

[124] Speech by Chefarzt Ritter in: Nietner, Zur Tuberkulose-Bekämpfung (1913), pp. 21–33, here p. 28.

[125] Staatsarchiv Amberg, Regierung der Oberpfalz, Kammer des Inneren 12,661, Städtisches Armen- und Krankenhaus in Stadtamhof, 1811–1897, medical certificate for the cancerous Mittermaierin, 1811.

[126] Axel Hinrich Murken, Vom Armenhospital zum Großklinikum. Die Geschichte des Krankenhauses vom 18. Jahrhundert bis zur Gegenwart, Cologne: Dumont 1991, p. 19.

[127] John Howard, Nachrichten von den vorzüglichsten Krankenhäusern und Pesthäusern in England, Leipzig: Göschen 1791, p. 150.

[128] Langrieger, Medizinische Versorgung (2010).

[129] C[arl] A[nton] Ewald, Über Alter und Sterben, Vienna: Hölder 1913, p. 30.

[130] See also Nolte, Todkrank (2016).

[131] Pastoret, Rapport (1816), p. 255, referring to article 25 of the edict of May 1707.

thought that family members rarely gave their consent to dissection, the Cologne hospital St. Revilien, in 1774, announced "as a decided rule that the body of anyone admitted here without charge will be dedicated to anatomy after death and, if requested, shall be delivered there. This is considered a condition for admittance, and family members have no right to object." Moreover, the physicians in the hospitals were increasingly interested in determining through autopsy what had caused the fatal outcome, hoping to improve their understanding of the nature of diseases and, as a result, their treatment.[132]

Among ordinary people, however, the dissection of bodies was regarded with aversion and the wish for a proper Christian burial was strong. Those who had no relatives or friends nearby to look after the burial and to protect the deceased from the doctors' grasp might try to employ their modest savings to buy "safety from the knives of the students."[133] In some towns, they could even regularly pay small amounts into a kind of burial fund which, in the case of death, paid out the sum necessary for a good Christian burial.[134] At the Nuremberg hospital Hundertsuppe, the question of who would pay for the burial if the patient died was taken so seriously that notes about a patient's participation in a burial fund, or else information about relatives, guild members or fellow citizens who would pay for the burial usually took up an equal amount of space in the admissions books as the patient information and diagnosis.[135]

While the fatally ill patients themselves thus had good reasons to avoid admission to a hospital, for some poor families it was a welcome relief when a dying family member was cared for and possibly buried at public expense. A Salzburg craftsman, for example, complained in April 1812 that his wife had been "bedridden with hectic fever" for more than 6 months. He had "so far nursed her with the utmost effort, diligence and patience and supplied her with the necessary medication." But now he was no longer in a position to do this, not least of all because nursing was very expensive. Therefore, he wanted to take her to the Salzburg Johannisspital.[136] Some institutions used this point explicitly in their advertising. For example, the Royal Hospital for Incurables announced that patients were "spared from being a burden upon relatives who in some cases might be anticipating what is called 'a happy release'."[137]

It stands to reason that quite a number of seriously ill patients who spent their last days in a hospital or a home for incurables did so rather involuntarily or out of

132 Stadtarchiv Köln, Best 160 St. Revilien Ka 55 Nr 191 1774–90; the ruling was repeated November 24, 1786.

133 Stöhr, Handbuch (1882), p. 290.

134 Ernst Vesper, Die Sterbekassen in alter und neuer Zeit. Posthumous edn by P. Braeß, Berlin: Duncker & Humboldt 1966.

135 Stadtarchiv Nürnberg C 23/I 2.

136 Stadtarchiv Salzburg, Älteres Städtisches Archiv, Pezoltakten 57, Leprosenhaus 1805–1816, supplication for admission, April 14, 1812.

137 J. C. Parkinson, Gordon Calthrop and anonymus, Three visits to the Royal Hospital for Incurables, West Hill, Putney Heath, London: Board of Management 1870, p. 22.

consideration for their impoverished or overwhelmed families. As Mohr's account of 1832 about 24-year-old Elisabetha H. has it, for example, she had "despaired of her recovery or convalescence" a few weeks before her death and pleaded more urgently every day to be released from the Würzburg Julius-Spital. But faced with the "unwillingness of her relatives," she had to resign herself to remaining at the hospital.[138] As we can see, for their inmates these institutions were not always a welcome last refuge.

138 Bernhard Mohr, Beiträge zur Kenntniss der organischen Hirnkrankheiten, Würzburg: Gedruckt bei C. W. Becher's Witwe 1833, pp. 7–21, cit. p. 19.

The Time After 1945

11

The time after the World War II was a period of profound change in terms of how the needs of terminally ill and dying patients were addressed. Developments in medicine and changes in society ultimately resulted in the emergence of the modern hospice movement, in different forms of palliative medical care for outpatients and inpatients and in the institutionalization of palliative medicine as an independent medical subdiscipline.

However, the road that led there was not as straight and even as might seem at a glance, and comparing different Western industrialized countries, we also discover considerable differences. The rise of the hospice system and of palliative medicine in many respects was interrelated in complicated ways with contemporary processes of change that took place in medicine, in healthcare and in society, and initially these processes tended to lead toward a further marginalization of hopelessly ill and dying patients.

What needs to be mentioned first in this context are the many medical innovations of the postwar period. New diagnostic processes opened up hitherto unimagined possibilities of detecting illness early and with precision, a prerequisite for precisely targeted treatment. New drugs were developed for many common diseases. For the first time, infectious diseases, which had by far been the most frequent cause of death for centuries, could now be treated effectively with antibiotics. Antibiotics did much to take the old fear out of tuberculosis, even if the disease had become considerably less significant even before. New medication for diabetes, hypertension and other widespread chronic complaints increased life expectancy for many people and improved quality of life in a way that one had not dared to hope for in earlier times. New surgical procedures—going as far as transplantation medicine—and a steadily improving intensive-care medicine made it possible to keep people alive who in the past would have soon succumbed to their illness.

The new diagnostic and therapeutic capacities, the successful battle against infectious diseases, and above all improved living and nutritional conditions for the vast majority of the population caused the average life expectancy for adults to rise further in most industrialized countries and, as a result, brought a change in the

M. Stolberg, *A History of Palliative Care, 1500–1970*, Philosophy and Medicine 123,
DOI 10.1007/978-3-319-54178-5_11

spectrum of "killer diseases". While consumption declined sharply, more and more people now died after prolonged suffering from one of the chronic diseases typically associated with late life. Cancer as well as cardiovascular diseases and their resulting conditions, including chronic cardiac insufficiency and stroke, became the leading causes of death in industrialized countries. In the 1980s, AIDS began to take its terrible toll, especially among the younger age groups.

The medical improvements and the associated, at times almost limitless, hopes of patients and their families further strengthened the significance of the hospital as the central medical facility, to which more and more patients turned in hope for a cure, when they became seriously ill. Much less than in previous centuries, death was readily accepted as the inevitable end of human life. Even with patients at a very advanced age, it became nearly automatic in the decades following the Second World War, to seek admittance to a hospital no matter how little hope was left. Moreover, due to changing family structures, there were now many more elderly people who had no one willing or in the position to care for them for an extended period of illness.

This meant that the percentage of people whose lives ended in the hospital increased significantly once again. For the sick this was not necessarily a blessing. Usually after having been admitted and released several times, they ultimately died in an expensive institution characterized by a high degree of labor division, whose very identity and mandate was to cure patients and restore their health. This also changed the image of dying—for the public and in everyday culture. Dying became strongly associated with impersonal and technological death in the hospital, with tubes and ventilators. The powerlessness in the face of physical decline and inescapable death was accompanied by a powerlessness in the face of apparatuses and the hospital as an institution.

Initially the marginalization of death and dying in the healthcare of the day corresponded with a tabooing of the subject in the public and in mass media. Soon after World War II, a growing countercurrent can be discerned however, first and foremost in the English-speaking world. Growing attention was paid to the grave deficiencies in the prevailing treatment of terminally ill and dying patients in hospitals.[1] The criticism was aimed for one thing at the insufficient mental and emotional support of dying patients by doctors, who really preferred to give them a wide berth. "Physicians have been taught to cure," David Shepard complained as late as the 1970s; "when they realize that cure is no longer possible, their own insecurities concerning death prevent them from comforting their patients and supporting them in ways that are not clinical."[2] Further, medical treatment itself was described as insufficient. Vogler was only one of many critics; regarding cancer patients he cautioned in 1951, "If we want to spare the patient unnecessary suffering, we must demand of this care that it be carried out from a scientific perspective until the very

[1] Field, Palliative medicine (1994).

[2] David A. E. Shepard, Terminal care: towards an ideal, in: CMA Journal 115 (1976), pp. 97–8.

last moment."[3] Dozens of articles and books appeared as early as the 1950s, treating different aspects of medical, nursing and pastoral care for terminally ill patients.[4]

In the 1960s, the subject of dying and death became increasingly discussed also in the wider public and in the media. A key figure in this development was the Swiss doctor Elisabeth Kübler-Ross.[5] In 1969, she published the results of her conversations with dying people in her book *On Death and Dying,* which became an international bestseller. Kübler-Ross decidedly opposed the denial and repression of death in modern, and especially in US society: "The more we are making advancements in science, the more we seem to fear and deny the reality of death."[6] In great detail, she described the mental states and hardships of the terminally ill. Dying in a modern hospital, she lamented, is "lonely and impersonal" and the severely ill are "often treated like a person with no right to an opinion."[7] "He may cry for rest, peace, and dignity, but he will get infusions, transfusions, a heart machine, or tracheostomy if necessary."[8]

The social and cultural upheavals of the 1960s fueled this development. The criticism of conventional norms, of traditional authority and hierarchies also applied to the medical world and its patriarchal "gods in white coats."[9] Alternative medicine and esoteric movements went in search of alternatives to scientific medicine and the dominant ways of addressing (or not addressing) the emotional and spiritual needs of sufferers. The ideal of the responsible and self-determined citizen—and patient—gained central importance. A growing number of researchers studied how the terminally ill themselves, their families, but also how contemporary society as a whole

---

[3] Paul Vogler, Hospitalitenkrankenhäuser, in: idem and Gustav Hassenpflug (eds), Handbuch für den Neuen Krankenhausbau, Munich–Berlin: Urban & Schwarzenberg 1951, pp. 36–41, here p. 37.

[4] A cursory look of the titles shows the range of issues approached: *The act of dying* (1948), *Dying of cancer* (1949), *Care of the dying* (1952), *Psychosocial aspects of cancer: professional attitudes and terminal care* (1952), *The use of heroin in therapeutics* (1953), *Case work in terminal illness* (1954), *Integrated services for the terminally ill cancer patient and his family* (1956), *The patient with incurable cancer* (1956), *Psychotherapy for the dying* (1957), *Care of the dying* (1957), *On death* (1958), *The dying* (1959), *Care of the dying* (1959), *Nursing the late cancer patient at home. The family's impressions* (1959), *A survey of the social needs of patients with incurable lung cancer* (1959), *The management of cases in the terminal stages of malignant disease* (1959), *The meaning of death* (1959).

[5] Cicely Saunders also credited Kübler-Ross' work with great influence on the developments in the US; the two met for the first time in 1966, at Yale University; cf. Historical Library of the Medical School, Yale University, New Haven, Grace Goldin collection, Cicely Saunders, Hints about the story of St. Christopher's, typescript, dated in handwriting spring 1979 (in what follows: Saunders, Hints (typescript)).

[6] Kübler-Ross, On death (1969), pp. 6–7.

[7] Ibid., p. 7.

[8] Ibid., p. 8.

[9] Illich, Limits (1977).

experienced death and dying, how they envisaged a "good" death, and to what extent these ideas and wishes were at variance with reality.[10]

These developments were reflected in a growing number of publications in which terminally ill patients and their families described their personal experiences.[11] Death and dying became subjects one could openly talk about, and people wanted to communicate about them publically—a development that has gained further momentum in recent times. In these personal accounts, we find a broad spectrum of responses to the process of dying and approaching death, ranging from despondency, withdrawal and depression to rebellion and anger, against the illness but also against doctors, nursing professionals and hospitals. Each story, each narrative, is unique but even a cursory reading of this literature reveals several basic response patterns, patterns that then resurface in the depiction of terminal illness in the mass media.

First, many authors describe a heroic "battle" against the illness. Until the bitter end the terminally ill face their disease with optimism and courage, they refuse to let it get them down, or else—and this seems to be the philosophical variant—they are determined to look death in the eye with Stoic equanimity. At the same time there are those who describe how their façade begins to crumble with the progression of their illness. "At the beginning, more than two years ago," as Harold Brodkey, suffering from AIDS, put it, "I thought it a matter of etiquette and of courtesy to be publicly brave about this illness, but is has become more difficult as time passes. Ego has resurfaced and so has bad temper."[12]

Struggling with an illness commonly is connected in second place with a search for the deeper meaning behind the illness. Ever new variations of this narrative

[10] Seminal contributions were Barney G. Glaser and Anselm L. Strauss, Awareness of dying, Chicago: Aldine 1965; Herman Feifel, Perception of death, in: Annals of the New York Academy of Sciences 164 (1969), pp. 669–77; Kübler-Ross, On death (1969); Ann Cartwright, Lisbeth Hockey and John L. Anderson, Life before death, London: Routledge & Kegan Paul 1973; in more recent times numerous publications have approached this issue; see e.g. Elsbeth Voogt et al., Attitudes of patients with incurable cancer toward medical treatment in the last phase of life, Journal of clinical oncology 23 (2005), pp. 2012–19; on the experiences of the relatives see e.g., A. Perreault, F. Fothergill-Bourbonnais and V. Fiset, The experience of family members caring for a dying loved one, in: International journal of palliative nursing 10 (2004), pp. 133–43; on the nurses' perspective see e.g., Nicholas Eschenbruch, Nursing stories. Life and death in a German hospice, New York: Berghahn 2007; on the wishes and expectations among the general public see e.g., Judith A. C. Rietjens et al., Preferences of the Dutch general public for a good death and associations with attitudes towards end-of-life decision-making, in: Palliative medicine 20 (2006), pp. 685–92.

[11] See the seminal work by Hawkins, Reconstructing illness (1993), esp. pp. 91–124 and the fairly recent survey by Jane E. Schultz and Martha Stoddard Holmes (eds), Cancer stories (= Literature and medicine 28/2), Baltimore–London: Johns Hopkins University Press 2010; see also Moamai, Krebs schreiben (1997); Stéphane Grisi, Dans l'intimité des maladies. De Montaigne à Hervé Guibert, Paris: de Brouwer 1996; on autobiographical writings by AIDS-patients see Beate Schappach, "Es war als hätte das Virus mich geschwängert". Vertextungsformen in AIDS-Autobiographien, in: Philipp Osten (ed.), Patientendokumente. Krankheit in Selbstzeugnissen. Stuttgart: Steiner 2010, pp. 143–59.

[12] Harold Brodkey, This wild darkness. The story of my death, London: Holt 1988, p. 153.

describe how a disease confronts patients with something that is of central importance in their lives, leading them to the essence, to the root of their existence and making them reconsider the "value of our life," as Arthur W. Frank put it, having experienced a heart attack and a cancer.[13] Thus, while those affected may experience many restrictions, they may also find that their lives have been enriched due to the illness, which could entail, as in the case of Fritz Angst alias Fritz Zorn, a painful coming to terms with one's own biography.[14] Just how deep-seated this need for making meaning is in many people is further shown in the enduring success of popular science titles such as *The Healing Power of Illness.* "There are no meaningless illnesses," Thorwald Dethlefsen wrote, summarizing the message of his highly successful books. "They show us where we got off course, put an end to a path wrongly taken, force us to ask questions."[15] Susan Sontag, drawing on her personal experience, underlined the ideological component and the negative consequences that these forms of meaning making have for those who have fallen ill.[16] Yet, for some people who have themselves to blame for their illness, this appears to be more bearable than regarding themselves as the victims of blind chance.[17]

Third, the battle against illness in many of the stories is also a battle against medicine, against hospitals, doctors and nursing personnel. This battle is sometimes described as grueling and demoralizing.[18] Yet, as Arthur Frank put it, experiencing the necessity to fight back against alienation and paternalism may be a precondition for an "authentic" experience of illness and dying for some patients.[19] The well-known Swiss lawyer Peter Noll, having considered the foreseeable restrictions and the decrease in his quality of life as well as the uncertain success of treatment, rejected bladder surgery to treat his cancer and decided to die his death very consciously, reflecting on it as he went along.[20]

---

[13] Frank, At the will of the body (1991), p. 1.

[14] Fritz Zorn, Mars, Munich: Kindler 1977.

[15] Thorwald Dethlefsen, Schicksal als Chance. Esoterische Psychologie, das Urwissen zur Vollkommenheit des Menschen, Munich: Bertelsmann 1979, cit. p. 146; idem and Rüdiger Dahlke, Krankheit als Weg. Deutung und Be-deutung der Krankheitsbilder, Munich: Bertelsmann 1983.

[16] Sontag, Illness (1978).

[17] In AIDS-(auto)pathography the quest for meaning can go hand in hand with the question of guilt, the guilt of the one by whom the patient was infected as well as the guilt of the patient himself who may already have transmitted the virus to others; cf. Hélène Laygues, SIDA. Témoignage sur la vie et la mort de Martin, Paris: Hachette 1985.

[18] This is a major theme, e.g., in Aleksandr Isaevič Solženizyn, Cancer ward, London: Bantam Books 1968; see also Huldrych M. Koelbing, Medizin, Arzt und Patient in Solschenizyns "Krebsstation", Zürich: Juris 1973.

[19] Arthur W. Frank. Tricksters and truth tellers: Narrating illness in an age of authenticity and appropriation, in: Jane E. Schultz and Martha Stoddard Holmes (eds), Cancer stories (= Literature and medicine vol. 28, n° 2), Baltimore – London: Johns Hopkins University Press 2010, pp. 185–99; see e.g., Audre Lorde, The cancer journals (special edition), San Francisco: aunt lute books 1997.

[20] Noll, Diktate (1984).

In summary, most (auto)pathographies ultimately reveal the patient's deeply felt need for control, a need that frequently appears to have been what compelled them to write down their experiences in the first place. By turning themselves into active, heroic fighters against their sicknesses, by lending the illness deeper meaning and even by rebelling against the illness and medicine, asserting their subjective perception and experience over the interpretive power of conventional medicine, the terminally ill counter to some degree the overwhelming, destructive power of death and dying.

There is a partial but not complete overlap between the depictions found in modern (auto)pathographies and the images generated by the media and the tabloids in particular of famous terminally ill people, especially cancer patients. Both depictions are characterized by the recurring theme of the heroic battle against the illness. In the privileged mass-media mode of presentation, celebrities suffering from cancer, to a certain extent anyway, set an example of the norms and ideals of a modern *ars moriendi*. However, in the depictions of the mass media much more than in (auto)pathographies, the theme of the heroic battle takes on tragic elements. As with the heroes in the dramas of antiquity, blind fate causes the rich and famous cancer sufferers to fall that much farther than ordinary people. In this way, the readers are served an intensive emotional experience. They can witness a celebrity's death and at the same time, as in a medieval death dance, they are reassured that those who are at the very top quite often fall all the farther in the end, while they themselves—for the time being—may live on.

11.1 Cicely Saunders and the Beginning of the Modern Hospice Movement

At around the time when Kübler-Ross brought the plight of dying patients to the attention of the general public, Cicely Saunders took decisive steps toward founding a modern hospice for the dying in England. This was to be a hospice that would satisfy the particular medical, emotional and nursing requirements of terminally ill and dying patients in a comprehensive way. Saunders described the path that led her there several times, including a detailed personal account that she wrote for Grace Goldin.[21]

Following back surgery and a religious awakening in 1945, she began work as a medical social worker at London's St. Thomas Hospital in 1947. She cared for seriously ill patients, supporting them after their release and sometimes to the very end. From 1948 to 1955, she volunteered once or twice a week at St. Luke's and gathered experience in the treatment of terminally ill patients, particularly in pain management. She completed her medical training, and with a research grant, transferred to

[21] Saunders, Hints (typescript); see also eadem, A personal therapeutic journey, in: British medical journal 313 (1996), pp. 1599–1601; eadem, The evolution of palliative care, in: Journal of the Royal Society of Medicine 94 (2001), pp. 430–2; for a detailed biography see Du Boulay, Cicely Saunders (1984).

St. Joseph's, another London hospice for the dying, in 1958. There she introduced what she had learned at St. Luke's—an approach that is widely established today—namely to keep administering pain medication in regular doses rather than wait until the effects wears off and patients ask for more. Before long, she was in charge of 45 of 150 beds for terminally ill patients. In subsequent years, she gave more and more talks and published contributions on the treatment of terminally ill patients. In the summer of 1959, she began developing plans to open her own hospice for the dying and ultimately succeeded in collecting the necessary funds to purchase a property and have a new hospice built. St. Christopher's, operating under the medical direction of Saunders, was inaugurated in 1967.

The same year, Saunders published a summary of her ideas in a small, practice-oriented handbook entitled *The Management of Terminal Illness,* which likely also served as a guideline for work at St. Christopher's.[22] She demanded that an unfavorable prognosis be communicated openly and that symptoms be controlled in a sophisticated manner, adapted to the situation of the individual patient as necessary. In this, she stated, doctors would be well advised to take the advice of experienced nurses.[23] In pain therapy, a specific, custom selection and precise dosing of medication was not the only important thing. Another matter was to allay patients' fear of future pain, as the fear in itself could be a significant source of suffering. As a tried and tested standard, she recommended the above-mentioned Brompton Cocktail, a combination of a morphine preparation, cocaine and alcohol, to which, in her experience chlorpromazine or prochlorperazine could be added which acted as tranquilizers and antidepressants and would also serve to alleviate nausea and vomiting as necessary. Powerful sedation was to be avoided if possible, as it made most patients uncomfortable. Patients were to be allowed to drink alcohol as much as they liked, as it promoted pain therapy in excellent ways.[24] Further, Saunders put a strong emphasis on the emotional and spiritual needs of the terminally ill and on the significance of close personal attention and affection.[25]

The founding of St. Christopher's was a milestone but in some respects the house must also be seen as part of a longer tradition that had produced a broad spectrum of institutions, especially in England. London's St. Luke's Home for the Dying, by Saunders's own indication, was an important model for St. Christopher's.[26] And since the opening of St. Luke's in 1893, further institutions had been established in the United Kingdom whose important if not essential function was to care and support the terminally ill and dying. Sylvia Lack, the medical director of the New Haven Hospice and a pioneer of the hospice movement in the USA, visited and described a number of these British institutions in the 1970s.[27] In Glasgow the

---

[22] Saunders, Management (1967).

[23] Ibid., pp. 5–10.

[24] Ibid., pp. 13–20.

[25] Ibid., pp. 21–5.

[26] Goldin, A protohospice (1981), p. 393.

[27] Historical Library of the Medical School, Yale University, New Haven, Grace Goldin collection, typescript travel account by Sylvia Lack. This account stands at the centre of a medical dissertation Anna Mauerhöfer, Würzburg, is in the process of completing.

Sisters of Charity opened the St. Margaret's Hospice in 1950, where in 1952, in three converted private homes, a total of 38 patients, all of them terminally ill, were cared for. After the Second World War, Marie Curie Nursing Homes were established in quite a few places, serving predominantly cancer patients and, like the older cancer hospitals, typically combining curative and palliative approaches.[28] Founded in 1954 in a splendid location overlooking the city of Glasgow, Strathclyde House had 15 beds for terminally ill patients and 15 for patients receiving radiotherapy. Between three and four patients died every week. In the same year as Strathclyde House, Conrad House in Newcastle upon Tyne opened its doors, offering 43 beds, 12 of which were reserved for patients receiving radiotherapy; here there were two to five deaths every week. Simply spectacular accommodation was offered at the first Marie Curie Home in the manor house Hill of Tarvit, 3 miles outside of Cupar. The house had belonged to the National Trust since 1948 and inmates lived among valuable antiques. However, it was difficult to reach and continued to be considered a "death house," and so, unsurprisingly, only half of the beds were occupied when Sylvia Lack visited. Easy to reach and located in an attractive area of Liverpool, Sunnybank Home by contrast had a long waiting list. In 1964, at around the same time as St. Christopher's, the Copper Cliff Nursing Home opened in Brighton. The driving force behind it was Dr. de Winter, the local head of the National Society for Cancer Relief. The 21 beds were reserved for patients with an estimated life expectancy of 6 weeks.[29]

The idea for St. Christopher's did not develop out of thin air then but had a range of predecessors and models. Yet it was Cicely Saunders, who, through her publications and talks as well as through the exemplary work done at St. Christopher's, helped establish on a broad basis the conviction that the dying required special institutions which offered the best possible nursing, sensitive care and best possible symptom control and also met the religious or spiritual needs of patients. Also, the opportunity for clinical research in this setting was taken from the start.[30]

St. Christopher's became a model for many more institutions of this kind in Europe and around the world.[31] They grew somewhat haltingly at first but then began to multiply within a short time. In the 1980s, the United Kingdom could already boast around 100 hospices. With some delay, the idea of the hospice also took root with similar speed in the United States.[32] By 1985, the USA had around 1500 hospice institutions. This was a development that was promoted decisively by

[28] See also Clark, From margins (2007), p. 433.

[29] In actual practice, however, the home also accepted patients with longstanding cancer, who needed special medical and nursing care.

[30] Cf. Clark, From margins (2007), p. 432.

[31] For overviews of the development of palliative care services in the first decades see Hayley and Sachs, A brief history (2005), and, for North America, Britain, Australia and New Zealand Lewis, Medicine (2007), pp. 121–158.

[32] Overview in Siebold, Hospice movement (1992).

legislation passed in 1982, which made hospice care refundable for terminally ill patients with a remaining life expectancy of less than 6 months as part of Medicare.[33]

11.2 The First Palliative Care Units: The Royal Victoria Hospital in Montreal

One essential objection to the establishment of independent hospices for the dying was and still is that they tend to promote the marginalization of dying. The concern has been that if the care of the dying is delegated to autonomous institutions, this might result in a failure to exert the necessary pressure on the medical world to develop new, more appropriate ways of dealing with death and dying, and indeed hospices might become ghettos for the dying. The combination of end-of-life care with a curative approach, which was the underlying principle of the Marie Curie Nursing Homes, promised a possible way out of this dilemma. However, experience showed that the population often nevertheless tended to perceive and fear these institutions as places of death.[34]

A second issue—which continues to cause tension and spawn debate today—was the question of whether an autonomous hospice, possibly under clerical direction, would be able to offer the necessary diagnostic and therapeutic competencies and the technology needed for professional palliative medical care. For many hospice initiatives, medical care provided by doctors was not the main priority from the outset, and critics were concerned that dying patients might receive inadequate symptom control and, in particular, insufficient pain medication.[35]

In light of this, palliative care units or wards within hospitals were an important institutional alternative to founding an autonomous hospice for the dying. There were historical precursors, such as the cancer unit at the Middlesex Hospital. The idea was that by creating these structures within a general hospital with a curative mandate, palliative medical care would be established at the very heart of health care. Care for terminal patients would profit from both the personnel resources and from the technical capacities of a highly developed and specialized hospital and at the same time satisfy the particular medical, emotional and spiritual needs of the terminally ill.

The Royal Victoria Hospital in Montreal played a pioneering role in achieving this vision when the first palliative care unit in the world was established there under the direction of Balfour Mount.[36] Following a panel discussion about death and dying in February 1973, a task force and the Ad Hoc Committee on Thanatology

---

[33] Connor, Development (2007).

[34] Historical Library of the Medical School, Yale University, New Haven, Grace Goldin collection, typescript travel account by Sylvia Lack (around 1974).

[35] Klaschik and Nauck, Historische Entwicklung (1998), p. 622.

[36] Balfour M. Mount, The Royal Victoria Hospital Palliative Care Service. A Canadian experience, in: Cicely Saunders and Robert Kastenbaum (eds): Hospice care on the international scene, New York: Springer 1997, pp. 73–85.

were formed with the goal of examining the care of terminally ill patients and their families and identifying deficiencies. Patients, doctors and paramedical personnel were given questionnaires.[37] As summarized by Mount, the results of the study were devastating: Dying patients at the Royal Victoria Hospital suffered unnecessarily—physically, mentally, interpersonally and spiritually—and the medical personnel were neglectful in taking their needs seriously.[38] Subsequently, a small group went to London to visit St. Christopher's, though the aim was not simply to copy Saunders' approach. Rather, the question was how to achieve similar care within a general hospital. In June 1974 an application for a "palliative care unit" that would be focused on the palliative care of cancer patients was filed at the Royal Victoria Hospital. The pilot project was successful. Its final report concluded "that the care of the dying and their families can be greatly improved. The cost involved is minimal—insignificant in the light of the suffering alleviated. There is, in fact, a saving in costs per patient treated."[39] Work could go on.

The reports written about the first years of the palliative care unit at the Royal Victoria Hospital stressed the need for interdisciplinary cooperation. Doctors and psychiatrists, social workers, physiotherapists, occupational and music therapists, dieticians, chaplains, receptionists and secretaries as well as volunteers together realized the concept of "total care" in this hospital unit of 12 beds. This was truly comprehensive care that also included spiritual needs.[40] The goal was to improve the patients' quality of life and help maintain their dignity.[41] Determined steps were taken to abolish the dominant practice of concealing a fatal prognosis from the patient: "The conspiracy of silence which too frequently surrounds the terminally ill heightens anxiety, strains relationships, enhances isolation and prevents communication with loved ones."[42] Paramount importance was given to an effective control of symptoms.[43] Pain management in particular was considered "the key to good palliative care."[44] Based on the positive experience in England, the use of the Brompton Cocktail was adopted. In addition, great attention was paid to the adequate interaction and communication with the dying and very hands-on, practical advice was given to the doctors involved in palliative care. This went as far as suggesting that doctors sit on the edge of the patient's bed, to address a patient by his or her name, to sometimes put one's professional role aside for a moment and to

[37] Osler Library, McGill University, Montreal, Royal Victoria Hospital, Montreal. Palliative care service/Service de soins palliatifs. Pilot project/Projet pilot, Jan. 1975 – Jan. 1977, Montreal 1976 (typescript.), preface and summary, pp. 59–60.

[38] Ibid., preface by Balfour M. Mount.

[39] Ibid.

[40] Ibid., esp. p. 35 (see also Ajemian and Mount, R.V.H. manual (1980)).

[41] Ibid., p. 36 (on this point see also Balfour M. Mount, The problem of caring for the dying in a general hospital; the palliative care unit as a possible solution, in: CMA Journal 115 (1976), pp. 119–121).

[42] Ibid., p. 22.

[43] Ibid., p. 66: "Before all else, palliative care must mean excellent symptom control."

[44] Ibid.

keep one's sense of humor.[45] The manifold challenges that can emerge for palliative medical care from patients' diverse cultural backgrounds—extensively discussed today and yet still underestimated in today's practice—were addressed in Montreal early on, for example the case of a man from Pakistan who might find it very difficult to have his personal hygiene attended to by a female nurse.[46]

The idea of a palliative unit integrated in a general hospital was soon emulated in numerous places around the world.[47] In 2007, there were more than 2500 hospital beds reserved for palliative medical care.[48] Nearly one in three hospitals in the USA included specialized palliative medical care in their services by 2005.[49]

11.3 Outpatient Care

A third institutional form of support and palliative medical care for terminally ill patients was outpatient care provided in the patients' own houses. Today, there is a broad spectrum of services. It ranges from support by volunteer members of hospice associations to highly professionalized services of mobile palliation teams.

The idea of outpatient care for terminal patients has a long history. In 1789, Lampe justified the founding of an outpatient infirmary saying that thanks to this institution, incurable patients were able to spend their final days in dignity, in good medical care surrounded by their family.[50] The Kaiserswerth deaconesses of the nineteenth century devoted much of their time to the home care of the sick and dying.[51] The municipal policlinics that were founded in the nineteenth century and which facilitated many home visits to offer medical students practice-oriented training were also a help to the terminally ill and dying. And the early specialized hospitals for cancer patients, too, combined inpatient and outpatient services. In Glasgow, for example, bedridden "policlinical" patients who had not been admitted to the city's Cancer Hospital profited from regular visits.[52] Considering the spread of cancer illnesses and the fact that they were usually fatal at the time, this seemed the only way of providing adequate care. In this sense, Rosa Goldblum-Abramowicz in 1908 claimed that it would never be possible to provide a bed in an appropriate

[45] Balfour M. Mount, Caring in today's health system (= offprint from CMA Journal 119 (1978)).

[46] Ajemian and Mount, R.V.H. manual (1980), pp. 47–60, "Cultural considerations in palliative care"; on this issue see e.g., Margaret Pabst Battin, Ending life. Ethics and the way we die, Oxford: Oxford University Press 2005.

[47] For an overview of the developments in the UK, the USA, Australia and New Zealand see Lewis, Medicine (2007), pp. 121–58.

[48] Derek Doyle, Palliative medicine in Britain, in: Omega 56 (2007), pp. 77–88.

[49] Connor, Development (2007), p. 93.

[50] Lampe, Nachricht (1789), p. 10.

[51] Karen Nolte, Dying at home: nursing of the critically and terminally ill in private care in Germany around 1900, in: Nursing inquiry 16 (2009), pp. 144–54.

[52] Goldblum-Abramowicz, Versorgung (1908), p. 22.

cancer asylum for every cancer patient, and on this basis called for an "organization of doctors and nurses" which would care for the diseased in their homes.[53]

In the USA, the very first efforts to develop modern palliative medical care even relied chiefly on outpatient solutions.[54] Here, Hospice Inc. in New Haven, Connecticut played a pioneering role. Cicely Saunders had lectured there at Yale University in the 1960s, at a time when the concept of the hospice was still hardly known in the United States. A more detailed exploration of the situation of the dying began in New Haven, and in 1971, an institution providing outpatient hospice care under the medical direction of the above-mentioned Sylvia Lack was able to begin operation. Lack, who was firmly rooted in Christian faith, had worked in hospitals in London and had seen how doctors on their rounds steered clear of the hopeless cases in the beds at the very end of the hall and how insufficient therapy and care had compounded the suffering of the terminally ill.[55]

[53] Ibid., p. 16.

[54] Connor, Development (2007).

[55] Stoddard, Hospice movement (1992), pp. 146–80; Siebold, Hospice movement (1992), pp. 97–100; Sylvia A. Lack, First American hospice: Three years of home care, New Haven: Hospice Inc. 1974.

Part III

Conclusion

12 Continuity and Change

12.1 The Long History of Palliative Care

Palliative medicine and end-of-life care look back on a centuries-old tradition. Ancient authors recommended and illustrated the use of symptom-alleviating *paregorica* and *prainonta* when a cure seemed impossible. In the Middle Ages, Latin as well as vernacular works referred explicitly to "palliative" treatment. In the sixteenth and seventeenth centuries, this *cura palliativa* was widely described and discussed as an autonomous and important form of medical practice. In the mid-seventeenth century, the medical support and care specifically of terminally ill and dying patients began to receive increased attention. Using terms such as *euthanasia palliativa, euthanasia medicinalis* and—prevailing in the nineteenth century—*euthanasia medica,* dozens of authors explored the specific physical and emotional needs of the terminally ill and dying. They formulated detailed recommendations for doctors and nursing personnel, urging them to help patients die as gently as possible and without suffering unbearable pain. With the homes for incurables and, beginning in the nineteenth century, the early hospices for the dying, institutions were created whose primary focus was palliative treatment.

In essence, many of the ideals and goals formulated in the past remain valid today: the value assigned to the alleviation of the suffering of the dying as an eminent objective, the warning against excessive curative zeal, the great attention given to the quality of nursing, the aspiration of caring for patients in a way that is personal and adapted to the individual (combined with the criticism of doctors who "believe that they have to concern themselves only with the illness and not with the human being"), an appreciation of spiritual needs and emotional and mental states, and the involvement of relatives in the process. In short, much of what is today referred to by the term "total care," the ideal of a comprehensive physical, emotional and spiritual support of the dying and their families, was demanded again and again in the medical literature for centuries.

However, the value attached to palliative care has varied significantly in theory and in practice throughout history. By no means can we trace a linear increase in

M. Stolberg, *A History of Palliative Care, 1500–1970*, Philosophy and Medicine 123,
DOI 10.1007/978-3-319-54178-5_12

appreciation; rather, we can identify a large undulating movement. While the doctor's duty to care for the dying was undisputed in the late Middle Ages and at the beginning of the early modern period, the professional situation of many doctors in the healthcare market was precarious. In this period, as each doctor treated disease in his way and both favorable and unfavorable developments were attributed to his skill—or lack thereof—a fatal outcome potentially threatened his reputation or even his professional existence. Therefore, those who sought to stand their ground against the competition—against other medical doctors, less educated barber surgeons and non-licensed healers—had good reason to hesitate when it came to supporting a patient until his death, leave alone when it came to taking on a new patient who was already moribund. Under these circumstances, there was little room for a dedicated exploration of medical end-of-life care.

In the course of the early modern period, as doctors, at least among the upper classes, became more established as the principal contact and trusted supporter at the sickbed, the professional risk involved in treating a patient whose prognosis was unfavorable decreased. Also, the gradual loss of religious certainties started to undermine the meaning of the physical suffering of dying as a divine test or as punishment. In fact, regarding it as such became scandalous from the viewpoint of enlightened humanitarianism. A new field of activity began to open for doctors with the care of the severely ill and dying, and because it involved intensive care, it was potentially very lucrative. This development reached its first summit toward the middle of the nineteenth century.

In the late nineteenth and early twentieth centuries, medical interest in palliative care dwindled as a growing optimistic belief in progress took hold. Hospitals above all, becoming increasingly central in the provision of medical care, no longer made much room for the inevitable natural end of every human life and for an appropriate support of the dying. The few institutions that were founded here and there specifically for the care of the terminally ill and dying were groundbreaking, yet in this initial phase they met only a fraction of the actual need for end-of-life care.

This marginalization of dying in medicine lasted for almost a century and was only reversed, in a decisive way, in the 1960s and 1970s, with the impetus coming from a few progressive thinkers such as Cicely Saunders and Balfour Mount, and it was supported by a growing criticism of medicine, which combined an appreciation of the autonomy and individuality of the experiencing patient with an outrage about the omnipotent demeanor of medical "thanatocrats."[1] A period of about 100 years, during which the palliative care of the severely ill and dying had faded into the background and much of the accumulated knowledge had sunk into oblivion, came to an end.

[1] Ziegler, Les vivants (1975).

12.2 Medicalization

At a more theoretical and generalizing level, three dimensions of nursing and medical care for dying patients can be discerned that are central to an understanding of the long-term historical developments and of the present situation. In what follows I want to discuss them under three headings or terms borrowed from sociology and cultural anthropology, namely "medicalization," "taboo" and "stigma."

Historians have dated the beginnings of a medicalization of dying to different points in time, to the late eighteenth century, to the late nineteenth century or even to the decades after World War II. The answer will depend to some degree on what we mean by "medicalization" in fact. "Medicalization" is a scintillating and multi-layered concept.[2]

If we speak of "medicalization" in the commonly used meaning of a process in which certain social areas or practices become defined as "medical" subjects or tasks and are consigned to medical expertise, then the medicalization of end-of-life care goes back very far. Numerous doctors, as we have seen, explored and discussed the topic in great detail already in the early modern period, applying procedures to incurable and dying patients that were explicitly denoted as "palliative."

A related meaning has us understand "medicalization" in relative terms as a process in which medicine usurps competing interpretations and interpretive entities. An illustrative example of this can be seen in the ideas about signs thought to announce that death was near. The art of early modern doctors who identified the signs of a person's approaching death in the urine or in bodily changes offered an alternative to the ideas and practices known by contemporary lay culture. According to Lehmann's account of 1685, the populace considered for example dark dreams, apparitions, the call of the screech owl or howling dogs harbingers of death.[3] The religious interpretation of the dying process, in particular, and the religious practices connected with it slowly started to lose ground to the medical approach. As we have seen, however, the assumption that doctors in the eighteenth and nineteenth centuries in a sense pushed chaplains off their traditional seat in order to sit there themselves proves too simple a view. Spiritual, religious and medical support were not and are not mutually exclusive. With patients who were able to afford medical care, doctors played an important role next to the chaplain already in the early modern period. As far as we can tell from case histories and funeral sermons, physicians,

---

[2] See the influential analysis by Peter Conrad and Joseph W.Schneider, Deviance and medicalization: from badness to sickness, St. Louis: Mosby 1980; on the history of the term and its different uses see Michael Stolberg, Heilkundige. Professionalisierung und Medikalisierung, in: Norbert Paul and Thomas Schlich (eds), Medizingeschichte. Aufgaben, Probleme, Perspektiven, Frankfurt: Campus 1998, pp. 69–85; Francisca Loetz, "Medikalisierung" in Frankreich, Großbritannien und Deutschland, 1750–1850. Ansätze, Ergebnisse und Perspektiven der Forschung, in: Wolfgang U. Eckart and Robert Jütte (eds), Das europäische Gesundheitssystem. Gemeinsamkeiten und Unterschiede in historischer Perspektive, Stuttgart 1994: Steiner, pp. 123–61.

[3] Lehmann, De moribundorum regimine (1685), p. 7; Lehman considered the latter notion to be plausible because animals with their more acute sense of smelling might be able to perceive the altered, pathological emanations which exuded from the bodies of the dying.

even in the sixteenth and seventeenth centuries, were for the most part in control of the situation, stepping back only, if at all, when the hour of death was near. When doctors, compared to the chaplains, gained significance over the following centuries, the main reason was not so much the increasing intensity of the medical care as the relative loss of significance of pastoral support, which for its part was due to the hour of death losing its meaning as a key moment determining a person's fate in the afterworld. At the same time the declining place of religious belief and of hopes for the afterworld removed from the suffering of dying people the deeper meaning of a divine trial. This lent medicine and its remedies all the more importance because medical treatment was at least able to ease the suffering that had become meaningless.[4]

A final understanding of medicalization sees it as a process in which medical practices, techniques and institutions obtain increasingly more significance in culture and society at large. Especially in hospitals, where more and more people were dying, medical and institutional constraints, both real and ostensible, became more decisive in the dying process. The anonymous and emotionally sterile atmosphere of hospitals was bemoaned as early as around 1900 as something that, as German poet Rainer Maria Rilke put it, robbed the dying of their "own" death. Uprooted from their familiar setting, without the support of family and friends who had commonly stood by at the sickbed and the deathbed, people dying in a hospital came to be much more at the mercy of doctors and nursing personnel. In the worst case, they had to endure many a questionable therapeutic attempt. In the 1960s and 1970s, this modern, "medicalized" form of dying came increasingly under criticism. Dying in the intensive care unit amongst tubes and apparatuses became the byword for an inhumane modern medical practice.[5] However, this was a medicalization of dying only in a very broad, not-strictly-accurate sense. The point of criticism was precisely that patients were not treated as dying human beings but as evidence of therapeutic failure and that their particular needs and hardships were insufficiently taken into account. Dying was shaped to a high degree by medical interventions, but these interventions were anything but aimed at supporting and shaping the process of dying. Rather, they were aimed at preventing a fatal outcome until the bitter end.

Only recently, over the last decades, has the medicalization of dying in the true sense of the word entered a new phase. End-of-life care has become widely recognized in medicine and in the public sphere as an important task of doctors and nurses, and it has been professionalized and institutionalized to an unprecedented degree. By alleviating physical suffering effectively and taking the emotional and spiritual needs of dying patients and their families seriously, a palliative medicine that has become increasingly specialized and founded on expert knowledge has, at least to some extent, taken hold of the reins on the traumatic experience of dying.[6]

---

[4] Jalland has arrived at the same conclusion for late Victorian England (Jalland, Death (1996), p. 52).

[5] Illich, Limits (1977), pp. 179–211.

[6] Cf. Seale, Constructing death (1998), esp. pp. 48–9 and p. 118–21.

12.3 Taboo

A second long-term development that has been described and discussed often when talking about dealing with the dying is the tendency to taboo and repress death. In former times, as Geoffrey Gorer summarized his findings in 1956, death was "mostly no secret," but part of everyday life. In the twentieth century, he argued, a "hitherto unnoticed shift in the area of prudery took place." While "the act of mating appears to be becoming an increasingly more acceptable topic of discussion by the day, the natural occurrence of death is becoming something 'unspeakable' to an ever greater degree."[7] In his studies on the history of death, Philippe Ariès also found a long-ranging process of repression to be at work. He mentioned the "tamed death" of earlier centuries and the "old attitude in which death was both familiar and near, evoking no great fear or awe," as a stark contrast to the modern situation, "where death is so frightful that we dare not utter its name."[8] Joachim Pfeiffer, in 1993, even went so far as to declare that "death is one of the great taboos of our society."[9]

For various reasons this conclusion does not stand up to closer scrutiny. First of all: Not only is unnatural, violent death not tabooed in the Western societies of the twentieth and twenty-first centuries, it is in fact ubiquitous. Gorer himself, in the 1950s, lamented a modern "pornography of death."[10] And the presence of violent death in the media has since reached wholly new dimensions. On any given day, scores of television shows confront audiences with dozens if not hundreds of murder scenes, and in the news, too, viewers now encounter images of corpses on a regular basis. And even with regard to the dying and "natural" death of terminally ill patients we can speak about "taboo" only to a very limited extent. The hospice movement, the impressive rise of palliative medicine, a broad public discussion about assisted suicide and other ethical questions related to death and dying, the millions of people who draw up an advance directive, thus addressing and dealing with their own death—all this goes to show that it is certainly possible today to speak about death and dying privately and publically.[11]

At the same time there is room for doubt about whether death and dying in former times were really as taken for granted, as familiar and comparatively free from fearful associations, as Ariès claims in his romanticizing view of the past. With good reason, early-modern authors such as Guazzus declared that nothing was more frightening than speaking about death, that the very word caused people to go pale

[7] Gorer, Pornographie (1956), p. 60.

[8] Ariès, Western attitudes (1974), p. 13.

[9] Joachim Pfeiffer, Die Sprache und der Tod. Zum Todesmotiv in den autobiographischen Schriften Thomas Bernhards und Josef Winklers, in: Bärbel Götz, Ortrud Gutjahr and Irmgard Roebling (eds), Verschwiegenes Ich. Vom Un-Ausdrücklichen in autobiographischen Texten, Pfaffenweiler: Centaurus 1993, pp. 109–23, cit. p. 109.

[10] Gorer, Pornographie (1956).

[11] Hugger already wondered about the strategic function of this claim that death was a taboo (Hugger, Meister Tod (2002), p. 16).

and freeze as if turning to ice.[12] The final months and weeks in a terminally ill person's life—this has become abundantly clear in this study—were often accompanied by unspeakable torment and horrors. Delius explained in 1769 that being afraid of death was only natural if someone had witnessed the respiratory distress of a dying person, the wheezing, the contorted lips, the trembling tongue, the sunken, glassy eyes, the bluish-gray color of face and skin.[13] In earlier times, many people experienced these or similar things in their immediate family, or with relatives, friends or acquaintances.

The widespread assumption that people then talked openly with the terminally ill about their approaching death, which often accompanies the thesis that death is increasingly tabooed, is almost completely at variance with the historical circumstances. As we have seen, the inevitable fatal outcome was regularly and systematically concealed from patients throughout most of the dying process, in fact even as late as their hour of death.

Ariès is certainly right, on the other hand, in saying that during the past 200 years dying has receded more and more into the background in many parts of everyday social life. Increasing mobility, the fragmentation of families and communities, an increasing life expectancy and the growing number of people who live in old-age and nursing homes—all this has effectively meant that in the twentieth century, there were more and more people who grew up never having experienced a dying relative or having seen a dead person. The rituals of a communal, public farewell at the deathbed were lost.[14] Concerned for the tender soul of children, parents or relatives began to keep them away from the dying. Thus, there are good reasons for stating, as Norbert Elias did, that there is "a maximal expulsion of death and dying from people's communal life in society."[15]

The most striking manifestation of this repression of dying can be seen in medicine and healthcare. Until the mid-nineteenth century, death and dying had their place and were recognized in medical literature and practice, although it was common practice even then for doctors to leave no stone unturned until the bitter end. Then, with the rise of modern medicine during the late nineteenth century, death as the inevitable end of every human being was almost completely pushed to the margins, a development that reached its highpoint after World War II. The therapeutic possibilities of modern medicine caused death and dying, especially in a hospital setting, to be seen increasingly as an accident, as an expression of failure. Death and dying were an affront to modern medicine's narcissistic sense of omnipotence.[16]

---

[12] Stephanus Guazzus, Euthanasia, Das ist: Ein lehrreich, nütz- und sehr tröstliches Gespräche, wie man nemlich christlich leben und seliglich sterben soll. Transl. by Melchior Wisaeus, Leipzig: Bey Abraham Lamberg 1625, p. 6.

[13] Delius, De vultu sereno (1769), p. VI.

[14] See also Ziegler, Les vivants (1975).

[15] Elias, Einsamkeit (1982), p. 39.

[16] In Germany, a very outspoken and influential proponent of this idea was the psychoanalyst Horst-Eberhard Richter; see his Der Gotteskomplex. Die Geburt und die Krise des Glaubens an die Allmacht des Menschen, 2nd edn, Munich: Econ Taschenbuch Verlag 2001, esp. pp. 173–4.

And the diminishing willingness of the modern medical community to accept its own limitations was mirrored in society by the growing expectations on the part of the population. It became ever more common to hospitalize patients, even when they were very old and a fatal outcome was more than predictable, the moment their health took an acute turn for the worse. This is still common practice today and it is based on the justifiable hope of being able to secure several more weeks or months of life. At some point however, during one of perhaps a whole series of hospital stays, all attempts to save a person fail and he or she dies a death that is thought of as unallowable.[17]

Only in recent times has the pendulum begun to swing in the direction of an increased acceptance of death and dying as the unavoidable end to every human life, and medicine is taking on the dying process in such a way that it aims to command and give shape to this process of dying rather than ignore it.

12.4 Stigma

A third dimension that is central to how incurable and dying patients were treated historically is their social stigmatization, something that has been far from adequately addressed in research.[18] Speaking generally, stigmatization is based on signs or characteristics that signal to others that a person is dangerous, immoral or impure. As a result that person is excluded from the rest of society as "different."[19] In this way, dying and especially the physical changes that come with dying have had a highly stigmatizing effect throughout long periods of European history.

To understand this better, we must remind ourselves of how drastically the physical appearance of many patients was transformed as they approached death. In the course of the illness, the patient's outward appearance and physical boundaries would often change in ways that we rarely encounter today in western industrial countries. Dropsy caused the extremities, the abdomen and the face to swell monstrously and sometimes made the skin literally burst open. Consumptives produced large amounts of foul-smelling sputum. They sometimes suffered from massive

[17] My own first encounter with a dying patient in 1977 during a nursing internship (which is required in Germany for medical students) in a small rural Bavarian hospital offered me some first-hand experience with the difficulty many physicians had, at the time, to accept the limits of what was medically possible. One of our patients was an elderly man with a severe heart condition. He was a charismatic, educated man with fine facial features. When I had time, I would visit him and we would talk. But his condition grew worse every day. Even I as a novice could see that death was written in his ashen, sunken face. Yet there was no talk of dying and death when doctors came to him on their rounds. Instead, when they were not able to place an i.v.-needle in the collapsed veins, the doctors decided in favor of a phlebotomy, i.e. a surgical opening of a vein under local anesthesia. While the sick man lay on the operating table with his arm open and bloody, he lost consciousness and died before our eyes. I liked the two doctors, was thankful for what they were teaching me, but in that moment they seemed to me like two barbaric butchers.

[18] An important recent exception is Szabo, Incurable (2009).

[19] See the seminal analysis by Goffman, Stigma (1963); for a fairly recent, critical survey of the wide range of definitions of and ideas about stigma see Green, End of stigma (2009), pp. 13–32.

diarrhea and in the end their body substance seemed to be literally dissolving in the typically plentiful perspiration, which soaked their nightgowns. Cancer in those times was usually first diagnosed only when the cancerous tumor had ulcerated and was discharging malodorous secretions.

These drastic symptoms were not only perceived as disgusting. They also had a specific and from the perspective of the bystanders mostly negative meaning in the context of the dominant concepts of the body and disease. Until well into the nineteenth century, both physicians and laypeople believed that sputum, secretions, skin rashes and tumors served to free the body from impure, morbid matter. They were the physical proof of the abundance of impure matter that accumulated in the body.

Early modern personal testimonies allow us to discern to what extent those affected experienced skin alterations and secretions as stigmatizing. When Johann Georg Bövingh began to suffer from favus of the scalp he in his own words kept "to himself like a leper" and was ashamed "to come before the eyes of others."[20] Indeed, sick people with visible "impure" changes in the face or hands could expect to be confronted with open expressions of revulsion and disgust. Young Marie Thérèse Dumoulin experienced this in the early eighteenth century when she had on her cheek a festering, inflamed growth from which blood and secretions oozed. She recounted that this "caused such a great revulsion" in visitors that many of them did not dare come too close to her or did so only "with the greatest aversion."[21]

What this meant for cancer sufferers, whose skin was affected to a far greater extent, often literally eaten up, can only be surmised.[22] Emotional agony consorted with the physical pain of a decaying body for these people, as Jean-Louis Alibert put it, who experienced the suffering of many dying cancer patients in the Hôpital Saint Louis. "These unfortunate people are perpetually agitated by the fear of being an object of disgust and repugnance for the people who give them their final care."[23] With good reason the admission policy guidelines of the Würzburg Kreisverpflegungsanstalt für Unheilbare, a home for incurables, named in 1859 all forms of cancer as first among the diseases that made patients suitable for admission, "but especially and above all cancer of the face."[24] When the face was affected, the sight could be terrifying. For example a doctor described in 1814 how the nose of his patient Theresa Riederin, who was suffering from "bone cancer," had caved in, and "ugly crusts spread from the forehead over the nose and down, with knots

[20] Johann Georg Bövingh, Die Lebensbeschreibung des Johann Georg Bövingh (1676–1728). Ed. by Elfriede Bachmann, in: Rotenburger Schriften 48/49 (1978), pp. 92–181, cit. p. 121.

[21] Relation de la maladie et de la guérison miraculeuse de Mlle Dumoulin operée par l'intercession de M. de Paris, sine loco 1735, p. 4.

[22] See also Stolberg, Metaphors (2014).

[23] Jean-Louis Alibert, Nosologie naturelle ou les maladies du corps humain distribuées par familles, Paris: Chez Caille et Ravier 1817, p. 543.

[24] Statuten der Würzburger Kreisverpflegungsanstalt für Unheilbare von 1859, 11a (my thanks to Hannes Langrieger who pointed this source out to me).

appearing over the collarbone and chest, a repulsive manure [sic] flowed from the cankerous tumors."[25]

Cancerous tumors and comparable physical disfigurements were not just ugly and revolting. According to widespread belief, they also posed a physical threat to those who got close to them. Looking at them necessarily aroused strong negative emotions. And strong, negative emotions, as we saw when discussing the concealment of an unfavorable prognosis, were feared as a powerful cause of illness. With pregnant women, a further concern was the effect of imagination: According to the traditional teaching, if pregnant women encountered people with disfigurements, the children growing in their wombs were at risk of being born with the same disfigurements.[26] Even the deaf posed a danger because, as O. Floß explained in 1737, they "could cause [through] the contortions in their faces and gestures a good deal of harmful apprehension and damage in pregnant women."[27] This explains why those in charge at the Dublin home for incurables wanted to admit especially those incurables who, as it was put, put themselves on show in the streets and in this way offended the eyes of those around them and put pregnant women at risk.[28] And for the same reason, the decision was made in Bamberg to admit all those to the infirmary for women, the Frauen -Siechhof, "whose physical affliction is monstrous to all foreigners and natives, and could make the most harmful impression on pregnant women who catch sight of them."[29]

Additionally, cancer sufferers as well as consumptives often exuded a revolting and sometimes utterly unbearable stench. In the case of women with uterine cancer, even doctors were sometimes pushed to the limits of what they could bear. In the advanced stage, wrote A. Gessner in 1899, there was often nothing more one could do to effectively fight the "revolting smell" of the excretions and it became "an agony for the patient and even more so for bystanders." He continued, "For the family, caring for a person with such an illness is truly one of the most difficult tasks, and it poses the greatest challenges to one's self-denial."[30] As a young doctor, Léon Daudet (1867–1942), who later became a writer, learned how difficult it was to get used to such things. His very first patient suffered from severe fistulas in her lower belly and which he was supposed to treat locally: "During the first attempt I thought I would have to vomit. The rotten smell was terrible." He was told that he would become hardened in the face of such things, but this was resoundingly not the case:

---

[25] Stadtarchiv Salzburg, ÄStA, Pezoltakten 57, Leprosenhaus 1805–1816, report by the police physician Oberlechner August 2, 1814.

[26] Stefanie Zaun, Daniela Watzke and Jörn Steigerwald (eds), Imagination und Sexualität. Pathologien der Einbildungskraft im medizinischen Diskurs der frühen Neuzeit, Frankfurt: Klostermann 2004.

[27] Stadtarchiv Augsburg, St. Servatius 22.

[28] Gentleman's and citizen's almanack 1755, p. 70.

[29] Lammert, Zur Geschichte (1880), pp. 139–40.

[30] A. Gessner, Palliative Behandlung des inoperablen Carcinoms, in: J. Veit (ed.), Handbuch der Gynäkologie, vol. 2, part 2, Wiesbaden: Bergmann 1899, pp. 461–87, cit. p. 484.

"Still today it happens that I dream of that bed, that drainage, that stench from which I would have preferred to flee."[31]

Moreover, for hundreds of years, phlegm, tumors, secretions and sweat were not only experienced as disgusting. They were also feared as a source of contagion. Experience taught that impure morbid matter could be passed on to other people through direct contact, making them sick. As late as 1908, Rosa Goldblum-Abramowicz, writing about cancer sufferers, noted that "Coming into contact with the sanious, terrible-smelling secretions is revolting and also harbors a danger for those nearby."[32] Indeed, according to the old doctrine of miasms, the foul stench that exuded from the sick and their secretions was evidence of a dangerous "infection" of the surrounding air: Volatile, impure morbid matter made its way through the air into other people's bodies via the pores or respiration, with devastating consequences. In earlier centuries, long before the discovery of the tubercle bacillus, consumptives with their transpiration, their typically plentiful perspiration and their foul-smelling sputum, were widely considered a danger to those around them. Even more so, the mere presence of those suffering from breast or uterine cancer signaled mortal danger to those around them because of the foul or sanious stench. Therefore, vigorous efforts were sometimes made to isolate those affected. 82-year-old Elisabeth Seiwaldin, for example, was admitted to the Salzburg home for lepers in 1784 for "open cancer wounds" because "she is not only terrible to behold, but also the people looking after her are exposed to the danger of contagion."[33] Similarly, the admittance in 1791 of 9-year-old Gertraud Mooserin, who was sick with bone cancer, was based on her being "marked with an extraordinary and contagious stench," so much so that she and her mother "would be tolerated nowhere."[34] In the case of 69-year-old Barbara Neumayr, the widow of a master brewer, the surgeon found that the "cankerous tumors" on her left upper jaw with her "foul-smelling and contagious transpiration" were the reason why her two children were ailing. She was to be admitted to a home because in the town "due to her contagious disease" no one would want to or be allowed to take her into their dwelling anymore.[35]

The disgust felt for cancer patients and the concern for the health of the population could even have effects on urban topography. From the beginning, the plan for the cancer hospital in Reims—the oldest known institution dedicated specifically to cancer—was that it would be opened on the outskirts of the city, in the middle of gardens. Nevertheless, residents in the area protested vigorously, fearing contagion, and even turned to the king for help. The authorities rejected the protests, but orders were nevertheless given that the bedding of the institution was to be used exclusively for cancer patients and in no way would be mixed up with that of the Hôtel

[31] Daudet, Devant la douleur (1915), p. 59.

[32] Goldblum-Abramowicz, Versorgung (1908), p. 12.

[33] Stadtarchiv Salzburg, NStA 243–3, commission report, May 22, 1840, extract from the protocol of April 27, 1784.

[34] Ibid., extract from the protocol of April 20, 1791.

[35] Stadtarchiv Salzburg, ÄStA, Pezoltakten 57, Leprosenhaus 1805–1816, Febrary 12, 1805.

Dieu . And in the end, in 1778, the institution was moved to a building outside the fortification walls.[36]

Even institutions for the sick, the incurable and the contagious sometimes found it difficult to deal with cancer sufferers and other "disgusting" patients. In Stadt am Hof a woman with cancerous tumors was not admitted to an institution in 1811 because "it must be feared that from these kinds of cancerous fumes a further spreading among the inmates, who are already in a miserable enough condition, will take place."[37] In the hospices for the dying, too, there were times when the situation seemed unmanageable. For example, in 1904, a man with cancer had to be released from St Luke's because, in the words of the doctor, he "caused such a terrible smell that no one but the doctors could bear him." Even the nurses shrank from entering the room.[38] Often an effort was made to separate such patients spatially from other residents. For instance, the cancer wards in the Hospital for Incurables in Donnybrook in the nineteenth century were moved to a remote part of the building "in consideration of the state of health in the institution."[39] At the Anstalt für männliche Unheilbare (Institution for Male Incurables) in Attl segregation was explicitly codified in the statutes, which stipulated the creation of a "special department" for all patients "who are marked by serious, disgusting or revolting conditions of the kind that preclude cohabitation in the home."[40] At the Toronto Home for Incurables as well, the need for sequestered rooms for cancer patients was soon felt: Due to the "offensive nature of the disease," these patients had to be separated from the other residents.[41]

Based on this imagery of contagion, impurity and the destruction of the body surface cancer was, for centuries, perceived as similar to a number of other stigmatizing diseases. Cancer, the French disease or syphilis and leprosy and to some extent also consumption and scabies shared an overarching semantic network, a mesh of terms, concepts and visual associations.[42] Ideas of inner filth and contaminating morbid secretions and transpirations were linked to images of repulsive changes or destruction inside the body, accompanied at times with the accusation of moral misconduct. In German-speaking areas, these conditions and the patients who suffered from them were summarily labeled—even in the medical literature and in

[36] Pol Gosset, L'hôpital des cancérés. Fondation du chanoine Godinot (1740), in: Union médicale du Nord-Est (1926), pp. 17–26.

[37] Staatsarchiv Amberg, Regierung der Oberpfalz, Kammer des Inneren 12661, Städtisches Armen- und Krankenhaus in Stadtamhof, 1811–1897, medical certificate for the cancerous Mittermaierin, 1811.

[38] Annual report of *St Luke's* 1904, p. 57, cit. in Goldin, A protohospice (1981), p. 397.

[39] Brady, History (1875), p. 33.

[40] Staatarchiv Regensburg, ZR I, 10347, Statutes of the Anstalt für männliche Unheilbare in Attl, Munich 1874, 64–5 (my thanks to Hannes Langrieger who pointed this source out to me).

[41] 9th annual report of the Toronto Home for Incurables (1883).

[42] Cf. Stolberg, Metaphors (2014).

official statements—as "disgusting" and "disgust-provoking" until well into the nineteenth century.[43]

The perception of cancer patients as belonging to the same category as patients with other illnesses thought to be "impure," repulsive and contagious is well illustrated by the fact that they were often housed together in institutions that marginalized them. The "Blatternhaus" in Landshut, for example, following an ordinance of 1560, was destined for people with *Blattern* or pox, in other words for those suffering from the French disease, as well as for those with a "tumor" and "open wounds and afflictions" that were also typical of cancer.[44] As late as the nineteenth century, the large, newly-built Swiety Lazarz in Warsaw admitted cancer patients alongside syphilitics and scabies-sufferers.[45] But what is especially noticeable here is the association with lepers. The numerous medieval hospitals for lepers or leprosaria were more or less the prototype of institutions for the accommodation and isolation of "impure" and incurable patients on a long-term basis. With the decline of leprosy in western Europe, some of these leprosaria were simply repurposed to become institutions for syphilitics, cancer sufferers and other patients with "disgusting" symptoms.[46] As early as the sixteenth century, the Feld- und Sondersiechenhaus in Stuttgart, for example, which was originally set up for lepers, accepted patients who were "marked by the French, the evil pox, ruptured nerves, and cancer, by fistulas and unclean wounds of burning scabies, by falling sickness and other abhorrent illnesses, those who have been excluded from the common bath."[47] The leprosy house in Mülln on the outskirts of Salzburg, according to a commission's report of 1840, chiefly served to accommodate poor people "who, due to an incurable, revulsion-causing or contagious evil, must be isolated from social life."[48] As we have seen, the Augsburg home for incurables also emerged from a former lazar house, St. Servatius. In other cities similar developments can be seen. For example in Straubing, after the extinction of leprosy, the local lazar house was opened to patients with other disgusting, incurable or infectious diseases. In the early nineteenth century, the house

[43] Carl Richard Hoffmann, Das Civil-Medizinal-Wesen im Königreiche Bayern mit den dermalen in Wirksamkeit stehenden Medizinal-Verordnungen, vol. 3: Die Medizinalpolizei (Fortsetzung), Landshut: Thomann 1863, p. 336, ordinance of the Regierung von Unterfranken und Aschaffenburg, April 19, 1859 on the Kreisverpflegungsanstalt zu Würzburg für Unheilbare und mit eckelerregenden Krankheiten Behaftete.

[44] Lammert, Zur Geschichte (1880), p. 172.

[45] Lorenz Köstler, Die Spitäler zu Warschau (= Beilage zu Heft 42 der Oesterreichischen medicinischen Wochenschrift (1842)), pp. 7–12.

[46] Langasco, "Ospedali degli incurabili" (1938), p. 58; Lammert, Zur Geschichte (1880), p. 225.

[47] Quoted by Lammert, Zur Geschichte (1880), p. 226; Lammert does not provide any more specific information on his source.

[48] Stadtarchiv Salzburg, NStA 243–3, commission report May 22, 1840. On the history of that institution see Peter F. Kramml and Sabine Veits-Falk, Die medizinische Versorgung der Stadt Salzburg am Ausgang des Mittelalters und zu Beginn der Frühen Neuzeit: Ärzte, Apotheker, Bader und Wundärzte sowie Hebammen—Spitäler und Lazarette, in: 54. Paracelsustag 2005, Salzburg: Internationale Paracelsusgesellschaft 2006, pp. 85–137, here pp. 123–5.

was largely shut down. Those, however, who were marked by cancerous wounds, had to remain at the lazar house.[49]

With the development of bacteriology, the historical fear of a miasmatic contamination of the air through tumors, secretions, expectoration or perspiration retreated to the background. But in its place, the discovery of the tubercle bacillus in 1882 renewed the fear of infection from consumption. Now, even more than the cancer patient, the person with open tuberculosis came to be feared as a great threat to those around him. The sheer number of sufferers made mandatory quarantine impossible, but in Germany, toward the end of the Weimar Republic and in the Nazi period, attempts were made to intern at least some of them. Under Wilhelm Frick, the Nazi Minister of the Interior, those suffering from tuberculosis in Thuringia could be forced into isolation in hospitals or special homes as early as 1930. If those affected remained in their own houses, these had to be marked, in an act of symbolic stigmatization, with large letters, similar to how "Jewish" businesses were soon marked.[50] Under the Nazi regime, exclusion and ostracism intensified dramatically and with deadly consequences. Thousands of people suffering from open tuberculosis were declared "asocial" and forcibly admitted to sanitariums. Faced with inadequate care, insufficient nutrition and forced into physical labor, many of them died or were murdered.[51]

In the nineteenth and twentieth centuries, cancer and consumption were also increasingly associated with moral impurity and depravity. The "romantic" perception of consumption as a medium of spiritualization, as we know it from sanitarium literature, was largely confined to educated patients. In the late eighteenth century, Johann Peter Frank had already expressed his outrage about the poor living conditions of many labourers which he saw as a major cause for consumption.[52] This notion was revived by the social hygienists of the early twentieth century, but in the nineteenth and twentieth centuries, consumption came to be denounced above all as a self-imposed affliction of the extravagant, bibulous, weak-willed and uncivilized proletariat.[53] Along similar lines, uterine cancer was ascribed in part to women's

[49] Lammert, Zur Geschichte (1880), p. 255; ordinance by the Landesdirektion Bayern, September 14, 1803, cit. in Max Josef Fuchs, Die Geschichte der Krankenanstalten und der Krankenpflege in Straubing, Munich: typescript med. diss. 1954, p. 93; see also Stadtarchiv Landshut, Bestand 1, 734 "Register der Personen im Blatternhaus 1598–1676", which also lists patients who were to be transferred to the leprosarium.

[50] Wolters, Tuberkulose (2011), pp. 64–5. In Nazi Germany, it was also proposed that the patients—like the Jews—should wear an armlet or some other warning sign.

[51] Ibid., pp. 66–93.

[52] Johann Peter Frank, Akademische Rede vom Volkselend als der Mutter der Krankheiten, Pavia 1790 (repr. Leipzig: Barth 1960).

[53] Vera Pohland, From positive-stigma to negative-stigma. A shift of the literary and medical representation of consumption in German culture, in: Rudolf Käser and Vera Pohland (eds), Disease and medicine in modern German cultures. Ithaca, N.Y.: Cornell Studies in International Affairs. Western Societies Papers 1990, pp. 144–68.

immoral sexual behavior, associated with masturbation and prostitution.[54] Today, particularly those who are HIV-positive or suffer from AIDS are faced with moral stigma, whereby, especially in conservative, religious circles, the infection is seen in connection with homosexuality and patients are blamed for their illness.[55]

In the twentieth century, an additional source of stigmatization arose from the side effects of medical treatment. Hair loss from chemotherapy, the maiming of mastectomy, scars from operations and skin alterations following radiotherapy were and are frequently experienced as jeopardizing patient's sense of self, his or her identity.[56] "Coming home from the hospital, it was hard not to feel like a pariah," wrote Audre Lorde, who suffered from breast cancer. "There were people who avoided me out of their own pain or fear." She found that this "status of untouchable is a very unreal and lonely one."[57]

Thanks to improved therapies, to an increasingly confident patient movement, and to the advocacy work done for example by performance artists and photo models who very consciously show themselves to the public with breast amputations,[58] the stigmatization of cancer patients and, to a lesser extent, of AIDS patients has decreased significantly in recent years, at least in cases where the disease hardly shows from the outside. Today, remarkably open and detailed reports about politicians' and artists' battles with cancer appear in the media, and this is not felt to be offensive or damaging to their reputations. Neither has the stigmatization of cancer patients as psychologically and emotionally deficient,[59] which was criticized by Susan Sontag, maintained its cultural potency. Yet, with a small number of terminally ill and dying patients it is still not possible to prevent to any level of satisfaction the physical decay, the destruction of physical boundaries, the discharge, the stench. Some terminally ill cancer and AIDS patients suffer from massive diarrhea or become unable to control their excretions. Others are severely disfigured by cancerous tumors, their face or head deformed. Others still, through the wheezing and rattling in their air passages, through constant coughing or expectoration, cause an involuntary physical, bodily empathy in those around them. As the British anthropologist Julia Lawton has explained, such phenomena involving the violation or dissolution of physical boundaries are experienced by the relatives, doctors and

---

[54] Karen Nolte, Carcinoma uteri and "sexual debauchery". Morality, cancer and gender in the nineteenth century, in: Social history of medicine 21 (2008), pp. 31–46.

[55] See the various contributions in Journal of HIV/AIDS & social services 6 (2007), n. 3 (special issue).

[56] Frank, At the will of the body (1991), p. 93; cf. Goffman, Stigma (1963).

[57] Audre Lorde, The cancer journals (special edition), San Francisco: aunt lute books 1997, p. 49; see also Suzette A. Henke, Shattered subjects. Trauma and testimony in women's life-writing, Basingstoke: Macmillan 1998, pp. 113–19.

[58] See e.g., Maren Klawiter, The biopolitics of breast cancer. Changing cultures of disease and activism, Minneapolis–London: University of Minnesota Press 2008.

[59] Sontag, Illness (1978).

nurses as a threat to their own physical boundaries, almost as if the smells, transpiration and secretions were seeping or flowing into their own bodies.[60]

Gorer, in 1956, established that "The natural processes of deterioration and decay have become sickening to us."[61] They were sickening and frightening in earlier times as well, in many ways. But truly, it seems that for many people in western societies it is more difficult than ever to be with those terminally ill and dying, in whom even modern medicine cannot prevent drastic disfigurements and physical disintegration. If we follow Norbert Elias and his analysis of the civilizing process in the Western world, this phenomenon is the consequence of a centuries-long development in which dealing with the elementary, animalistic aspects of the human being—especially, dealing with human excretions—was increasingly subjected to and normalized by social rules, and internalized in the form of rules of conscience.[62] According to Elias's somewhat controversial but certainly inspiring analysis, this development culminated in the modern *homo clausus* who—in opposition to the pre-modern body that was always in a state of exchange with its surroundings—is characterized by the clear, impenetrable boundaries of its body, exercising a permanent control over its bodily functions and especially over its excretions.[63] Seen this way, the deteriorating body of the cancer or AIDS patient, which decomposes, so to speak, into stinking secretions or diarrhea, is the stark counter-image to the modern body ideal. According to Julia Lawton's research, it is, significantly, often not so much foreseeable death that leads to the decision to have the terminally ill treated in a palliative care facility, but rather the "unbounded body," the decomposing body especially of cancer patients, which pushes the families of the ill to the limits of the subjectively bearable.[64] Palliative medicine, as John F. Scott put it polemically in 1994, referring to the etymological root of "palliative" as "cloaking," had become a shroud or cloak with which our society covered up the horrors of death.[65]

Looked at this way, the modern hospices for the dying and other palliative medical facilities do not in the eyes of the historian stand in the tradition of the medieval pilgrims' hospice, but rather at best follow from those lazar houses and homes for incurables which offered lepers and other "disgusting" patients a refuge and a certain measure of medical care and nursing, and at the same time were meant to protect the rest of society from the revolting sight of them, from their frightening presence. Today, hospices for the dying and palliative medicine do an incredible

[60] Lawton, Contemporary hospice care.

[61] Gorer, Pornographie (1956), p. 60.

[62] Elias, Einsamkeit (1982), p. 39.

[63] Norbert Elias, The civilizing process, Oxford: Blackwell 1994 (German orig. 1939); see also Seale, Constructing death (1998), pp. 118–9 and p. 150.

[64] Lawton, Contemporary hospice care.

[65] John F. Scott, More money for palliative care? The economics of denial, in: Journal of palliative care 16 (1994), pp. 35–8.

amount of good. They help many people die a "good death," the death that previous generations could often only dream of. Developing palliative medical care further is among the most important desiderata of today's healthcare politics. Yet dealing adequately with the danger of unintentionally excluding, indeed stigmatizing, the dying—and especially those whose physical boundaries appear to be dissolving—remains one of the great challenges for the future.

Selected Bibliography

Ackerknecht, Erwin W. 1968. Death in the history of medicine. *Bulletin of the History of Medicine* 42: 19–23.

Ajemian, Ina, and Balfour M. Mount. 1980. *The R.V.H. manual on palliative/hospice care: A resource book*. New York: Arno Press.

Alberti, Michael. 1722a. *De abstinentia a medicis et medicamentis morbos mortemque interdum avertente*. Resp. Joh. Christ. Zeys. Halle/Magdeburg: Hendel.

———. 1722b. *De religione medici*. Subm. Johann Friedr. Broesike. Halle/Magdeburg: Henckel.

Anonymus. 1806. Vom Verhalten der Ärzte gegen unheilbare Kranke und Sterbende. In *Allgemeine medizinische Annalen des neunzehnten Jahrhunderts*, cols. 537–546.

———. 1838. Der Arzt und die Euthanasie. Von einem Arzte. In *Deutsche Vierteljahrs-Schrift*, 226–239. Stuttgart: J.G. Cotta.

Ariès, Philippe. 1974. *Western attitudes toward death: From the Middle Ages to the present*. Baltimore: Johns Hopkins University Press.

———. 1977. *L'homme devant la mort*. Paris: Seuil.

Augenius, Horatius. 1602. *Epistolarum et consultationum medicinalium prioris tomi libri XII*. Venice: Apud Damianum Zenarium.

Bächtold-Stäubli, Hanns (ed.). 1937. Handwörterbuch des deutschen Aberglaubens, vol. 8. Berlin/Leipzig: Gruyter.

Baltes, Wilhelm. 1842. *De euthanasia*. Berlin: Nietack.

Beier McCray, Lucinda. 1989. The good death in seventeenth-century England. In *Death, ritual and bereavement*, ed. Ralph Houlbrooke, 48–61 and 212–213 (notes). London/New York: Routledge.

Benzenhöfer, Udo. 2009. *Der gute Tod? Geschichte der Euthanasie und Sterbehilfe*. Göttingen: Vandenhoeck & Ruprecht.

———. 2010. *Euthanasia in Germany before and during the Third Reich*. Münster/Ulm: Klemm + Oelschläger.

Bergdolt, Klaus. 2004. *Das Gewissen der Medizin. Ärztliche Moral von der Antike bis heute*. Munich: Beck.

Berridge, Virginia, and G. Edwards. 1987. *Opium and the people. Opiate use in nineteenth-century England*. 2nd ed. New Haven/London: Yale University Press.

Beschuetz, Ludwig. 1832. *De euthanasia medica*. Berlin: Nietack.

Bichat, Xavier. 1800. *Recherches physiologiques sur la vie et la mort*. Paris: Brosson and Gabon.

Binding, Karl, and Alfred Hoche. 1920. *Die Freigabe der Vernichtung lebensunwerten Lebens. Ihr Maß und ihre Form*. 2nd ed. Leipzig: Meiner.

Binet-Sanglé, Charles. 1919. *L'art de mourir. Défense et technique du suicide secondé*. Paris: Albin Michel.

Bloch, Oskar. 1908. *Vom Tode. Eine gemeinverständliche Darstellung*. 2 vols. Stuttgart: Juncker.

Boerhaave, Herman. 1721. *Institutiones medicae in usus annuae exercitationis domesticos digestae*. 4th ed. Leiden: Van der Linden.

M. Stolberg, *A History of Palliative Care, 1500–1970*, Philosophy and Medicine 123,
DOI 10.1007/978-3-319-54178-5

Boudewijns, Michael. 1666. *Ventilabrum medico-theologicum, quo omnes casus cum medicos tum aegros aliosque concernentes eventilantur, et quod SS. PP. conformius, scholasticis probabilius, & in conscientia tutius est, secernitur*. Antwerp: Apud Cornelium Woons.

Brady, Cheyne. 1875. *The history of the hospital for incurables*, With a sequel by C. R. T. Dublin: Browne & Nolan.

Brand, Ulrich. 1977. *Ärztliche Ethik im 19. Jahrhundert. Der Wandel ethischer Inhalte im medizinischen Schrifttum – ein Beitrag zum Verständnis der Arzt-Patient-Beziehung*. Freiburg: H. F. Schulz.

Brockerhoff, Heinrich. 1843. *De euthanasia medica*. Berlin: Nietack.

Brodie, B.C. 1847. *Vorlesungen über wichtige Gegenstände der therapeutischen und operativen Chirurgie*, ed. Friedrich J. Behrend. Leipzig: Kollmann.

Browne, Oswald. 1894. *On the care of the dying. A lecture to nurses*. London: George Allen.

Buck, Katharine Joy. 2005. *Rights of passage. Reforming care of the dying 1965–1986*. PhD thesis, University of Virginia, School of Nursing.

Bullar, Joseph. 1856. On the use of small doses of opium in the act of dying from phthisis. Association Medical Journal 4 (new series): 268–269.

———. 1866. Chloroforme in dying. *British Medical Journal* 2: 10–12.

Burney, Fanny. 1975. *The journals and letters of Fanny Burney* (Madame d'Arblay), ed. Joyce Hemlow, vol. 6. Oxford: Oxford University Press.

Cabanis, P.J.G. 1791. *Journal de la maladie et de la mort d'Honoré-Gabriel-Victor Riquetti Mirabeau*. Paris: Grabit.

Cabrol, Bartholomé. 1604. *Alphabeton (graece) anatomikon, hoc est anatomes elenchus accuratissimus, omnes humani corporis partes, ea qua solent secari methodo, delineans*. Geneva: Chouët.

Callegari, Paulus. 1828. *De cura palliativa*. Padua: Typis Seminarii.

Capellmann, C[arl]. 1895. *Pastoral-Medicin*. 10th ed. Aachen: Barth.

Cardano, Girolamo. 1536. *De malo recentiorum medicorum medendi usu libellus*. Venice: N.N.

Carol, Anne. 2004. *Les médecins et la mort. XIXe-XXe siècle*. Paris: Aubier.

Castro, Roderigo da. 1662. *Medicus-politicus: sive de officiis medico-politicis tractatus*. Hamburg: Hertelius.

Cavina, Marco. 2015. *Andarsene al momento giusto. Culture dell'eutanasia nella storia europea*. Bologna: Il Mulino.

Chartier, Roger. 1976. Les arts de mourir, 1450–1600. *Annales E.S.C* 31: 51–75.

Chaunu, Pierre. 1978. *La mort à Paris. 16e, 17e, 18e siècles*. Paris: Fayard.

Choulant, Ludwig. 1836. *Anleitung zur ärztlichen Praxis*. Leipzig: Voss.

Clark, David. 1999. Cradled to the grave? Terminal care in the United Kingdom 1948–67. *Mortality* 4: 225–247.

———. 2007. From margins to centre: A review of the history of palliative care in cancer. *Lancet Oncology* 8: 430–438.

Clark, David, and J. Seymour. 1999. *Reflections on palliative care*. Buckingham: Open University Press.

Codronchi, Baptista. 1591. *De christiana ac tuta medendi ratione*. Ferrara: Apud Benedictum Mammarellum.

Collner, Joh. 1799. *Eric: Specimen academicum de cura moribundorum*. Praes. Joh. H. Engelhart. Lund: Litteris Berlingianis.

Connor, Stephen R. 2007. Development of hospice and palliative care in the United States. *Omega* 56: 89–99.

Cook, Gordon C. 2006. *The incurables movement: An illustrated history of The British Home*. Oxford: Radcliffe.

Daudet, Léon. 1915. *Devant la douleur. Souvenirs des milieux littéraires, politiques, artistiques et médicaux de 1880 à 1905. Deuxième série*. Paris: Nouvelle Libraire Nationale.

de Graffigny, Françoise. 1985–2016. *Correspondance,* ed. J.A. Dainard et al. 15 vols. Oxford: Oxford University Press.

de Chauliac, Guy. 1976. *Chirurgia magna*. Darmstadt: Wissenschaftliche Buchgesellschaft. (orig. 1585)

de Necker, Suzanne Curchod. 1780. *Einrichtungen und Anstalten in dem Hospice de Charité zu Paris*. Leipzig: Weidmanns Erben und Reich.

de Pastoret, Claude Emmanuel Joseph Pierre. 1816. *Rapport fait au conseil général des hospices, par un de ses membres, sur l'état des hôpitaux, des hospices et des secours à domicile à Paris, depuis le 1. janvier 1804 jusqu'au 1. janvier 1814*. Paris: Huzard.

Delius, Heinrich Friedrich. 1769. *De vultu sereno morientium*. Erlangen: Apud J. D. M. Camerarium.

Detharding, Georg Christoph. 1723. *De mortis cura*. Praes. Georg Detharding. Rostock: Adler.

Dieffenbach, J[ohann] F[riedrich]. 1832. *Anleitung zur Krankenwartung*. Berlin: Hirschwald.

Dietrich-Daum, Elisabeth. 2007. *Die "Wiener Krankheit". Eine Sozialgeschichte der Tuberkulose in Österreich*. Munich: Oldenbourg.

Dowbiggin, Ian. 2005. *Life unworthy of life. A concise history of euthanasia*. Lanham: Rowman & Littlefield.

Doyle, Derek, Geoffrey Hanks, and Nathan I. Cherny, eds. 2005. *Oxford textbook of palliative medicine*. 3rd ed. Oxford: Oxford University Press.

Du Boulay, Shirley. 1984. *Cicely Saunders. The founder of the modern hospice movement*. London: Hodder and Stoughton.

Elias, Norbert. 1982. *Über die Einsamkeit der Sterbenden in unseren Tagen*. Frankfurt: Suhrkamp.

Elkeles, Barbara. 1979. *Aussagen zu ärztlichen Leitwerten, Pflichten und Verhaltensweisen in berufsvorbereitender Literatur der Frühen Neuzeit*. Med. Diss. Hannover: Typescript.

———. 1989. Die schweigsame Welt von Arzt und Patient. Einwilligung und Aufklärung in der Arzt-Patienten-Beziehung des 19. und frühen 20. Jahrhunderts. *Medizin, Gesellschaft und Geschichte* 22: 197–211.

Ernst, Katharina. 2003. *Krankheit und Heilung. Die medikale Kultur württembergischer Pietisten im 18. Jahrhundert*. Stuttgart: Kohlhammer.

Fabry, Wilhelm. 1652. *Wund-Artzney, Gantzes Werck, und aller Bücher, so viel deren vorhanden. Welche theils vor diesem getruckt, theils anjetzo erst an das Tagliecht kommen*. Frankfurt: Beyer.

Falk, Cornelia Maria. 1983. *Geschichte und Bedeutung der Euthanasia medica des 19. Jahrhunderts und ihr Einfluß auf die spätere Euthanasiediskussion und Ausübung der Sterbehilfe*. Med. Diss. Marburg: Typescript.

Favre, Robert. 1978. *La mort dans la littérature et la pensée françaises au siècle des Lumières*. Lyon: Presses Universitaires de Lyon.

Fearon, Henry. 1790. *Abhandlung vom Krebse nebst einer neuen Methode zu operiren, insonderheit bey Krebsen an den Brüsten und Hoden*. Duisburg: Helwingsche Universitäts-Buchhandlung.

Ferriar, John. 1798. On the treatment of the dying. In *Idem: Medical histories and reflections*, vol. 3, 191–208. London: Cadell and Davis.

Field, David. 1994. Palliative medicine and the medicalization of death. *European Journal of Cancer Care* 3: 58–62.

Fleming, Natalie A. 2005. *The care of the dying. A turn-of-the-century phenomenon*. Dissertation. London: Typescript.

Franck, Rudolf. 1926. *Moderne Therapie in innerer Medizin und Allgemeinpraxis. I. und II. Teil*. Leipzig: Vogel.

Frank, Johann Peter. 1788. *System einer vollständigen medicinischen Polizey, vol. 4: Von Sicherheits-Anstalten, so weit sie das Gesundheitswesen angehen*. Mannheim: Schwan und Götz.

Frank, Arthur W. 1991. *At the will of the body. Reflections on illness*. Boston: Houghton Mifflin.

Friese, Ernestus Theophilus. 1723. *De vehementia aegrotandi et facilitate moriendi hominum robustorum prae imbecillioribus, occasione proverbii: Die gesundesten Leute sterben am ersten*. Königsberg: Reusner.

Fye, W. 1978. Bruce: Active euthanasia. A historical survey. *Bulletin of the History of Medicine* 52: 492–502.

Gleixner, Ulrike. 2005. *Pietismus und Bürgertum. Eine historische Anthropologie der Frömmigkeit. Württemberg 17.–19. Jahrhundert*. Göttingen: Vandenhoeck & Ruprecht.

Gmelin, Ferdinand G. 1830. *Allgemeine Therapie der Krankheiten des Menschen*. Tübingen: Osiander.

Goetz, Jakob. 1841. *De euthanasia, qualis medicorum est*. Diss. med. Rostock: Adler.

Goffman, Erving. 1963. *Stigma: Notes on the management of spoiled identity*. New York: Prentice-Hall.

Goldblum-Abramowicz, Rosa. 1908. *Die Versorgung der unheilbaren Krebskranken*. Diss. med. Berlin: Siebert.

Goldin, Grace. 1981. A protohospice at the turn of the century. St. Luke's House, London, from 1893 to 1921. *Journal of the History of Medicine and Allied Sciences* 3: 383–413.

Gorer, Geoffrey. 1956. Die Pornographie des Todes. *Der Monat* 8: 58–62.

Gossweiler, Joseph C. 1838. Erinnerungen an die Sorge für einen ruhigen und leichten Tod (Euthanasie) (lecture abstract). *Schweizerische Zeitschrift für Natur- und Heilkunde* 3: 35–36.

Gottstein, Adolf. 1926. *Das Heilwesen der Gegenwart. Gesundheitslehre und Gesundheitspolitik*. 3rd ed. Berlin: Deutsche Buch-Gemeinschaft.

Green, Gill. 2009. *The end of stigma? Changes in the social experience of long-term illness*. London: Routledge.

Gregory, John. 1772. *Lectures on the duties and qualifications of a physician*. London: Strahan and Cadell.

Grote, Katja. 1996. *Der Tod in der Literatur der Jahrhundertwende. Der Wandel der Todesthematik in den Werken Arthur Schnitzlers, Thomas Manns und Rainer Maria Rilkes*. Frankfurt: Peter Lang.

Grübler, Gerd (ed.). 2007. Quellen zur deutschen Euthanasie-Diskussion 1895–1941. Berlin: LIT-Verlag.

———. 2011. *Euthanasie und Krankenmord in der deutschen Literatur 1885–1936*. Marburg: Tectum-Verlag.

Guttstadt, A. 1900. *Krankenhauslexikon für das Deutsche Reich*. Berlin: Reimer.

Haeberlin, Carl. 1919. *Vom Beruf des Arztes*. Frankfurt: Minjon.

Halford, Henry. 1842. On the deaths of some eminent persons of modern times. In *Idem: Essays and orations*, 215–255. London: John Murray.

Harraden, Beatrice. 1894. *Ships that pass in the night*. Leipzig: Tauchnitz. (orig. 1893).

Hauffe, Fridericus Timotheus. 1843. *De euthanasia*. Diss. med. Würzburg: Zürn.

Hawkins, Anne Hunsaker. 1993. *Reconstructing illness. Studies in pathography*. West Lafayette: Purdue University Press.

Hayley, Déon Cox, and Greg A. Sachs. 2005. A brief history and lessons learned from twin efforts to transform medicine. *Clinics in Geriatric Medicine* 21: 3–15.

Healy, Tim M. 2004. *125 years of caring in Dublin: Our Lady's Hospice, Harold's Cross, 1879–2004*. Dublin: Farmar.

Heberden, William. 1802. *Commentaries on the history and cure of diseases*. London: [Payne].

Heer, Henricus ab. 1645. *Observationes medicae oppido rarae in Spa & Leodii animadversae, cum medicamentis aliquot selectis, & ut volunt secretis*, ed. Joannis Michaelis. 2nd ed. Leipzig: Kühn.

Heinzelmann, Richard. 1845. *De euthanasia medica*. Diss. med. Berlin: Schäde.

Hellwag, Otto. 1841. *De euthanasia*. Diss. med. Berlin: Typis fratrum Schlesinger.

Hennemann, W. 1830. Kakothanasie. *Beiträge Mecklenburgischer Ärzte zur Medicin und Chirurgie* 1: 175–180.

Hennig, Karl Christian. 1735. *De dysthanasia medica. Vom schwehren Todt*. Praes. Michael Alberti. Halle/Magdeburg: Hendel.

Heyn, [Med.-Rat]. 1921. Ueber Sterbehilfe (Euthanasie). *Zeitschrift für Medizinalbeamte* 34: 253–263, 273–281.

Heyse, Paul. 1886. Auf Leben und Tod. In *Idem: Himmlische und irdische Liebe – F.V.R.I.A. – Auf Tod und Leben. Novellen (= Achtzehnte Sammlung der Novellen)*, 2nd ed., 229–316. Berlin: Hertz.

Hoffmann, Friedrich. 1738. *Medicus politicus sive regulae prudentiae secundum quas medicus juvenis studia sua & vitae rationem dirigere debet, si famam sibi felicemque praxin & cito acquirere & conservare cupit*. Leiden: Bonk.

Hoffmann, Christoph. 1969. *Der Inhalt des Begriffes "Euthanasie" im 19. Jahrhundert und seine Wandlung in der Zeit bis 1920*. Med. dissertation. Berlin: Typescript.

Hornemann, Emil. 1881. *Vom Zustande des Menschen kurz vor dem Tode*. Gotha: Schloessmann.

Houlbrooke, Ralph. 1998. *Death, religion and the family in England, 1480–1750*. Oxford: Clarendon Press.

Hufeland, Christoph Wilhelm. 1806. Die Verhältnisse des Arztes. *Journal der praktischen Arzneykunde und Wundarzneykunst* 23: 5–36.

———. 1837. *Enchiridion medicum oder Anleitung zur medizinischen Praxis*. 3rd ed. Berlin: Jonas.

Hugger, Paul. 2002. *Meister Tod. Zur Kulturgeschichte des Sterbens in der Schweiz und in Liechtenstein*. Zürich: Offizin.

Hughes, Nic, and David Clark. 2004. "A thoughtful and experienced physician": William Munk and the care of the dying in late Victorian England. *Journal of Palliative Care* 5: 703–710.

Humphreys, Clare Joanne. 1999. *"Undying spirits": Religion, medicine and institutionalized care of the dying 1878–1938*. PhD thesis, Sheffield.

Humphreys, C[lare Joanne]. 2001. "Waiting for the last summons". The establishment of the first hospices in England 1878–1914. *Mortality* 6: 146–166.

Husson, Armand. 1862. *Étude sur les hôpitaux*. Paris: Dupont.

Illich, Ivan. 1977. *Limits to medicine. Medical nemesis: The expropriation of health*. Harmondsworth: Penguin. (orig. 1976)

Irmak, Kenan H. 2002. *Der Sieche. Alte Menschen und die stationäre Altenhilfe in Deutschland 1924–1961*. Essen: Klartext-Verlag.

Jäger, C[arl] C[ornelius]. 1840. *De euthanasia*. Diss. med. Dresden: Ramming.

Jahn, Jakob Dietrich Ludwig. 1839. *De euthanasia*. Diss. med. Kiel: Mohr.

Jalland, Pat. 1996. *Death in the Victorian family*. Oxford: Oxford University Press.

Jentink, Andreas. 1840. *De promovenda euthanasia*. Utrecht: Ex Officina Paddenburgii.

Käser, Rudolf. 1998. *Arzt, Tod und Text. Grenzen der Medizin im Spiegel der deutschsprachigen Literatur*. Munich: Fink.

Kellehar, Allan. 2007. *A social history of dying*. Cambridge: Cambridge University Press.

Kessler, Friedrich. 1828. *De euthanasia medica sive de moribundorum adjuvandorum ratione*. Diss. med. Berlin: Typis Feisteri et Eisersdorffi.

Klabund [aka Alfred Henschke]. 1917. *Die Krankheit. Eine Erzählung*. Berlin: Erich Reiß.

Klaschik, E[berhard], and F[riedemann] Nauck. 1998. Historische Entwicklung der Palliativmedizin. *Zentralblatt für Chirurgie* 123: 620–623.

Klohss, Karl Ludwig. 1835. *Die Euthanasie oder die Kunst den Tod zu erleichtern*. Berlin: Reimer.

Knefelkamp, Ulrich. 2005. Über die Pflege und medizinische Behandlung von Kranken in Spitälern vom 14. bis 16. Jahrhundert. In *Matheus, Funktions- und Strukturwandel*, 175–194.

Kortum, Carl Theodor. 1800. Kleine Aufsätze. *Journal der praktischen Arzneykunde* 10, H. 2: 21–64.

Koslofsky, Craig M. 2000. *The Reformation of the dead. Death and ritual in early modern Germany, 1450–1700*. Basingstoke: Macmillan/St. Martin's Press.

Krecke, Albert. 1932. *Vom Arzt und seinen Kranken*. Munich/Berlin: Lehmanns Verlag.

Krügelstein, Franz Christian Karl. 1807. *Handbuch der allgemeinen Krankenpflege. Zum Gebrauch für Aerzte und Familienväter*. Erfurt: Henningssche Buchhandlung.

Krünitz, Johann Georg. 1773–1858. *Oeconomische Encyclopädie oder allgemeines System der Land-Haus- und Staats-Wirthschaft in alphabetischer Ordnung*. 242 vols. Berlin: Pauli.

Kselman, Thomas. 1993. *Death and the afterlife in modern France*. Princeton: Princeton University Press.

Kübler-Ross, Elisabeth. 1969. *On death and dying*. New York/Toronto: Macmillan et al.

Küchler, Elias. 1692. *De cura palliativa*. Praes. Henricus Christophorus Alberti. Erfurt: Typis Joh. Henr. Groshii.

Kümmel, Werner Friedrich. 1984. Der sanfte und selige Tod. Verklärung und Wirklichkeit des Sterbens im Spiegel lutherischer Leichenpredigten des 16. bis 18. Jahrhunderts. In *Leichenpredigten als Quelle historischer Wissenschaften*, ed. Rudolf Lenz, vol. 3, 199–226. Köln: Marburg.

Lachmund, Jens, and Gunnar Stollberg. 1995. *Patientenwelten. Krankheit und Medizin vom späten 18. bis zum frühen 20. Jahrhundert im Spiegel von Autobiographien*. Opladen: Leske und Budrich.

Lammert, G[ottfried]. 1880. *Zur Geschichte des bürgerlichen Lebens und der öffentlichen Gesundheitspflege, sowie insbesondere der Sanitätsanstalten in Süddeutschland*. Regensburg: Wunderling.

Lampe, Johann Georg. 1789. *Nachricht von der Stiftung und Einrichtung der Krankenanstalt in St. Petersburg*. St. Petersburg: Schnoor.

Langasco, P. Cassiano da. 1938. *Gli "ospedali degli incurabili". Un istituto della restaurazione cattolica*. Genua: Dissertazione per la Laurea nella Facoltà di Storia Ecclesiastica della Pontificia Università Gregoriana.

Langrieger, Hannes. 2008. Ein Platz für Sterbende? Das Unheilbarenhaus in der vormaligen freien Reichsstadt Regensburg. *Würzburger medizinhistorische Mitteilungen* 27: 105–163.

———. 2010. Die medizinische Versorgung Unheilbarer und Sterbender in Bamberg um 1800. *Würzburger medizinhistorische Mitteilungen* 29: 73–117.

Laqueur, Thomas W. 1989. Bodies, details, and the humanitarian narrative. In *The new cultural history*, ed. Lynn Hunt, 176–204. Berkeley: University of California Press.

Lavi, Shai J. 2005. *The modern art of dying. A history of euthanasia in the United States*. Princeton/ Oxford: Princeton University Press.

Lawton, Julia. 1998. Contemporary hospice care. The sequestration of the unbounded body and "dirty dying". *Sociology of Health and Illness* 20: 121–143.

Lebrecht, Leo. 1821. *Der Arzt im Verhältnisse zur Natur, zur Menschheit und zur Kunst*. Mainz: Kupferberg.

Lehmann, Christoph. 1685. *De moribundorum regimine*. Praes. Joh. Daniel Maior. Kiel: Joachim Reumann.

Lewis, Milton J. 2007. *Medicine and the care of dying. A modern history*. Oxford: Oxford University Press.

Linkenheld, J. 1894. Palliative Operationen. In *Fünfzig Beiträge aus dem Gebiete der gesammten Medicin. Festschrift zur Feier des fünfzigjährigen Jubiläums des Vereins der Ärzte des Regierungsbezirks Düsseldorf*, 416–419. Wiesbaden: J. F. Bergmann.

Lister, Martin. 1698. *Octo exercitationes medicinales de quibusdam morbis chronicis*. Amsterdam: Gallet.

Ludwig, Christian Gottlieb. 1772. Oratio de officio medici erga moribundos. In *Idem: Adversaria medico-practica*, vol. III, part 1, 169–188. Leipzig: Apud Haeredes Weidmanni et Reich.

Lund, Edward. 1880. *Palliative medicine and palliative treatment in surgical cases. Address delivered at the meeting held in Manchester*. London/Manchester: J. & A. Churchill/J. E. Cornish.

Maeterlinck, Maurice. 1913. *Vom Tode*. Trans. Friedrich von Oppeln-Bronikow[s]ki. Jena: Diederichs.

Mann, Thomas. 1929. *The Magic Mountain*. Trans. H. T. Lowe-Porter. London: Martin Secker.

Marx, K[arl] F.H. 1827. Ueber Euthanasie. *Litterarische Annalen der gesammten Heilkunde* 7: 129–151. (orig. 1924).

Matheus, Michael (ed.). 2005. *Funktions- und Strukturwandel spätmittelalterlicher Hospitäler im europäischen Vergleich*. Stuttgart: Steiner.

Max, Katrin. 2008. Literarische Texte in der Medizingeschichte. Klabunds Erzählung "Die Krankheit". *Würzburger medizinhistorische Mitteilungen* 27: 164–202.

———. 2013. *Liegekur und Bakterienrausch: literarische Deutungen der Tuberkulose im "Zauberberg" und anderswo*. Würzburg: Könighausen & Neumann.

Mayer, Ingrid. 1982. *Euthanasie in der medizinischen Diskussion und Schönen Literatur um 1900*. Med. Diss. Heidelberg: Typescript.

McManners, John. 1981. *Death and the enlightenment. Changing attitudes among Christians and unbelievers in eighteenth-century France*. Oxford: Oxford University Press.
Meisner, Christianus. 1705. *De incurabilibus affectibus*. Praes. Georg Ernst Stahl. Halle/ Magdeburg: Henckelius.
Mendelsohn, Martin. 1897. Ueber die Euthanasie. *Zeitschrift für Krankenpflege* 19: 1–7, 36–39.
Mendelsohn, [Martin]. 1898. Euthanasie. In *Encyklopaedie der Therapie*, ed. Oscar Liebreich, vol. 2, 245–250. Berlin: Hirschwald.
Mielke, Leonie. 2006. *Sterben und Tod im modernen Wohlfahrtsstaat: dargestellt an der deutschen Hospizbewegung*. Phil. Diss. Berlin: Typescript.
Mischke, Marianne. 1996. *Der Umgang mit dem Tod. Vom Wandel in der abendländischen Geschichte*. Berlin: Reimer.
Moamai, Marion. 1997. *Krebs schreiben. Deutschsprachige Literatur der siebziger und achtziger Jahre*. St. Ingbert: Röhrig.
Moll, Alfred. 1902. *Ärztliche Ethik. Die Pflichten des Arztes in allen Beziehungen seiner Thätigkeit*. Stuttgart: F. Enke.
Müller, Theophilus. 1675. *De aegro agonizante*. Altdorf: Heinrich Meyer.
Müller, Petrus. 1778. *Meletemata circa morbos quosdam incurabiles*. Copenhagen: N. Müller.
Munk, William. 1887. *Euthanasia: Or, medical treatment in aid of an easy death*. London: Longmans, Green, and Co.
Murphy, Caroline C.S. 1989. From Friedenheim to hospice. A century of cancer hospitals. In *The hospital in history*, ed. Lindsay Granshaw and Roy Porter, 221–241. London/New York: Routledge.
Mursinna, Christian Ludwig. 1801. Etwas über den Gebrauch des Cosmischen Mittels und dessen Wirkung. *Journal für die Chirurgie, Arzneykunde und Geburtshülfe* 1: 440–479.
Nassauer, Max. 1911. *Sterben...ich bitte darum! In: Idem: Sterben...ich bitte darum!* 27–132. Munich: Gmelin.
Nietner, [Johann] (ed.). 1912. *Zur Tuberkulose-Bekämpfung 1912. Verhandlungen des Deutschen Zentral-Komitees zur Bekämpfung der Tuberkulose*. Berlin: Deutsches Zentralkomitee zur Bekämpfung der Tuberkulose.
——— (ed.). 1913. *Zur Tuberkulose-Bekämpfung 1913. Verhandlungen des Deutschen Zentral-Komitees zur Bekämpfung der Tuberkulose*. Berlin: Deutsches Zentralkomitee zur Bekämpfung der Tuberkulose.
Noll, Peter. 1984. *Diktate über Sterben & Tod*. Zürich: Pendo.
Nolte, Karen. 2006a. Vom Umgang mit Tod und Sterben in der klinischen und häuslichen Krankenpflege des 19. Jahrhunderts. In *Pflege – Räume, Macht und Alltag. Beiträge zur Geschichte der Pflege*, ed. Sabine Braunschweig, 165–174. Zürich: Chronos.
———. 2006b. Wege zu einer "Patientengeschichte" des Sterbens im 19. Jahrhundert. *BIOS* 19: 36–50.
———. 2010a. Ärztliche Praxis am Sterbebett in der ersten Hälfte des 19. Jahrhunderts. In *Ärztliches Ethos im Kontext. Historische, phänomenologische und didaktische Analysen*, ed. Walter Bruchhausen and Hans-Georg Hofer, 39–57. Bonn: Bonn University Press.
———. 2010b. Pflege von Sterbenden im 19. Jahrhundert. Eine ethikgeschichtliche Annäherung. In *Transformationen pflegerischen Handelns. Institutionelle Kontexte und soziale Praxis vom 19. bis zum 21. Jahrhundert*, ed. Susanne Kreutzer, 87–107. Osnabrück: V&R unipress.
———. 2016. *Todkrank. Sterbebegleitung im 19. Jahrhundert. Medizin, Krankenpflege und Religion*. Göttingen: Wallstein.
Oberlin, Caspar Heinrich. 1752. *De opio in medicina adhibendo*. Strasbourg: Typis haeredum Pauschingerianorum.
Oetheus, Jakob. 1574. *Gründtlicher Bericht, Lehr unnd Instruction von rechtem und nutzlichem brauch der Artzney, den Gesunden Krancken und Kranckenpflegern [...]*. Dillingen: Sebald Mayer.
Oppert, Franz. 1872. *Hospitäler und Wohlthätigkeits-Anstalten*. 3rd ed. Hamburg: Meissner.

Ossberger, Josef. 1955. *Das Euthanasieproblem in den letzten 150 Jahren auf Grund der Autobiographie von Ärzten*. Med. Diss. Munich: Typescript. LMU München.
Ostermann, Artur. 1928. *Krankenpflegelehrbuch*. 10th ed. Berlin: Springer.
Paradys, Nikolaus. 1796. Rede von Nikolaus Paradys, Professor in Leyden, über das, was die Arzneiwissenschaft vermag, den Tod leicht und schmerzlos zu machen. *Neues Magazin für Aerzte* 18: 560–72. (orig.: Oratio de euthanasia naturali et quid ad eam conciliandam medicina valeat, Leiden: H. Mostert 1794)
Paul, Astrid. 2005. *Der Tod in der Literatur um 1900. Literarische Dokumentationen eines mentalitätsgeschichtlichen Wandels*. Marburg: Tectum.
Percival, Thomas. 1803. *Medical ethics, or, a code of institutes and precepts, adapted to the professional conduct of physicians and surgeons*. Manchester: J. Johnson/R. Bickenstaff.
Pfeiffer, Carl. 1839. *De euthanasia medica*. Diss. med. Berolini: Berlin.
Pfeiffer, Joachim. 1997. *Tod und Erzählen. Wege der literarischen Moderne um 1900*. Tübingen: Niemeyer.
Piller, Gudrun. 2007. *Private Körper. Spuren des Leibes in Selbstzeugnissen des 18. Jahrhunderts*. Cologne/Weimar/Vienna: Böhlau.
Pohl, Klaus-Peter. 1982. *Unheilbar Kranker und Sterbender – Problemfälle ärztlicher Deontologie. Stellungnahmen aus dem 18. Jahrhundert und ihre historischen Voraussetzungen*. Med. diss. Münster: Typescript.
Pohland, Vera. 1984. *Das Sanatorium als literarischer Ort. Medizinische Institution und Krankheit als Medien der Gesellschaftskritik und Existenzanalyse*. Frankfurt: Lang.
Porter, Roy. 1998. Death and the doctors in Georgian England. In *Death, ritual and bereavement*, ed. Ralph Houlbrooke, 77–94 and 216–220 (notes). London/New York: Routledge.
Porter, Roy, and Dorothy Porter. 1988. *In sickness and in health*. London: Fourth Estate.
Puchelt, Friedrich August Benjamin. 1826. *Umriss der allgemeinen Gesundheits-Krankheits- und Heilungslehre. Part 1*. Heidelberg: Mohr.
Putz, Franz Xaver. 1843. *De euthanasia*. Diss. med. Vienna: Überreuter.
Questel, Caspar. 1678. *Dissertatio academica de pulvinari morientibus non subtrahendo, von Abziehung der Sterbenden Haupt-Küssen, ex moralibus, divinis, juris item ac artis medicae principiis methodice proposita, et exemplis rarioribus illustrata*. Jena: Johannes Gollner.
Reil, Johann Christian. 1816. *Entwurf einer Allgemeinen Therapie*. Halle: Curt.
Reimann, [Dr.] [...]. 1843. *Über die Schädlichkeit euthanasischer Handlungsweisen am Krankenbett für das ärztliche und nichtärztliche Publikum*. Berlin: Stuhr'sche Buchhandlung.
Rey, Roselyne. 1998. *The history of pain*. Cambridge: Harvard University Press.
Richter, H.E. 1841. Euthanasia. In *Encyklopädie der gesammten Medicin*, ed. Carl Christian Schmidt, vol. 2, 363–367. Leipzig: Wigand.
Richter, Isabel. 2010. *Der phantasierte Tod: Bilder und Vorstellungen vom Lebensende im 19. Jahrhundert*. Frankfurt: Campus.
Riva-Rocci, [Scipione]. 1896. La cura dell'agonia. *Gazzetta medica di Torino* 47: 464–471.
Roelcke, Volker. 2006. "Ars moriendi" und "euthanasia medica": Zur Neukonfiguration und ärztlichen Aneignung normativer Vorstellungen über den "guten Tod" um 1800. In *Sterben und Tod bei Heinrich von Kleist und in seinem historischen Kontext*, ed. Lothar Jordan and Kleist-Museum Frankfurt a. d. Oder, 29–44. Würzburg: Königshausen & Neumann.
Rosa, Georg Ludwig. 1742. *De curatione palliativa*. Praes. Andreas Elias Büchner. Erfurt: Typis Heringii.
Salzmann, C[hristian] C[arl]. 1835. *De euthanasia medica*. Diss.med. Berlin: Nietack.
Sander, Friedrich. 1875. *Ueber Geschichte, Statistik, Bau und Einrichtung der Krankenhäuser. Nebst einem Bericht über das Krankenhaus der Stadt Barmen*. Cologne: Dumont-Schauberg.
Saunders, Cicely. 1967. *The management of terminal illness*. London: Hospital Medicine Publications.
———. 1988. The evolution of the hospices. In *The history of the management of pain: From early principles to present practice*, ed. Ronald D. Mann, 167–178. London: Parthenon.
Schaffrath, Heinrich Daniel. 1869. *Die Euthanasie*. Diss. med. Bonn: J. F. Carthaus.

Schalle, Eduard. 1832. Zur Psychologie und Euthanasie. *Archiv für medizinische Erfahrung*. 278–302.

Schalle, Eduard Wilhelm. 1839. *De euthanasia*. Diss. med. Leipzig: Typis Staritzii.

Scheffler, W. 1900. Bericht über die englischen Cancerhospitäler. *Verhandlungen der Deutschen Gesellschaft für Chirurgie* 2: 17–22.

Scheidhauer, Moritz Wilhelm. 1831. *De cura moribundis adhibenda*. Diss. med. Leipzig: Ex Officina Gust. Naumanni.

Schilling, Katharina. 2011. *„Ach gib mir doch nur etwas Luft, Du hast der Luft so viel!" Pallativmedizin im frühen 19 . Jahrhundert*. Cologne: WiKu-Verlag (= Diss. med., Würzburg 2010).

Schleiner, Winfried. 1995. *Medical ethics in the renaissance*. Washington, DC: Georgetown University Press.

Schnitzler, Arthur. 1961. Sterben. In: *Idem: Die erzählenden Schriften*, vol. 1, 98–175. Frankfurt: S. Fischer. (orig. 1892)

Scholand, J.M. 1837. *Der Menschenfreund, oder Anleitung zur zweckmäßigen Pflege und Behandlung der Kranken. Sterbenden, Todten und Scheintodten, sowie auch Gedanken zur Besiegung der Todesfurcht und des Schmerzes beim Ableben der Unsrigen. Part 2: Anleitung zur zweckmäßigen Pflege und Behandlung der Sterbenden, Gestorbenen u. Scheintodten*. Magdeburg: W. Heinrichshofen.

Schriever, Wilhelm. 1836. *De euthanasia*. Diss. med. Berlin: Nietack.

Schulz, Zacharias Philipp. 1735. *De euthanasia medica, vom leichten Todt*. Praes. Michael Alberti. Halle/Magdeburg: Typis Joh. Christiani Hendelii.

Seale, Clive. 1998. *Constructing death. The sociology of dying and bereavement*. Cambridge: Cambridge University Press.

Seidel, Bruno. 1662. *Liber morborum incurabilium causas, mira brevitate, summa lectionis jucunditate exhibens*. Leiden: Apud Petrum Hackium.

Seitz, Oliver, and Dieter Seitz. 2002. *Die moderne Hospizbewegung in Deutschland auf dem Weg ins öffentliche Bewußtsein. Ursprünge, kontroverse Diskussionen, Perspektiven*. Herbolzheim: Centaurus Verlag.

Sicard, Emile. 1913. *Essai sur l'euthanasie*. Diss. med. Montpellier: Imprimerie Firmin et Montane.

Siebold, Cathy. 1992. *The hospice movement. Easing death's pains*. New York: Twayne.

Siena, Kevin. 2009. Suicide as an illness-strategy in the long eighteenth century. In *Histories of suicide: International perspectives on self-destruction in the modern world*, ed. John Weaver and David Wright, 53–72. Toronto: University of Toronto Press.

Snow, Herbert. 1890. *The palliative treatment of incurable cancer. With an appendix on the use of the opium-pipe. Being a lecture delivered at the cancer hospital*. London: Baillière, Tindall and Cox.

Sontag, Susan. 1978. *Illness as metaphor*. New York: Farrar, Straus und Giroux.

———. 1988. *AIDS and its metaphors*. New York: Farrar, Straus and Giroux.

Soutar, William. 1954. *Diaries of a dying man*, ed. Alexander Scott. Edinburgh/London: Chambers.

Spender, John Kent. 1874. *Therapeutic means for the relief of pain*. London: Macmillan.

Stahl, Georg Ernst. 1702. *Mortis theoria medica. Subm. Ernst Gottholdt Struve*. Jena: Zeitler.

Steingießer, Hildegard. 1938. *Was die Ärzte aller Zeiten vom Sterben wußten*. 2nd ed. Greifswald: L. Bamberg (orig. 1936).

Stoddard, S. 1992. *The hospice movement. A better way of caring for the dying*. New York: Vintage.

Stoddard Holmes, M. 2003. "The grandest badge of his art": Three Victorian doctors, pain relief, and the art of medicine. In *Opioids and pain relief. A historical perspective*, ed. Marcia L. Meldrum, 21–34. Seattle: IASP Press.

Stöhr, August. 1882. *Handbuch der Pastoralmedicin mit besonderer Berücksichtigung der Hygieine*. 2nd ed. Herder: Freiburg im Breisgau.

Stolberg, Michael. 2007a. Active euthanasia in early modern society. Learned debates and popular practices. *Social History of Medicine* 20: 205–221.

———. 2007b. „Cura palliativa ". Begriff und Diskussion der palliativen Krankheitsbehandlung in der vormodernen Medizin (ca. 1500–1850). *Medizinhistorisches Journal* 42: 7–29.

———. 2009. Europas ältestes Sterbehospiz? Das Nürnberger Krankenhaus „Hundertsuppe", 1770–1813. *Medizin, Geschichte und Gesellschaft* 28: 153–178.

———. 2011. *Experiencing illness and the body in early modern Europe*. Houndsmills/New York: Palgrave.

———. 2014. Metaphors and images of cancer in early modern Europe. *Bulletin of the History of Medicine* 88: 48–74.

Storm, Theodor. 1988. Ein Bekenntnis. In *Idem: Novellen 1881–1888*, ed. Karl Ernst Laage, 580–633. Frankfurt: Deutscher Klassiker Verlag. (orig. 1887)

Struve, Christian August. 1799–1801. *Die Kunst, das schwache Leben zu erhalten und in unheilbaren Krankheiten zu fristen. Three parts*. Hannover: Gebrüder Hahn.

Stubendorff, Julius. 1836. *De euthanasia medica*. Diss. med. Dorpat: Typis J. C. Schuenmanni.

Student, Johann-Christoph. 2007. Geschichte und Konzepte von Hospizbewegung und Palliative Care. In *Palliative care. Wahrnehmen – verstehen – schützen*, ed. *Idem* and Annedore Napiwotzky, 3–12. Stuttgart: Thieme.

Süß, Winfried. 2003. *Der "Volkskörper" im Krieg. Gesundheitspolitik, Gesundheitsverhältnisse und Krankenmord im nationalsozialistischen Deutschland 1939–1945*. Munich: Oldenbourg.

Sylvius, Franciscus. 1695. Praxeos medicae idea nova. In *Idem: Opera omnia*, 149–872. Utrecht/Amsterdam: G. van de Water and A. Schelte.

Szabo, Jason. 2009. *Incurable and intolerable. Chronic disease and slow death in 19th-century France*. New Brunswick: Rutgers University Press.

Thierfelder, [Johann Gottlieb]. 1843. Darf der Arzt dem Kranken die vorhandene unvermeidliche Gefahr des nahen Todes ankündigen, und unter gewissen Umständen das Leben absichtlich verkürzen? *Medicinischer Argos* 5: 148–162.

Upmarck, Johannes. 1760. *Dissertatio historico-philosophica de euthanasia*. Subm. Andreas Fellenius. Stockholm: Literis Werneri.

van der Linden, Johann Antonides. 1656. *Selecta medica et ad ea exercitationes batavae*. Leiden: Elsevir.

van Foreest, Pieter. 1601. *Observationum et curationum chirurgicarum libri quatuor posteriores, de vulneribus, ulceribus, fracturis, luxationibus*. Leiden: Raphelengius.

———. 1603–1606. *Observationum et curationum medicinalium libri XXXII*. Leiden: Raphelengius.

van Heurne, Johannes. 1590. *Praxis medicinae nova ratio, qua libris tribus methodi ad praxin medicam, aditus facillimus aperitur ad omnes morbos curandos*. Leiden: Raphelengius.

Vanderpool, Harold Y. 2015. *Palliative care. The 400-year quest for a good death*. McFarland: Jefferson.

Vigo, Giovanni da. 1543. *The most excellent workes of chirurgerye, made and set forth by maister John Vigon, heed chirurgie[n] of our tyme in Italie*. London: Edward Whytchurch.

Vogel, Rudolf Augustin. 1760. *Animadversiones super morbis incurabilibus*. Def. Joh. Wilhelm Janssen. Göttingen: Ex Officina Schulziana.

Vogel, [Dr.] [...] von. 1834. Euthanasia. In *Encyclopädisches Wörterbuch der medicinischen Wissenschaften*, ed. D.W.H. Busch et al., vol. 11, 598–603. Berlin: Veit & Co.

von Döbeln, Johann Jakob. 1700. *Liber de erroribus vulgi circa medicinam & medicos. D. i. Die vertheidigte Artzney-Kunst und der vertheidigte Artzt, wider die heutige Unart und Verächter derselben*. Lund: Abraham Haberegger.

von Haller, Albrecht. 1923. *Albrecht von Hallers Briefe an Johannes Gesner (1728–1777)*, ed. Henry E. Sigerist. Berlin: Weidmann.

von Krosigk, Ernestine. 1834. *Über den Umgang mit Leidenden. Seitenstück zu Adolph Freiherrn von Knigges Über den Umgang mit Menschen*. 2nd ed. Berlin: Sander'sche Buchhandlung.

Vovelle, Michel. 1983. *La mort et l'occident de 1300 à nos jours*. Paris: Gallimard.

Watson, Thomas. 1851. *Die Grundgesetze der praktischen Heilkunde*, vol. 1. Translated from the 3rd English edition by J. H. Steinau. Leipzig: Brockhaus.
Wedel, Georg Wolffgang. 1682. *Opiologia*. Jena: Sumptibus Johannis Bielkii.
———. 1703. *De cura palliativa*. Subm. Philipp Friedrich Schmeltzer. Jena: Litteris Christoph. Krebsii.
Williams, Samuel D. 1870. Euthanasia. In *Essays by members of the Birmingham Speculative Club*, 210–237. London/Birmingham: Williams & Norgate and Josiah Allen.
Wilson, Erasmus. 1845. *The history of the Middlesex Hospital during the first century of its existence*. London: Churchill.
Wolfart, K. Chr. 1819. Betragen am Sterbebette. *Jahrbücher für den Lebens-Magnetismus oder Neues Askläpieion* 1 n 2: 59–63.
Wolters, Christine. 2011. *Tuberkulose und Menschenversuche im Nationalsozialismus. Das Netzwerk hinter den Tbc-Experimenten im Konzentrationslager Sachsenhausen*. Stuttgart: Steiner.
Woyt, Johann Jakob. 1709. *Gazophylacium Medico-Physicum oder Schatz-Kammer, medicinisch- und natürlicher Dinge*. Leipzig: Lankisch.
Zacchia, Paolo. 1651. *Quaestiones medico-legales*. 3rd ed. Amsterdam: J. Blaeu.
Zach, Ignatius. 1792. *De cura, quam moribundis debent, qui aegrotis sunt a ministerio*. Apitz: Frankfurt an der Oder.
Zech, D[etlev]. 1994. Entwicklung der Palliativmedizin in Deutschland. In *Palliativmedizin heute*, ed. E[berhard] Klaschik and F[riedemann] Nauck, 85–102. Berlin/Heidelberg/New York: Springer.
Ziegler, Jean. 1975. *Les vivants et la mort*. Paris: Editions du Seuil.
Zielinski, Helmut R. 1993. *Palliative Therapie und Hospizbewegung in der Bundesrepublik Deutschland*. Saarbrücken: Scheidt.
Ziemssen, Wilhelm Ludwig. 1845. *De euthanasia medica*. Diss. med. Greifswald.
Zumstein, Hansjürg. 1986. Le débat sur l'euthanasie avant la deuxième guerre mondiale. Thèse de maîtrise, Université Paris IV, Paris.

Index

M. Stolberg, *A History of Palliative Care, 1500–1970*, Philosophy and Medicine 123,
DOI 10.1007/978-3-319-54178-5

Michael Stolberg

A History of Palliative Care, 1500–1970

Concepts, Practices, and Ethical Challenges

Springer

Michael Stolberg
Institut für Geschichte der Medizin
Universität Würzburg
Würzburg, Germany

Translated by Logan Kennedy and Leonhard Unglaub

ISSN 0376-7418 ISSN 2215-0080 (electronic)
Philosophy and Medicine
ISBN 978-3-319-54177-8 ISBN 978-3-319-54178-5 (eBook)
DOI 10.1007/978-3-319-54178-5

Library of Congress Control Number: 2017934070

Cover illustration: Louis Hersent (1777–1860), *The dying Bichat mourant assisted by his physicians Esparon and Roux* (courtesy of the *Musée de l'Histoire de la Médecine*, Paris)

Printed on acid-free paper

This Springer imprint is published by Springer Nature
The registered company is Springer International Publishing AG
The registered company address is: Gewerbestrasse 11, 6330 Cham, Switzerland

MIX
Papier aus verantwortungsvollen Quellen
Paper from responsible sources
FSC® C105338

If you have any concerns about our products,
you can contact us on
ProductSafety@springernature.com

In case Publisher is established outside the EU,
the EU authorized representative is:
Springer Nature Customer Service Center GmbH
Europaplatz 3, 69115 Heidelberg, Germany

Printed by Libri Plureos GmbH
in Hamburg, Germany